# 210° CELSIUS

## 16 WAYS THE TRUCKERS IGNITED CANADA FOR THE LONG HAUL

*Barry W. Bussey*

◆ FriesenPress

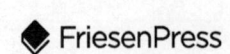

One Printers Way
Altona, MB R0G 0B0
Canada

www.friesenpress.com

**Copyright © 2023 by Barry W. Bussey**
First Edition — 2023

All rights reserved.

No part of this publication may be reproduced in any form, or by any means, electronic or mechanical, including photocopying, recording, or any information browsing, storage, or retrieval system, without permission in writing from FriesenPress.

ISBN
978-1-03-918475-6 (Hardcover)
978-1-03-918474-9 (Paperback)
978-1-03-918476-3 (eBook)

1. POLITICAL SCIENCE, POLITICAL FREEDOM & SECURITY

Distributed to the trade by The Ingram Book Company

"Through personal history and his academic credentials, Mr. Bussey weaves a fast-moving description of The Truckers' Convoy, its significance, and the assault on freedom that the Governments of Canada and The Establishment have unleashed. It is an open question whether our freedom can be restored." —**Honourable A. Brian Peckford P.C., last surviving first minister who was a signatory to The Patriation Agreement of 1981—the founding document to The Constitution Act of 1982, which includes The Charter of Rights and Freedoms**

"The Canadian truckers have earned a high place in the struggle for freedom in our time. They demonstrated great courage and persistence against all odds and in the face of astonishing smears. They further showed what it is going to take to reclaim our freedoms. Barry Bussey's book documents it all with great precision. This book is a service to the cause of freedom and to accurate historical documentations of our frightening times." —**Jeffrey Tucker, Brownstone Institute**

"Barry W. Bussey's incisive look into the Canadian government's handling of the Freedom Convoy provides an eye-opening perspective on power dynamics and governmental responsibility. Through a meticulous analysis of the Emergencies Act, Bussey unveils startling instances of overreach and the subsequent shortcomings of the Public Order Emergency Commission. His pragmatic suggestions pave the way for a more transparent and accountable framework. His work is not just an examination—it's a call to action. Bussey's take on the Freedom Convoy is a lesson in precision, advocating for democracy, civil liberties, and transparency. Every page reveals a commitment to truth, fostering a deeper trust in governance. This isn't merely a book; it's a roadmap for ensuring the vitality of our democratic values. An essential read for those who value a just and accountable society." —**Tom Marazzo, Canadian Veteran, MBA, CD1**

"Dr. Bussey does what few so far have done. He lays out what the Canadian experience of COVID crackdowns involved in 2020-2022: around the world coordinated lockdowns and harsh restrictions on key civil liberties such as speech, assembly, conscience, mobility and religion; and showed the corruption and/or incompetence of all sectors of society: politics, law, media, policing and medicine itself.

Big Pharma and Health Sector Regulators combined to repress information and formulate directives to push citizens towards drugs that were not fully tested, were experimental, and cooperated with the coercion, through mandatory vaccine orders, of whole sectors of the population against long-standing medical ethics framed around voluntary informed consent and doctor/patient confidentiality. The covid mandates were, in fact, in direct contravention of the Nuremberg Code and the Siracusa Principles, yet a complicit media failed in any properly investigative journalism to point this out.

The exaggerations and blatant manipulation of populations by fear-mongering lies and suppression of information showed the urgent need for deep reforms of Emergency powers and the legal frameworks to review them.

Barry Bussey's book details a large part of the Canadian story and will prove a most useful source of background information for domestic and international citizens and policy makers as they think through how to resist State over-reaches in the future for issues such as "climate-change" or further "pandemics" or whatever the globalist Controllers dream up next in their drives for greater centralised controls and increased global governance." —**Iain T. Benson, PhD, Professor of Law, University of Notre Dame Australia, Extraordinary Professor, University of the Free State, South Africa**

"In the life of a nation, some moments stand out. The Freedom Convoy was one of those moments. In compliant Canada, the Truckers shattered the COVID trance. From his front-row seat on Canada's descent into authoritarianism, lawyer, author, and freedom fighter Barry W. Bussey explains how the Truckers' peaceful presence in Ottawa has inspired Canadians to find their way out of the abyss." —**Bruce Pardy, professor of law, Queen's University**

"Canada's response to the pandemic was a trial by fire for its institutions and those we deem fit to lead them. Very few proved their mettle as admirably as Barry W. Bussey, who demonstrates his ample worth in this unflinching assessment of our manifold failures of the last three years. His account is notable for its unflinching truth telling, penetrating judgment, and great compassion for all those whom our institutions and leaders failed. A gripping yet easily digestible chronicle that leaves the reader well-informed and better engaged; a guide for the perplexed and a reminder that it is still possible that justice will be done." —**Ryan Alford, professor, Bora Laskin Faculty of Law, Lakehead University**

"Barry W. Bussey is a Supreme Court attorney with immense learning and experience in the areas of constitutional law and public policy. His latest book is an indispensable guide to understanding how the federal government betrayed democracy and the rule of law during the Trucker Protest." —**Michael Alexander—litigation lawyer with over thirty years of experience in advocacy before government tribunals and commissions, trial and appeal courts, and the Supreme Court of Canada**

"When Justin Trudeau invoked the Emergencies Act, he thought he'd rid himself of that turbulent truckers' convoy. But Barry W. Bussey insists passionately that the protest arose from deep, legitimate discontent about the direction in which our elites had been taking our country and is continuing to change Canada for the better." —**John Robson, is a journalist, history professor, filmmaker, and executive director of the Climate Discussion Nexus**

"Barry's captivating analysis goes beyond the emotional, sourcing scores of first-hand accounts from Freedom Convoy 2022. Digging into root causes, this sweeping account of a seminal season in Canadian history goes further than most; asking 'why?' and most importantly 'what is our responsibility for the years ahead?' *210 Celsius* captures the history, while delving into the future implications of what transpired and what we all need to do next. For those of who you care about remembering the past and guarding our future, this is a critical read." —**Greg Hill, founder and co-director of Free** to Fly, has had a distinguished thirty-year career in aviation, first in the military and then with a major Canadian airline, which sidelined him from flying and threatened termination in 2021 over health freedom.

"If truth prevails, the Freedom Convoy may be the most important event in Canadian history. With Canada teetering on the brink of totalitarianism, a few thousand truckers inspired a movement that fanned the flames of freedom, justice, rights and personal responsibility. Their efforts pulled Canada back from tyranny.

Bussey's *210° Celsius: 16 Ways the Truckers Ignited Canada for the Long Haul* masterfully documents how Canadians have been transformed by the adversity, and by the courage and integrity of the truckers who gathered in Ottawa in February 2022. In spite of all the hardship, abuse, discrimination and coercion, or rather maybe because of these hardships, Canada may be on a more solid foundation.

This historical event exposed the dearth of honesty, ethics and integrity, not only at the highest levels of government, but in virtually every institution in this country. The result is Canadians are ending their childish relationship with authority and learning that our survival requires an informed and vigilant electorate.

This is a story that needs to be told so that future generations may be prepared and eternally vigilant." —**Ted Kuntz, President, Vaccine Choice Canada**

"Barry W. Bussey's book represents a monumental and significant achievement of compiling and documenting so many important voices, perspectives and facts that have received little to no attention in mainstream media in relation to the Freedom Convoy. Barry's work represents an invaluable resource for anyone trying to gain a deeper and broader understanding of how the truckers transformed the Canadian political, social and legal landscape. A must-read for lawyers, academics, and all history buffs."—**Daniel Freiheit is an Ontario lawyer certified as a corporate commercial specialist by the Law Society of Ontario. After receiving numerous business and employment inquiries regarding COVID 19** vaccine mandates, Freiheit realized the importance of advocating for a fair, reasonable, and compassionate approach to vaccine mandates, and started Lion Advocacy, a personal advocacy social media platform (primarily on Twitter) dedicated to improving public policy regarding vaccine rollouts.

"Bussey provides an important heterodox view of the convoy phenomenon and the long-term political fallout. A must-read for anyone interested in better understanding a seismic event in Canadian political history." **—Aaron Wudrick, lawyer and the director of MacDonald-Laurier Institute's Domestic Policy Program**

"The Canadian government responded to the COVID pandemic by abridging human rights and restricting civil liberties, and most of us meekly went along with it. Canadian truckers were among the resisters. In his important new book *210° Celsius: 16 Ways the Truckers Ignited Canada for the Long Haul*, Barry Bussey isolates lessons from the truckers' protest that we had better study closely if we want Canada to be a democracy of free and equal people. Most of the lessons are painful or distressing (that both the media and the judiciary will toady for the government, for instance) but some give hope (that ordinary people are capable of heroism, for one). Bussey knows that Santayana is right: if we don't struggle to understand our recent history, we're in grave danger of repeating it." **—Mark Mercer, professor of philosophy and past president of the Society for Academic Freedom and Scholarship**

"As the Western world slides into an authoritarian, anti-scientific dark age, the Freedom Convoy of 2022 provided a brilliant glimpse of the peaceful individual resistance needed to restore reason and stability to society. Barry Bussey's book offers a vital documentation of this milestone in Canadian history." **—Joseph Hickey, BSc, MSc, PhD, executive director, Ontario Civil Liberties Association, president, Correlation Research in the Public Interest**

"Once started, this book is impossible to put down. Barry Bussey documents how the Truckers' Protest exposed and confronted tyranny at all levels of government and gave such hope and inspiration to millions of Canadians and others around the world. Bussey's insight and analysis is also focused upon how so many in academia, medicine, law enforcement, banking, and government service became weaponized against ordinary people—people who lost their jobs, businesses, homes, and families due to the tyrannical mandates. But most important, Bussey's analysis is convincing that the Truckers' Protest is not over. It started a fire that burns in the hearts of millions of Canadians who will never again submit to tyranny. A worthy and easy read." —**Donald Best—anti-corruption advocate, former Toronto Police detective. Sole recipient 2018 Ontario Civil Liberties Award**

"Dr. Bussey PhD is an attorney, among the topics addressed in this work he cross-examines healthcare and shows how it failed. Bussey offers a concise and provocative indictment we cannot ignore. A short read you will remember for a long time." —**Shawn Whatley MD, author of** *When Politics Comes Before Patients: Why and How Canadian Medicare is Failing,* **2020**

"I want to thank Barry Bussey for taking a stand in the midst of difficult and unrelenting opposition. This book will highlight the courage and heroic efforts that many Canadians displayed while their freedoms were being attacked." —**Pastor David Ripley, Grace Christian Fellowship, Creston BC**

"The title of Bussey's book is not just clever, but it says why the Trudeau government wants us to forget all about the most cataclysmic demonstration.

Without giving away that significance, so expertly and thoughtfully and incisively set out by Bussey, the Trucker Demonstration was the canary in the coalmine for Canada—it should be remembered and studied for what caused it and its long-term impact.

Anyone who ignores its significance to the future of Canadian politics and society does so at their peril." —**Stephen LeDrew, lawyer, broadcaster, and host of** *The LeDrew Three Minute Interview*. **www.stephenledrew.ca**

"Bussey has provided a well-researched and thoughtful treatise on the truckers' protest that happened in Canada during the winter of 2022. This type of book is important not only for all Canadians, but all countries where democracy is being eroded and citizens of the world are being duped by duplicitous leaders and paid-off media." —**Renata Jasaitis, College professor**

"The Freedom Convoy was a watershed moment in Canadian history. Controlled by no particular entity or group, it was the most independent and organic grassroots protest to date in our country. Barry W. Bussey, a lawyer noted for his freedom advocacy—including multiple times at the Supreme Court of Canada—and an academic noted for his scholarship on freedom of conscience, is precisely the kind of informed and analytical mind needed to digest this remarkable event. His book is straightforward, easy-to-read, and well documented. With the ever-present vitriol, hyperbole, and exaggerations on all sides, we need a keen and thoughtful account of this event and its ramifications. This book is that work. I highly endorse this book and wish our leaders would draw from this well of reason and common sense." —**Derek Sloan, former Canadian member of Parliament, author, and leader of the Ontario Party.**

"As Saruman ignored the peril of the awakening Ents, Trudeau underestimated the tsunami of protest unleashed by the truckers who sustain Canada's economy. In this accessible and engaging analysis, Barry W. Bussey uses his astute legal mind to expose the sources and enablers of the government overreach that precipitated this seismic event. Through primary sources, he also paints a profoundly sympathetic portrait of the protestors whose basic human and Charter rights were routinely violated. This book is call to action for those who want their first freedoms restored." —**Angus Menuge, PhD, professor and chair of philosophy, Concordia University Wisconsin, past president of the Evangelical Philosophical Society**

"Dr. Barry Bussey's book is a must-read for anyone genuinely interested in understanding the truth and impact of the Canadian truckers' convoy at a time when concerns loom about a potential second COVID PSYOP, including more mask mandates, social distancing, contact tracing, digital sign-ins, lockdowns, and a push towards further experimental vaccination. They have paved the way for future resistance to tyranny. Indeed, the Canadian truckers sparked demonstrations by Dutch farmers and other similar movements throughout the world.

In *210° Celsius*, Bussey, with his extensive knowledge of Canadian jurisprudence and his unwavering commitment to what is good and true, provides us with an invaluable resource that exposes the colluding corruption among the legacy media, governments, big pharma, big tech, and health organizations within Canada and throughout the globe. *210° Celsius* also shows how the truckers' convoy not only changed the world but can also function as a piece of historical knowledge with a template that will help prevent future tyranny, whether generations from now or in the immediate future." —**Scott D. G. Ventureyra, PhD, editor-in-chief of True Freedom Press, author and editor of** *COVID-19: A Dystopian Delusion*

"Through his academic training and wide experience in constitutional law and public policy, Barry Bussey is well qualified to address the issues discussed in this book. An important read for all Canadians who care about the future of our great nation!" —**Harold Albrecht, member of Parliament, 2006–2019**

"Barry's book is clearly written and accessible to every reader. I urge every Canadian to read this book if for no other reason, than to understand how our Charter of Rights and Freedoms was meant to work but was instead abused by state actors. The time for willful blindness is over." —**Leslie J. Smith, employment lawyer, Ontario, Canada.**

"As a practicing lawyer and practical academic, Barry Bussey has long committed himself as an active participant in the interaction between government and constitutionally guaranteed rights and freedoms. In *210°*

*Celsius* Dr. Bussey presents well-documented content and firsthand testimony essential to understanding the already secured place in Canadian History of the 2022 Freedom Convoy, a peaceful protest that ended with the Trudeau Government invoking the first-ever use of the Emergencies Act." —**Don Hutchinson (BA, JD, DMin), lawyer and author of** *Under Siege: Religious Freedom and the Church in Canada at 150 (1867–2017)*.

"*210° Celsius* is a magnificent portrait of the trucker convoy and its influence that remains living in our world. Bussey doesn't just concentrate on particular frames of the protest, he paints an entire picture. His newest contribution to history makes us aware of the freedom we have because of the truckers; it makes us aware of the freedoms we would've lost without them." —**Tanner Hnidey, economist, freelance speaker, social critic, and lay-theologian. He's the author and editor of TannerHnidey.com.**

# 210° Celsius:
# 16 Ways the Truckers Ignited Canada for the Long Haul

High pressured diesel sprayed into a truck engine with compressed air at 210° Celsius automatically roars the engine to life. The Canadian government's compression and suppression of freedom reached autoignition of the citizenry. Truckers crossed the country to Ottawa to say, "Enough is enough!" Tens of thousands joined the protest and its ramifications remain for the long haul.

# TABLE OF CONTENTS

| | |
|---|---|
| **PART ONE** | 1 |
| **PREFACE** | 3 |
| **INTRODUCTION** | 13 |
|    *Time to connect some dots:* | 31 |
|    *Two Views of the Same Reality* | 32 |
|    *Compelled to Write* | 35 |
| Chapter One: Setting the Stage | 39 |
| Chapter Two: The Election That Changed Canadians | 49 |
| Chapter Three: The Tribal Attack against Unvaccinated Canadians | 59 |
| Chapter Four: The Trucker Reaction: Not on Our Watch! | 75 |
| **PART TWO – 16 WAYS THE TRUCKERS IGNITED CANADA FOR THE LONG HAUL** | 91 |
| 1. Gave People Hope | 93 |
| 2. Broke Trudeau's Monopoly over the COVID Narrative | 99 |
| 3. Gave the Average Canadian a Voice | 109 |
| 4. Showed That Elites Can Push Only So Far | 115 |
| 5. Revealed the Steel Fist in a Tyrant's Velvet Glove | 125 |
|    *The Pre-Cursor—The SNC-Lavalin Affair* | 135 |
|    *The Trudeau Way* | 141 |
|    *Prime Minister Justin Trudeau's POEC Testimony* | 144 |
| 6. Exposed the Inhumanity of the Administrative State | 161 |

7. Revealed the Absolute Necessity of Justice Not Only Being Done but Seen To Be Done 169
   *Tamara Lich* 178
      *First Court Hearing* 180
      *Second Court Hearing* 182
      *Third Court Hearing* 184
      *June 16, 2022, JCCF Gala* 187
      *Fourth Court Hearing* 195
      *Fifth Court Hearing* 198
      *The Trial* 201
   *Conclusion* 202
8. Exposed the Failure of the Academics 205
9. Exposed the Utter Complicity of Mainstream Media 213
10. Exposed the Complicity of the Banks 229
11. Exposed the Complicity of the Healthcare System 239
12. Exposed the Complicity of the Police 249
13. Exposed the Complicity of Politicians 267
14. Exposed the Lies of the Prime Minister 277
15. Revealed That Non-Violent Protest Works 289
16. Awakened the People to Faith and Freedom 301

**CONCLUSION** 317

**EPILOGUE: TRYING TO MAKE SENSE OF CANADA AFTER ROULEAU** 325
   *Why Rouleau Didn't Have All the Information Needed to Rule on Emergencies Act Invocation.* 331

**ACKNOWLEDGEMENTS** 335

## DEDICATION

To all those who lost family, friends, and jobs because of human folly and hubris in the 2020–2022 COVID-19 pandemic. May the memories of your loss kindle compassion and concern still as we work together to make the world a better, not bitter, place to live that respects conscience and justice.

To my father, Henry Winston Bussey, a man who is true to his conscientiously held beliefs, though the heavens fall.

To my grandchildren, who will want to know when they are of age what my views were at this very troubled time in our nation's history.

# A book with a difference! Are you ready to accept the call to action?

This book is not meant to be read and put back on the shelf to collect dust. Barry invites you to join him in an ongoing conversation about our First Freedoms. He has recorded a video for each chapter so that you may continue the dialogue with your friends. A companion **210° Celsius Study Guide** is available at a nominal cost so that you and your friends can dig deeper into how we can flourish as a truly free and democratic society.

Simply scan this QR code with your smartphone or tablet and start a study group today and be ready to answer the call to change Canada for the better!

# PART ONE

# PART ONE

# PREFACE

IT SHOOK CANADA. It shook the world. The symbol of resistance against government abuse of power during the COVID-19 pandemic was The Trucker Freedom Convoy 2022 in Ottawa.

The mainstream media (MSM) downplayed the Convoy's significance. In fact, MSM hardly made a dissonant note from the Canadian Government's narrative. According to the government and the media, the protestors were a "fringe minority with unacceptable views." This book refuses to accept such a trite "soundbite." Rather, it takes a common-sense approach of the issues and argues that there was and is a lot more complexity to the protest that must not be overlooked.

Why would truckers instantaneously drop everything, get in their trucks, and drive to Ottawa in the bitterly cold 2022 winter? Not only is it important to hear directly from the truckers, but we must step back and consider the larger political and social context. We will examine the possible long-term implications of this dramatic grassroots uprising, unparalleled in Canadian history.

This book is not meant to be provocative for provocation's sake. Rather it is an honest attempt, based on experience and observation of this protest, to understand the motivation behind it and make a reasonable account of why the protest was so necessary and consider its far reaching consequences.

There are at least sixteen ways one could argue that the protest commenced a movement of people who are committed to resisting government abuse of individual freedom for the long haul. Many of these challenges remain with us still, but it is my position that the truckers had a huge role in opening the minds of Canadians, indeed the world, to not blindly go along with the government narrative. Questioning government authority to ask hard questions remains a bedrock principle of a free society if we are to keep it. Be wary of government that claims to help.

It must be said at the outset that it was not only Prime Minister Justin Trudeau who is to be blamed for the angst of the average Canadian that led to this protest. All governments—from whatever partisan stripe, whether they be Conservative, Liberal, or NDP, were complicit in limiting Canadian freedom. With each passing day and as more information is being revealed, we must ask, "Was this draconian treatment necessary?" "Could we have done better?" Unfortunately, no one political party or leader in power can be said to be a heroic champion of freedom during the COVID-19 era. All failed to provide the necessary leadership we so desperately needed and did not get.

At the centre of the newsreel during this dark time we can all certainly agree that Mr. Trudeau's statement that those who refused the experimental COVID-19 vaccine were "racist," "misogynist," and "anti-science"[1]— combined with his chilling words, "Do we tolerate these people?"[2]—was ominous. Then, during his testimony at the Public Order Emergency Commission in late 2022, he flatly denied that he had maligned the unvaccinated at all. This is but one illustration of leadership this country has been under during the last eight years.

"Disinformation!" screams Prime Minister Trudeau at the opposition. However, he has no shame regarding his own disinformation campaign. A former member of his cabinet said his penchant is to "casually lie" and "think he could get away with it."[3] Sadly, to date he has been able to get away

---

1 Matthew Miller, "Trudeau: Canadians who protested him are 'racist,' 'misogynistic,' 'anti-vaxxer mobs,'" *Washington Examiner*, September 8, 2021; accessed May 29, 2023, https://www.washingtonexaminer.com/news/justin-trudeau-protesters-anti-vaxxer-mobs-racist.

2 Licia Corbella, "Trudeau has forgotten the lesson of tolerance he learned at his father's knee," *Calgary Herald*, February 7, 2022; accessed May 29, 2023, https://calgaryherald.com/opinion/columnists/corbella-trudeau-has-forgotten-the-lesson-of-tolerance-he-learned-at-his-fathers-knee.

3 Jody Wilson-Raybould, *"Indian" in the Cabinet: Speaking Truth to Power* (Toronto, ON: HarperCollins Canada, 2021) [hereinafter, "Wilson-Raybould"], 229, Kindle Edition.

with it.[4] Is it not a fair statement to say that this is, at least partly, due to his government funding "Canadian" news outlets? Are we to be surprised that they would espouse what the government decides are "Canadian" values? Amazingly (or perhaps to be expected), former Justice Paul Rouleau gave Mr. Trudeau even more space to continue in his misinformative ways by stating that Trudeau met the threshold to impose the Emergencies Act, admitting others might come to a different conclusion.

However, despite his incredible string of good fortune in weathering scandal after scandal (and we will see what the Beijing electoral interference may yet bring, yes, even though The Right Honourable David Johnston gave him another pass), the Trucker Freedom Convoy put him on notice that it may not be so easy in the next election. (One must wonder whether he will face the electorate in 2025.) Indeed, the Trucker Freedom Convoy 2022 was a powerful pushback against a "sunny ways" prime minister who cynically took Canadians for granted. A pushback that is unprecedented in Canadian history.

We Canadians defer, to a fault, to our prime ministers. In a perfect world, such trust would be merited but our world is not perfect. The line between good and evil, as Aleksandr Solzhenitsyn observed, runs through every human heart.[5] That includes us and our prime ministers. Accountability is a must when holding power. Representative democratic societies require nothing less.

---

4   The Latin maxim comes to mind, "*Mundus vult decipi, ergo decipiatur,*" meaning "The world wants to be deceived, so let it be deceived."
5   Aleksandr I. Solzhenitsyn, *The Gulag Archipelago Two, 1918–1956*, (New York, Harper & Row, 1974)
    Part 4, Chapter 1, 615:
    It was granted me to carry away from my prison years on my bent back, which nearly broke beneath its load, this essential experience: how a human being becomes evil and how good ...
    Gradually it was disclosed to me that the line separating good and evil passes not through states, nor between classes, nor between political parties either—but right through every human heart—and through all human hearts. This line shifts. Inside us, it oscillates with the years. And even within hearts overwhelmed by evil, one small bridgehead of good is retained. And even in the best of all hearts, there remains ... an unuprooted small corner of evil.

The goodwill of the populace can never be taken for granted. It must be earned. There is a solemn obligation on those in power, to act as trustees, not to fritter away or mock such sacred trust obligations. In other words, public officials (elected or nonelected) are in a fiduciary relationship with the public they govern.[6] Such officials are in a superior position because they are on the inside of knowing what subjects are being debated that will affect the citizen. Such knowledge and the ability to decide what government policy will be implemented is power. Citizens delegate power to their political class to work in the public interest.

Political trust is the lifeblood of our country and the basis of our progeny's future. For they are the beneficiaries of our current society.

The more successful the devious politician is in deceiving the population from their beneficial interests of good government and sound public policy, the greater the harm to the peace of those he rules.

During the 2021 election, Trudeau openly threatened to take away the charitable status of pro-life groups that were involved in "disinformation." As we will see, unfortunately he and his government were and are the source of much "disinformation" while maintaining the uncanny ability to appear legitimate. As Katie Telford, the prime minister's chief of staff, observed with former attorney-general Wilson-Raybould: "We don't want to debate legalities anymore. If Jody is nervous, we would of course line up all kinds of people to write op-eds saying what she is doing is proper."[7]

The ability to control the propaganda is key to labelling the opposition as engaged in "disinformation." Saying that pro-life groups are engaged in "disinformation" reminded me of the 2018 Canada Summer Jobs scandal.[8] The Trudeau government required religious entities to "check the box" on the Summer Jobs application form for funding in order to hire summer students. The "box" indicated their agreement with his pro-choice views and other ideological commitments that ran contrary to their teachings

---

[6] The 1215 *Magna Carta*, clause 40, King John agreed, "To no one will we sell, to no one deny or delay right or justice."
[7] Wilson-Raybould, 214.
[8] Barry Winston Bussey, The Canada Summer Jobs Debate and the Democratic Decline (June 9, 2019). Available at SSRN: https://papers.ssrn.com/sol3/papers.cfm?abstract_id=3401591.

and understandings of life, as well as rights and freedoms guaranteed in the Canadian Charter of Rights and Freedoms.

It was the first time that Canadians were expected to acquiesce to government ideological commitments if they wanted to partake in a government program. Normally, government programs are designed for all citizens. Under Mr. Trudeau's administration government programs are increasingly the domain of only those citizens who agree with the government's ideological beliefs. Therefore, the most recent attacks against the unvaccinated were but the latest reiteration of his approach to governing—divide and conquer. We see the same with the new scandal of electoral interference by a foreign power, as he accuses any questions about the topic as "racist" and xenophobic.[9]

This type of governance from a Canadian prime minister is unprecedented and, in my view, dangerous. It's tribal. Citizens are no longer simply Canadians with equality. Now our ideological commitments determine our "have or have not" status regarding access to government programs and protections. The unwarranted travel vaccine mandate was just one example of egregious government punishment for the "wrong" views.

I took the leap to start a new non-profit[10] entity at a time when I should have been thinking about retirement, not starting a new entity to oppose government infringement on our first freedoms of speech of conscience and religion, and of inviolability of the person. We also advocate on the importance of the rule of law and democracy. A short time after our foundation launched, the Trucker Freedom Convoy was all over the news. I admired the courage of the truckers to stand up when everyone else had caved-in to the government dictates. The truckers, those "fringe minority," were saying (and represented everyday people in saying) "Enough is enough!"

---

9   Brian Lilley, "Trudeau warns journalists that questions about China's election interference are racist and should stop," *Toronto Sun*, February 28, 2023; accessed May 29, 2023, https://torontosun.com/opinion/columnists/lilley-trudeau-warns-journalists-that-questions-about-chinas-election-interference-are-racist-and-should-stop.
10  First Freedoms Foundation, https://www.firstfreedoms.ca

The prime minister belittled the truckers. He was obviously miffed, perhaps baffled, that anyone would dare hold a different view than his and do something about it. As expected, the mainstream media were there to join the mocking of the truckers. Supporting the truckers was then and continues to be for the members of "The Cathedral"[11] the new social taboo.

The truckers were the uneducated, or "terrorists," as Deputy Prime Minister Chrystia Freeland referred to them in her notes after talking with the Canadian bankers. They were the "fringe minority" with "unacceptable views," as the prime minister called them. The establishment were not in favour of the truckers and all they represented. Their actions challenged the "new normal" of government by fiat during the COVID-19 pandemic. Indeed, the pandemic was a catalyst for Mr. Trudeau to engage in implementing governance ideas gleaned from the World Economic Forum (WEF) connections.

The trucker convoy across the country was the "Canadian Paul Revere ride," warning us that our treatment at the hands of our government was unacceptable and the government had thrown away its right to the benefit of the doubt. It was a call that remains fixated in our minds—despite the "Tut tut!" of those in the Cathedral. The time had come for freedom, not "freedumb" (as the scornful mocked the truckers).[12]

No doubt in the minds of the government in Ottawa the truckers failed. They didn't get the federal government to back down; in fact, the government doubled down on their mandates and crushed the protest. At best, the government enjoyed only a pyrrhic victory. Prime Minister Justin Trudeau did an applause-worthy job in explaining his decision to invoke the Emergencies Act when he testified at the Public Order Emergency Commission hearings. It was by far his best performance. It appears our own "Teflon" prime minister has "done it again" with nothing to fear. Justice Rouleau sure helped. It might look that way, but I believe a major chink in his armour was revealed. He pushed too far, as we will discuss. Canadians now realize they have a voice, but only if they don't wait for

---

11  I define what I mean by this term on pages 21 and 22 below.
12  Just a Canadian, "The Day the FreeDUMB Died," YouTube, February 27, 2022, 8:46, https://www.youtube.com/watch?v=XboIVT3OiDw.

others to speak up. It is that willingness to push back that has changed Canada for the long haul.

I venture to say that while Mr. Trudeau may continue to "win" for a while yet—with the support of Mr. Jagmeet Singh and the NDP, he may end up being prime minister for another go—although I question that as his approval poll numbers continue to sink[13]—we are witnessing an accumulation of misdirected actions and misspeak concerning the truth that adds more weight against his political future. Even the recent revamping of the cabinet[14] may not change the trajectory that has taken years to develop. Think of Old Marley's ghost in Dickens' *A Christmas Carol*. Eventually, even precious metal tarnishes. The truckers may have saved Canadians from a naïve belief that government is always good. Although Mr. Trudeau is "absolutely, absolutely serene and confident" that he made the right choice in invoking the Emergencies Act,[15] many Canadians experienced "the same interactions [...] very differently from one person to the next."[16]

A suave politician with a history of scandals, coverups, and lies. A hard-working trucker and his big rig, driving through the Rockies and across the snowy prairies. A state-funded journalist looking for "dirt" to discredit the movement. A desperate family facing stacks of bills and an empty pantry. A maverick Albertan standing up against a coercive government and greedy corporations. A doctor under fire for challenging the medical establishment. These could be stock characters in a blockbuster movie. These individuals—and thousands like them[17]—were all part of an unfolding, real-life drama that gripped a bitterly cold Canada in January and February 2022.

---

13   https://angusreid.org/trudeau-tracker/ accessed July 27, 2023.
14   July 26, 2023, Prime Minister announces changes to the Ministry, https://www.pm.gc.ca/en/news/news-releases/2023/07/26/prime-minister-announces-changes-ministry
15   POEC,Volume31,p.68–69.Online:https://publicorderemergencycommission.ca/files/documents/Transcripts/POEC-Public-Hearings-Volume-30-November-24-2022.pdf
16   Obviously, a play on Mr. Trudeau's reaction to the groping allegations he faced. See *Toronto Star*, "Trudeau on Groping Allegation: 'I Did Not Act Inappropriately,'" YouTube, July 5, 2018, 2:21, https://www.youtube.com/watch?v=iuH0EKBEaFQ.
17   See Gabrielle Bauer, *Blindsight is 2020*, (Brownstone Institute, 2023), for a great presentation of many who stood up against the current.

The dramatic skills of Prime Minister Justin Trudeau, a former part-time actor and high school drama teacher, were on full display during the Freedom Convoy protests. He began by scoffing at the "fringe minority" approaching Ottawa. He ended by invoking the most extreme powers available to him through the never-before-used Emergencies Act.

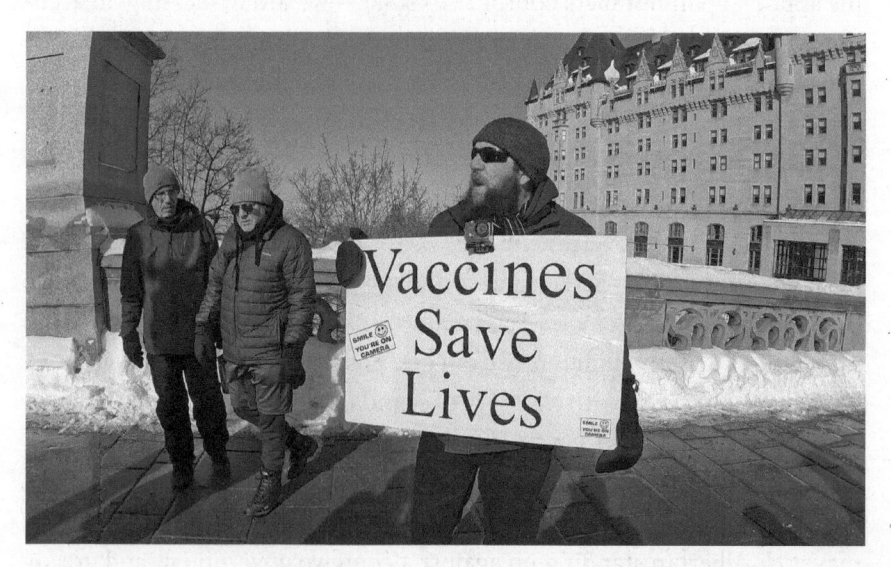

*A Vaccine Supporter At The Trucker Protest Let His Views Be Known*

On the surface, the protests failed. Trudeau refused to meet with the truckers. Federal vaccine mandates weren't lifted until June 20, 2022, and even then, they were only "suspended," not eliminated. Months after the convoy was forcefully—even brutally—cleared from the capital, the government scandals, coverups, and lies continue as inflation soars, the economy teeters on the verge of collapse, and a new scandal involving foreign electoral interference supporting the ruling Liberals emerges. The Public Order Emergency Commission (POEC) hearings held in November revealed that the prime minister had no evidence that the situation had met the conditions outlined by the Emergencies Act for invoking its powers. He was given a pass by Rouleau, but it was not a home run, as Rouleau stated, "I have done so with reluctance."[18]

Canadians are waking (even if ever so slowly) from their slumber. They've had enough of Trudeau's antics, and, thanks to the truckers, they're no longer willing to "go with the flow." They've seen the blatant biases of the media. Their eyes have been opened to the propaganda and political lies. Their sense of isolation and division has been replaced by a growing sense of unity and hope for the future—a future without politicians who use the currency of fear to divide opposition and therefore get their way.

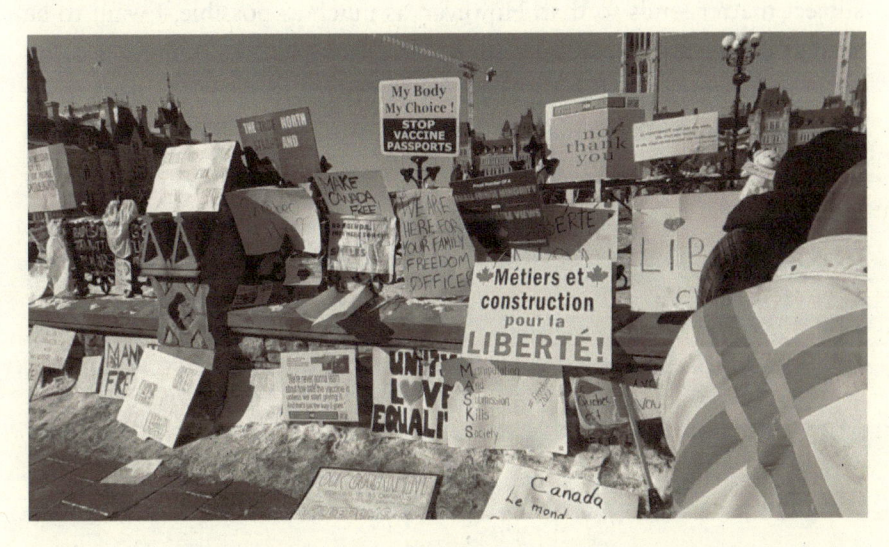

*Supporters Set Up A Freedom Memorial At Parliament Hill*

That is the real drama that this book will recount: how the truckers exposed the failures of elites while empowering ordinary Canadians to stand for faith, freedom, and hope. It's a book about the best of the Trucker Freedom Convoy and how we might use that positive spirit to make Canada a better place to live.

---

18  Public Order Emergency Commission, "Report of the Public Inquiry into the 2022 Public Order Emergency. Volume 1: Overview" (Ottawa, 2023), 247, accessed May 10, 2023. https://publicorderemergencycommission.ca/files/documents/Final-Report/Vol-1-Report-of-the-Public-Inquiry-into-the-2022-Public-Order-Emergency.pdf.

In recent years, most of my writing has been academic. This is my first major work meant for the general public. However, understand that as an academic and a lawyer, I don't want to state something as a fact that I can't back up, and I've used many citations so that you, the reader, will know that I'm not making it up. Many people were asked for their opinion on my drafts. It slowed me down but everyone who assisted me in reviewing this work has made it much better.

I give insights that I hope the reader will find helpful in understanding the concepts that politicians routinely use in debating public policy. Throughout this work, I do offer my opinions. That is as it should be. The subject matter lends to that. However, as much as possible, I want to be seen as having a reasonable opinion, even if the reader disagrees. I didn't write to be agreeable but to share my thoughts on what I believe to be a pivotal moment in Canadian political history—the Trucker Freedom Convoy 2022 and why I think the momentum it generated is for the long haul.

# INTRODUCTION

**WHY THIS BOOK?**

An acquaintance of mine recently said to me, "Barry, I admire your willingness to suffer personal cost for what you believe in. We often talk about taking a stand on issues, but how many do it? I totally disagree with you, but I admire you."

I appreciated his honesty, the frankness, and the willingness to talk to me directly.

During the years 2020–2022, we all suffered the "sudden friendship and family death syndrome." Those who you thought were friends struggled with your decision for or against the various governments' approach to the COVID-19 pandemic. The governments of Canada as a whole (provincial and national), regardless of party affiliation, failed the Canadian people. Their failures will reverberate for years to come. It wasn't simply the vaccine mandates, but their failures included the entire imposition of policies that removed basic human rights to speech, conscience, and inviolability of the person. Quite frankly the rule of law itself was challenged to a breaking point as we were governed increasingly by state bureaucrats rather than by our elected representatives. Those who stood against these measures were seen as nonconformists and troublemakers, defying a government that was "trying to do the right thing."

Many failed to recognize that questioning government policies that affect fundamental human rights is not only proper but the only way to maintain a "free and democratic" country. If we've learned anything from the last several years of government bungling, it's that we, the citizens, must, indeed we have a duty to speak out and question the government. Government must not be given the benefit of the doubt—period, and certainly not when they trample on our rights. We cannot give our political masters a free pass. We must challenge as never before.

Unfortunately, many of us were sideswiped by how quickly years-long friendships suddenly dried up because we dared to question the narrative. How could that be?

As a student of history, I understand vicariously how it works. Many in the past felt compelled by Providence or personal conscience to say, "I cannot go along with government and/or government policy." These individuals were willing to face whatever repercussions came for being true to conscience. Today, those who refuse the "COVID-19 vaccine" on conscience are compelled by the same kind of courage as those who stood in front of the tanks in Tiananmen Square, or who refused to offer the pinch of incense to Caesar. To the conscientiously convicted, going along with the crowd is a non-starter when their conscience fundamentally opposes forced action.

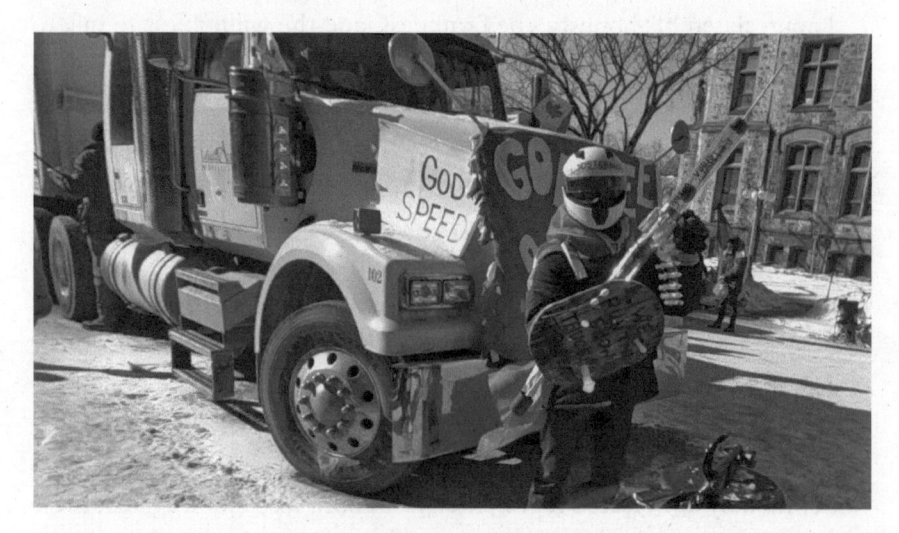

*Some Went To Great Creative Lengths To Make Their Point*

So convinced are these conscientious objectors that they're willing to pay the price. They are not provocateurs. They aren't interested in creating a scene for the sake of grabbing the spotlight. They simply cannot violate their conscience. And because of their conviction, they do end up creating a scene that causes their friends to simply shake their heads in disbelief and walk away. The loss of friends is at first a lonely experience, but in time solace is found when they bump into people on the same path and make new friendships.

Let me be clear: I am not saying that those who got the COVID-19 vaccine—without a tinge of conscientious objection—are somehow evil. Not at all. They followed what they thought to be right or did it to maintain their livelihood as most truckers did. As an aside, truckers had a higher vaccine rate than the general population.[19]

Others may have felt it would be unconscionable not to take the vaccine for valid reasons, such as protecting one's neighbour from a terrible disease. Nor am I trying to convince you, the reader, of what is appropriate for you to do, but I do hope that you appreciate that government coercive policies implemented during the pandemic were wrong.

No government has any business demonizing citizens for being faithful to their fully or partially informed conscientious opinion. The government stepped into a deeply spiritual, or metaphysical, realm in which they had no competence to interfere. It's this basic point that the Trucker Freedom Convoy came to represent.

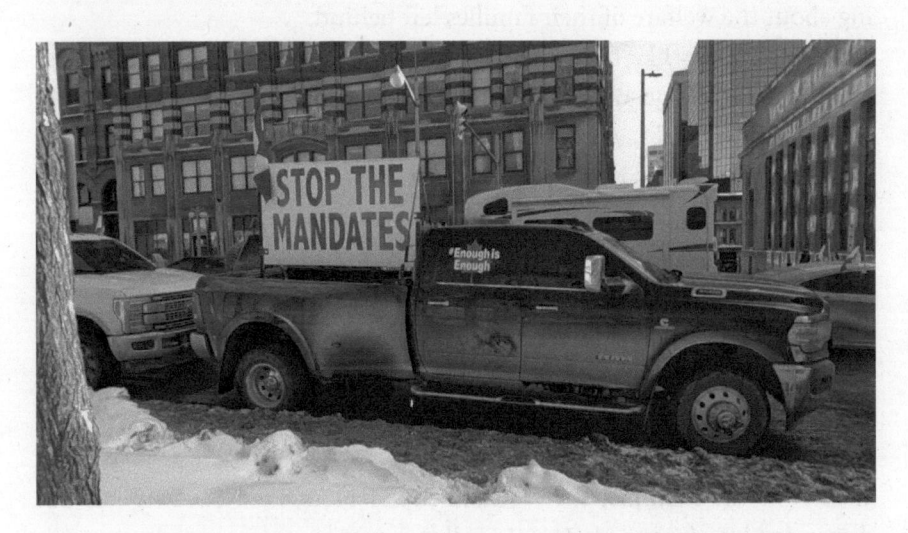

*Mud-laden Trucks Travelled Long Distances With A Short Message*

---

[19] Katherine Fung, "Canadian 'Freedom' Truckers Protest Vaccines As 90 Percent of Drivers Vaccinated," Newsweek, January 28, 2022, accessed September 5, 2023, https://www.newsweek.com/canadian-freedom-truckers-protest-vaccines-90-percent-drivers-vaccinated-1674109

Herein is the crux of the matter: as a society, we must allow individuals to follow the dictates of their conscience. We may not agree with what others choose, but we must respect the individual conscience as it expresses deep spiritual commitments.

Fourteen years ago, I travelled around North America interviewing Canadian men who were conscientious objectors and refused to bear arms in WWII. I plan to put together a documentary of their story and hope to finish this project someday before my sojourn on earth is done. These were once young men whose conscience did not allow them to join or accept conscription into the regular forces. The Canadian government established many work camps around the country for these objectors to serve their country for the same amount of time as regular conscripts. The inmates worked on public service projects such as building roads in Banff and Jasper; they cut "snags" in the forests of British Columbia; they logged or farmed in Ontario. They were paid half of what the military conscripts were paid. Some were married with children and owned a farm back home with mortgages to pay. I heard their stories of mental breakdowns worrying about the welfare of their families left behind.

Conscience is like that. It demands us to be true to convictions even when the state says otherwise. Even when family says otherwise. Even when the "experts" say otherwise. Even when refusing to accept the state directive comes at a huge personal cost. The objectors understand that there are certain hills we must be willing to die on. To the non-objector, such convictions are utter foolishness, and they have no sympathy for the consequences of the "choices" the conscientious make.

I also understand that when government takes upon itself draconian powers in times of "national emergency," it rarely lets them go. We need only to remember the powers the Canadian state and other Western democracies took for themselves in response to the 9/11 attacks in 2001. In the US for example, the Department of Homeland Security has not disbanded but expanded. The Canadian government gave itself sweeping powers with *The Anti-Terrorism Act*. Those powers remain. They haven't been cut back, but at every opportunity are expanded. Canada has the mechanisms for secret trials, pre-emptive detention, and surveillance to deal with "terrorism." And, of course, because of the "terrorist Trucker Freedom Convoy," they can now seize bank accounts.

Those in power redefine words to enable their continued hold on power. The word "terrorist" is malleable, as is any other word, by government say-so. We must hold government accountable to the misuse of language. "Terrorism" used in the context of the Freedom Convoy 2022 makes no sense. Consider the horrific acts of terror around the world. Think only of the October 7, 2023, Hamas raids on Israel that included the brutality upon innocent children in a kibbutz in the hundreds upon hundreds of innocent civilians massacred.[20] That is terrorism. What happened in Ottawa during the Freedom Convoy 2022 was not terrorism.[21] It was a peaceful protest. CBC news could not bring itself to call the Hamas attack on October 7, 2023 "terrorism"[22] but had no problem publishing stories from 'experts' that called into question the peaceful Canadian truckers.[23]

---

20  Lazar Berman, "'At least 40 babies killed': Foreign reporters taken to massacre site in Kfar Aza With terrorists' bodies still lying in the grass, international press witnesses firsthand the shocking aftermath of Hamas's slaughter of Israeli civilians," The Times of Israel, October 10, 2023, https://www.timesofisrael.com/israel-takes-foreign-journalists-to-see-massacre-site-in-kfar-aza/ "It's not a war," General Itai Veruv, head of the IDF's Depth Command, told reporters. "It's not a battlefield. You see the babies, the mothers, the fathers in their bedrooms, in their protection rooms, and how the terrorists kill them. It's not a war… it's a massacre."

21  Phil Gurski, "The 'truck convoy' is many things but it is not terrorism," Ottawa Citizen, Feb 03, 2022, https://ottawacitizen.com/opinion/gurski-the-truckers-convoy-is-many-things-but-it-is-not-terrorism

22  Marnie Cathcart, "CBC Leaked Email Tells Reporters Not to Use Term 'Terrorists' in Connection With Israel Attacks, The Epoch Times, October 8, 2023, https://www.theepochtimes.com/world/cbc-leaked-email-tells-reporters-not-to-use-term-terrorists-in-connection-with-israel-attacks-5506197; see @StopAntisemites https://twitter.com/StopAntisemites/status/1710862706914349283

23  Elizabeth Thompson, "Convoy protest could change the way money is monitored, says watchdog agency," CBC, February 10, 2022, https://www.cbc.ca/news/politics/truck-convoy-fundraiser-gofundme-1.6346639. Thompson went to some length to make a connection between the trucker protest and 'Ideologically Motivated Violent Extremism' as government monitored donations to the protest; Stephanie Hogan, "The Ottawa convoy has 'shattered norms' for protest in Canada. Will we see more of it?" CBC News, February, 19, 2022, https://www.cbc.ca/news/canada/trucker-freedom-

CBC was not alone – *Parliament Today* warned that those donating to the Convoy could be charged with supporting terrorism.[24]

Prime Minister Trudeau's invocation of the Emergencies Act gave him the ability to expand the Terrorist Financing Act rules to, in essence, declare those who gave money to the truckers' crowdfunding campaign as supporters of "terrorism." If you control the definitions of words, you control speech. If you control speech, then your views become truth.

In the same methodical manner, we saw the police move a half-step forward in a rhythmical beat during the final days of the Trucker Freedom Convoy. They marched on the peaceful protesters in front of the historic Chateau Laurier in Ottawa in February 2022. With each new "crisis," Canada is slowly changing its peaceful demeanour into a more authoritarian one. The incremental process is there for all to see. Every crisis is seen as an "opportunity" for further expansion of power. An expansion of the term "terrorism." The government takes one step at a time until it reaches the point of serious pushback by citizens. By that time, the government might have taken ten steps forward. At the pushback, it might give back two, but it keeps eight. The net effect is that we are less free, and the totalitarian advance may continue with the next "crisis."

That, in my view, is a process with perilous potential for totalitarianism.

---

convoy-new-normal-1.6355574, University of Ottawa Professor, Regina Bateson was quoted as saying, "What we've seen in Ottawa is something that had elements of a protest to start with, that then morphed into an illegal occupation, that now has significant foreign involvement, as well as more organized militia-style activity happening."

24 "Parliament Today deletes tweet suggesting donations to trucker convoy could be providing 'financial services' for 'terrorist activity'," https://web.archive.org/web/20230207160157/https://westphaliantimes.com/parliament-today-deletes-tweet-suggesting-donations-to-trucker-convoy-could-be-providing-financial-services-for-terrorist-activity/

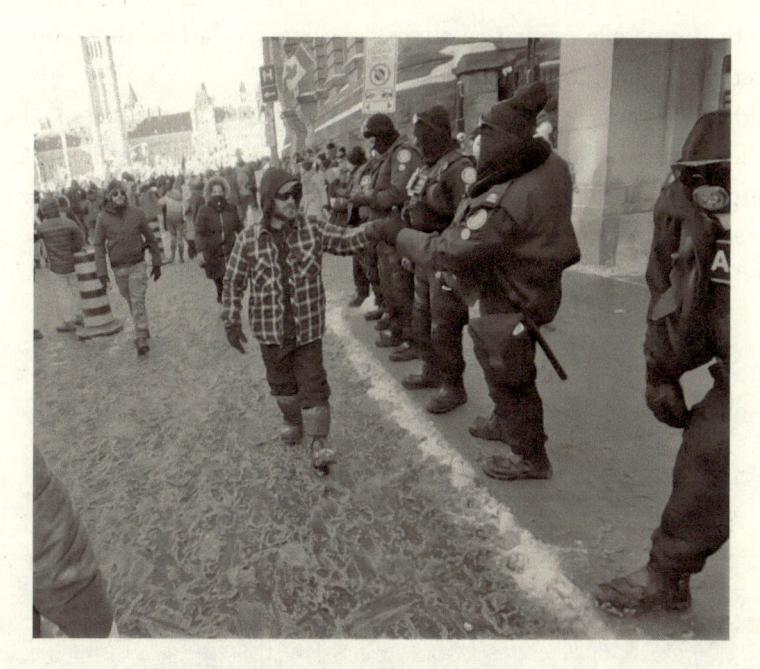

*Protesters Saw Police As Allies*

Canada's federal government is currently led by an ideologically driven executive willing to destroy our freedoms in pursuit of its utopian goals. It has little respect for the Constitution and our long political and social traditions. It wants to do things differently because it arrogantly claims to know more than those who built our country and whose cultural commitments made our institutions work. Our current executive is not unlike the youthful crypto currency manager who claimed an ability to defy all the rules of finance, known throughout the centuries, in the pursuit of a new buzz phrase: "effective altruism." His crypto was a fraud.[25] The rules of finance remain, but his crypto empire is crumbling.

This type of governance has a dark history throughout the millennia. Leaders fixated on their own objectives, at the expense of the law and their people, have destroyed entire civilizations. Their lack of empathy for the

---

25  Jonathan Hannah, "Sam Bankman-Fried's downfall is more than a black eye for Effective Altruism," *Philanthropy Daily*, November 18, 2022, accessed May 10, 2023, https://www.philanthropydaily.com/sam-bankman-frieds-downfall-is-more-than-a-black-eye-for-effective-altruism/.

pain of the people is seen as almost necessary to attain their "utopian" objectives deemed to be "for the collective good."

When the people rise up to confront the utopian madness,[26] they're labelled enemies of the state. The evidence revealed from the Public Order Emergency Commission clearly reveals the government's clandestine plan to create the narrative that the truckers were extreme even before they rolled into Ottawa.[27]

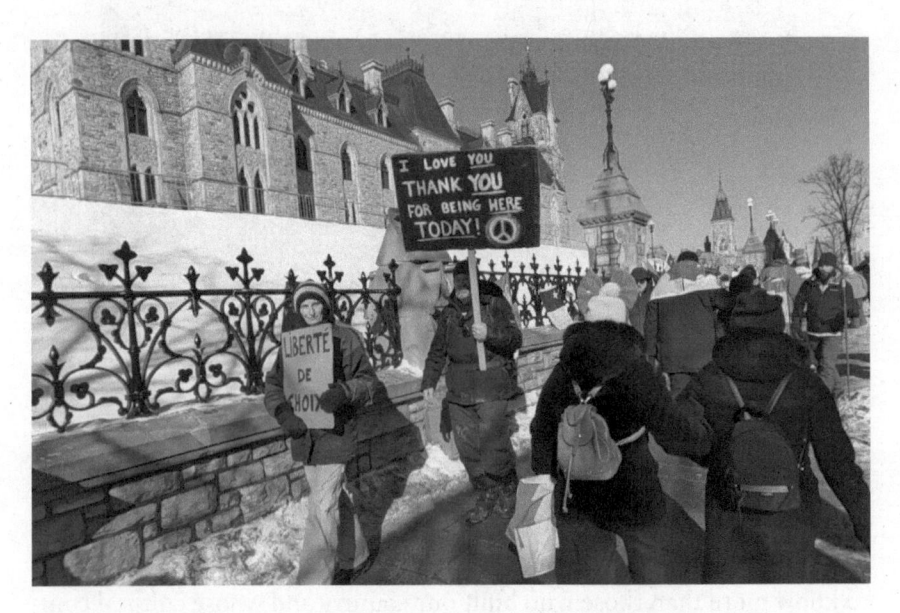

*Far From Extremists The Protesters Were Peaceful*

The Trucker Freedom Convoy struck a chord in the hearts of many Canadians who were sick and tired of the government mandates during the COVID-19 pandemic. The lost jobs, the broken homes, the constant messages of fear propagated throughout the mainstream media escalated when the prime minister declared an attack on the unvaccinated in 2021.

---

26  See Barry W. Bussey, "Utopian Danger—Interview with Professor Ryan Alford," First Freedoms Foundation, accessed May 10, 2023, https://firstfreedoms.ca/utopian-danger-freedom-feature-with-dr-ryan-alford/.

27  Andrew Lawton, "Mendicino's office wanted to keep 'crazies' in Freedom Convoy," *True North*, October 31, 2022, accessed May 10, 2023, https://tnc.news/2022/10/31/mendicinos-office-convoy/.

Up to and during the election, he and his political operatives took an aggressive turn for political purposes. Once the truckers got caught up in the political web, they took it upon themselves to push back against the government overreach. It was a spontaneous uprising of hurting people who could no longer stay quiet in the face of government lies and disinformation in its attempt to control an uncontrollable virus.[28] The ideas of those members of "the Cathedral" are at odds with those who are on the ground simply trying to earn a living and going about their daily affairs.

By "members of the Cathedral,"[29] I mean those "progressive" social influencers of the left, the "ruling class of government, big business, media, and academia," and they are nervous about populist movements like the Truckers' Convoy. I agree with Prof. Bruce Pardy, who points out

---

28  John Johnson and Denis Rancourt, "Lockdowns Did Not Save Lives," Brownstone Institute, September 6, 2022, https://brownstone.org/articles/lockdowns-did-not-save-lives/. It was found that the lockdowns were a massive experiment that "was a failure of public health policy and that lockdown measures should not be used during future disease outbreaks." Also see Drs. Neil Rau, Pooya Kazemi, Martha Fulford, and Jennifer Grant, "COVID measures were a mistake, let's not repeat them: It is time to accept that the virus cannot be stopped and will continue to evolve," *National Post*, September 14, 2022, accessed May 10, 2023, https://nationalpost.com/opinion/opinion-draconian-COVID-measures-were-a-mistake-lets-not-repeat-them.

29  I first thought that I would refer to this group as "the chattering classes"; however, I wasn't totally comfortable with that appellation, as it comes across as crass or pejorative. In a way, I want to be pejorative, but that defeats my purpose of trying to be reasonable. The term "chattering classes" has been around for a long time, although I thought I had coined the term! Nothing new under the sun, as Solomon said. Anne E. Kornblut's April 2, 2006 *The New York Times*, "The Peculiar Power of the Chattering Class," https://www.nytimes.com/2006/04/02/weekinreview/the-peculiar-power-of-the-chattering-class.html, provides a good description of what I wanted to get across by using the term, but again it has a negative connotation. As you will see, I'm a fan of Aleksandr Solzhenitsyn, who famously stated that we ought to "live not by lies." Then I came across John Pye's *Cathedral of Lies: The Art of Deception Is a Dangerous Game* (John Pye Books, 2013) and Steve Cortes "The Cathedral of Lies: A cascade of Falsehoods from the Ruling Class—on January 6th, Ukraine, & Inflation," March 7, 2023, https://stevecortes.substack.com/p/the-cathedral-of-lies. He provides a great description: "The Cathedral—an appellation for the Ruling Class of government, big business, media, and academia—clearly feels the growing power of the patriotic populist movement in America."

that they are not a "class" in the Marxist-Leninist sense. They are, using Pardy's words,

> ... civilized. The group that will take direction from the people of "expertise." [These are] the people who are educated. The people who live in cities. The people who work for institutions like the government. These are the "real" people. These are the "progressive" people. These are the "reasonable" people. These are the people who "make sense." And, if you don't go along with measures that are recommended by experts and that are designed by the common good then you are an unsophisticated redneck. And you deserve to be condemned.[30]

The ideological commitments of the Cathedral are currently dominant in our culture. This class includes the mainstream media, academia, most labour union leaders, most big tech oligarchs (Elon Musk being the exception, it seems, we shall see as time goes on), big business, and others who love to pontificate on how we all ought to live to support the "progressive" far left of centre agenda. They are the complex web that establishes society's current taboos. They claim ownership of our vocabulary and therefore seek to control our speech and our minds by default. Pushback against their worldview is met with an avalanche of vitriol. They label those who think differently with a slew of pejorative terms, such as "racist," "anti-science," "non-compassionate," "selfish," "uneducated," and "hurtful." Many more slurs can be added to the growing list.

I recognize that not everyone who is part of mainstream media, academia, labour-union leadership, big tech oligarchies, big business, etc., is speaking with the same voice. Not at all. There's considerable debate and discussion about a multitude of issues and concepts. Also, among these groups are those who disagree profoundly with the "accepted" opinions but refuse to speak out for fear of losing their jobs or positions or the berating and belittling they are subjected to.

---

30  Barry W. Bussey and Bruce Pardy, discussing the first day of hearings of the Public Order Emergency Commission, October 13, 2022, https://firstfreedoms.ca/day-one-public-order-emergency-commission/.

Despite this complexity, there is, in my view, a consensus on acceptable and unacceptable opinion and views, on what can and cannot be said and done in society-at-large, which is dominated by those in the Cathedral. In my analysis, the current prime minister personifies the goals and objectives of the members of the Cathedral. He is their spokesperson, and like all politicians, he plays to his base for political gain[31] and speaks the "woke" language to which this class has become so attuned.

To understand our prime minister and those around him, it's important that we try to "walk in his shoes" to make sense of his view of the world. We may pick up on his beliefs by the language he uses and by his actions. The two are not necessarily synonymous with the prime minister—he will say one thing to keep his support base on his side, but then do another. However, at times he is synchronised, and that's when we need to worry. Such commitments are leading this country into a horrendous mess financially, socially, and morally.

This "woke" language, no doubt, sounds odd to the average Canadian just trying to make ends meet. It is odd. Understanding the prime minister's use of "woke" terminology helps us make sense of his over-the-top response.

First, we need to understand the term "woke." As was pointed out to me recently, "Though you conservatives now like to use 'woke' as a slur, remember the root is being awake. Aware. Paying attention." Indeed, it is. What is it that the members of the Cathedral want us to be aware of? It's primarily our own inherent racism and bias supporting the "colonial" institutions that continually enforce our "White privilege."

Being aware of one's bias is helpful in trying to discover what is true. One must be aware that there are truths—objective truths. Take George Orwell's observation that 2 + 2 does not equal 5. It never has, nor will it, no matter how much those in power, as described in *1984*, seek to enforce

---

31 Pascale Dangoisse & Gabriela Perdomo, "Gender Equality through a Neoliberal Lens: A Discourse Analysis of Justin Trudeau's Official Speeches," Women's Studies in Communication," Taylor & Francis Online, July 16, 2020, https://www.tandfonline.com/doi/abs/10.1080/07491409.2020.1781315?journalCode=uwsc20..

their view that it does. It's here where the "woke" would argue that "you conservatives" are wrong. Let me explain.

The "progressive left" increasingly sees the world very differently from the "conservative right." It used to be that progressives were advocates of "secular liberalism," with a small "l." That's liberalism in a post-Enlightenment secular philosophy that supports individual freedom, separation of church and state, free enterprise, freedom of speech, freedom of conscience and religion, the inviolability of the person and the rule of law.

The Canadian Charter of Rights and Freedoms is a very "liberal" document with a few carry-overs of the mixing of church and state, such as in the education rights of Roman Catholics to receive public funding in certain provinces. For those in the Cathedral, at least from how I understand them, the Charter needs to be "updated" with the concept of "Charter values." The term "Charter values" is nowhere in the Charter. It's a recent judge-made concept that seeks to divine or figure out the spirit, or the essence, of the Charter that is applicable to the case in court. It's a vague concept with the horrendous outcome that individuals or entities with Charter rights are denied those rights because of so-called "Charter values."

For example, Trinity Western University (TWU), a Christian school, was denied the right to have a law school by the Supreme Court of Canada because it purportedly violated the "Charter value" of equality. TWU required students to commit to living the Christian teachings of the school. That was seen as not treating everyone equally. TWU had Charter section 2(a) right to freedom of religion, and section 15 right of equality, of which religion is one, so it should have been allowed to have its law school.[32] A Charter right was violated because of a "Charter value!" Does

---

[32] I acknowledge that it remains an open question as to whether a corporate entity has constitutionally protected rights. The Supreme Court of Canada opinion is divided on that point but the issue is in play and yet to be determined. See the reasoning of McLachlin C.J. and Rothstein and Moldaver JJ. at paragraphs 89–102 in Loyola High School v. Quebec (Attorney General), 2015 SCC 12 (CanLII), [2015] 1 SCR 613, <https://canlii.ca/t/ggrhf>, retrieved on 2023-09-05

that make sense to you? Not to me either. It's part of the "idiosyncrasies of the judicial mind."[33]

Not surprisingly, the most prominent "Charter value" of all, at least right now, is equality, but not equality as you would normally think of it. We often see equality as everyone being treated the same or having the same opportunity to make it in one's career, education, and so on. That is not what's being referred to. Instead, it's the *equality of outcome*, where everyone has exactly the same material or social goods.

The progressives moved our collective frame of reference, being "liberalism," further to the left with the adoption of postmodernism. Postmodern thought rejects the Enlightenment search for objective truth. It sees reason and individualism as Western patriarchal constructs that reinforce colonial institutions such as the monarchy, parliament, capitalist markets, the family, the Christian religion, and private property. Liberalism sought ongoing conversations in a "free and democratic society" to maximize individual freedom while maintaining social peace. Postmodernism rejects liberalism outright.

Postmodernism turns on the liberal democratic state and "deconstructs" the system to discover its winners and losers, its oppressors and its oppressed.[34] Everything is viewed through this zero-sum lens. It awakens, it makes everyone aware of the "inherent bias" of our liberal society based on group identities such as race, sex, and language. The number and scope of identities continue to be in flux. Conflict and oppression, communalism and egalitarian ideals are promulgated. With every liberal institution viewed as part of the colonial power structure, even science and technology are considered part of the oppressive system. It is a "cult of victimhood"

---

33 As per Justices Côté and Brown, in dissent of the SCC's decision *in Law Society of British Columbia v. Trinity Western University*, 2018 SCC 32 (CanLII), [2018] 2 SCR 293, accessed May 12, 2023, https://canlii.ca/t/hsjpr, at para. 308.

34 Stephen R.C. Hicks, *Explaining Postmodernism: Skepticism and Socialism from Rousseau to Foucault*, Expanded Edition ( Ockham's Razor Publishing, 2011).

wrapped in Marxist ideological analysis that foments a revolution against liberal society.[35]

The individual isn't seen as an individual but as a member of a group. The truckers aren't individuals but rather part of a group—White Canadians. As "White Canadians" (put in quotes because the truckers, their lead organizers, and their supporters were not all White), they have all kinds of "privileges," and during the convoy they were using their "colonial" power to take over the government (which is led by a White man of wealth and privilege) and discriminate against the various oppressed identity groups.[36]

This thinking also allows those in the Cathedral and government to justify the use of the Emergencies Act, even though the legislative conditions of the Act were not met. The rationale goes something like this: "Well, we may not have had the legal conditions to invoke the Act, but the Act is *outdated,* and it *should* allow us the ability to invoke it when there's *violence.*" Violence does not have to be "physical." It can be "verbal" too.

Therefore, by invoking the Act, the prime minister's office (PMO) could make the argument that the Act should be "read" as if the conditions were met. Why? Because of the *violence* of the words spoken by the truckers during their protest! We'll look at why all of this was not true, but that's the kind of thinking that has been going on within the Cathedral and the PMO's office.

To be "woke" then is to be aware of the fundamental identities of individuals that put them into a group that is oppressed. The goal of being "woke" is to challenge and fight the oppressors by ensuring there is "substantive equality." As noted above, this is not equality of opportunity but equality of outcome. Being judged by one's character, as the Rev. Martin

---

35  Bruce Bawer, *The Victims' Revolution: The Rise of Identity Studies and the Closing of the Liberal Mind* (New York: HarperCollins, 2012), xvi.
36  Nina Zajac wrote, "The Convoy of truckers occupying Ottawa since Jan. 28 is led by white supremacists. Not only is tolerance of the movement insulting to racialized Canadians, but it is also indicative of Canada's tolerance for racist actions." See Nina Zajac, "The Trucker Convoy demonstrates Canadians' tolerance of white supremacy," *The Charlatan*, February 15, 2022, accessed May 10, 2023 https://charlatan.ca/2022/02/15/opinion-the-trucker-convoy-demonstrates-canadians-tolerance-of-white-supremacy/.

Luther King, Jr. called for, is not the goal of this postmodern "woke" ideology. One's communal identity is the key, or at least plays a major role in advancing a person through whatever field of endeavour is pursued.

There's more.

The critical race theorists argue that there is a hierarchy of the oppressed that determines who is more deserving of advancement to ensure that equality of outcome is realized. Here we get another term: "intersectionality."[37]

Intersectionality argues that a person with more than one oppressed identity suffers oppression on a greater scale than a person with only one oppressed identity. For example, consider a man who belongs to an ethnic minority as being oppressed because of his ethnicity, but a woman who belongs to the same ethnic minority is oppressed doubly because she's also a woman. Therefore, the woman is more oppressed than the man. It gets more complicated with more identifiers, such as sexual orientation, disability, etc.[38]

By contrast, the "white, male, middle-and upper class, abled" persons are the ones who sit "at the tables of power."[39] They're the most "oppressive" of the lot. As Robin Diangelo describes, these oppressors may not have any idea that they are oppressors. "[A]ll humans have bias, inequity can occur simply through homogeneity; if I am not aware of the barriers you face, then I won't see them, much less be motivated to remove them. Nor will I be motivated to remove the barriers if they provide an advantage to which I feel entitled."[40]

When the White oppressors are "woke" to their racial bias, they must acknowledge their position of superiority and their inherent fragility

---

[37] Kimberlé Crenshaw has been credited with articulating the intersectional analysis in her piece, "Demarginalizing the Intersection of Race and Sex: A Black Feminist Critique of Antidiscrimination Doctrine, Feminist Theory and Antiracist Politics" (1989) University of Chicago Legal Forum, 139.

[38] Note that none of these categories take socioeconomic status into account; thus you end up with the implausible result that a homeless White man has more "privilege" than a Black lesbian woman who is a medical doctor.

[39] Robin Diangelo, *White Fragility: Why It's So Hard for White People to Talk about Racism*, (London, UK: Penguin, 2018), xvi.

[40] Ibid., ix.

toward any criticism, listen attentively to those aggrieved, never be defensive but reflect on the criticism, and work to change behaviour.[41] There is to be no discussion of why it is so. The focus is "on *how*—rather than *if*—our racism is manifest."[42]

Instead of being defensive over whether you're guilty of racism, you're to assume that racism is inevitable. Once you're aware, you can then make progress in removing racism from your life. For example, a White woman who cries in front of Black people triggers them because of the history of Black men being lynched after being falsely accused of rape by the crying White woman. "When a white woman cries, a black man gets hurt."[43] Therefore, a White woman who is now "woke" is never to cry among "racialized" people, because it will trigger harm. How does that fit with the truckers and Trudeau's response? We'll connect the dots shortly. In fact, this entire book will be connecting the dots on a whole lot of fronts.

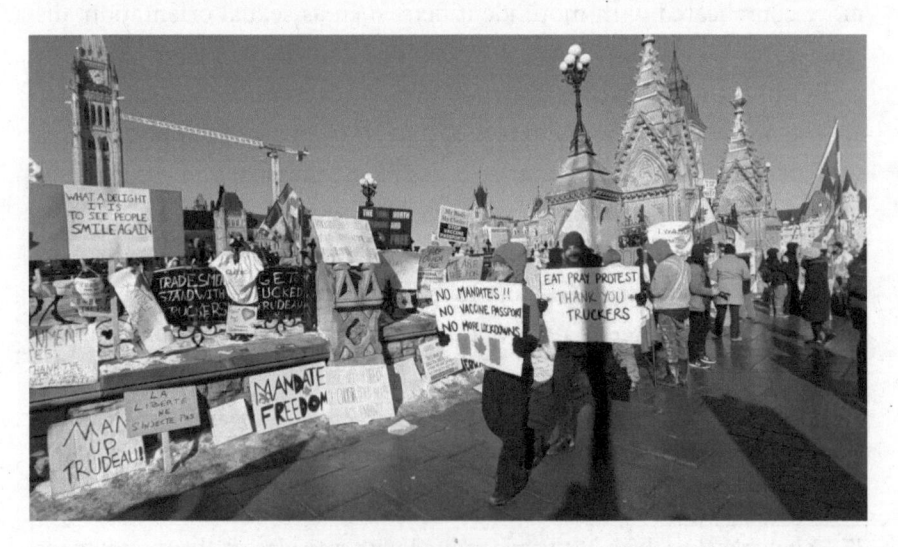

*The Winter Carnival-Like Atmosphere*

---

41   Ibid., 99–113.
42   Ibid., 129.
43   Ibid., 133.

Pluckrose and Lindsay share this description of the "woke" "scholar-activists":

> Not only do these scholar-activists speak a specialized language—while using everyday words that people assume, incorrectly, that they understand—but they also represent a wholly different *culture*, embedded within our own. People who have adopted this view may be physically close by, but intellectually, they are a world away, which makes understanding them and communicating with them incredibly difficult. They are obsessed with power, language, knowledge, and the relationships between them. They interpret the world through a lens that detects power dynamics in every interaction, utterance, and cultural artifact—even when they aren't obvious *or real*. This is a worldview that centers social and cultural grievances and aims to make everything into a zero-sum political struggle revolving around identity markers like race, sex, gender, sexuality, and many others.

Pay attention to what they have to say next, as it allows us to make sense of the hatred against the truckers:

> To an outsider, this culture feels as though it originated on another planet, whose inhabitants have no knowledge of sexually reproducing species, and who interpret all our human sociological interactions in the most cynical way possible. But, in fact, these preposterous attitudes are completely human. They bear witness to our repeatedly demonstrated capacity to take up complex spiritual worldviews, ranging from tribal animism to hippie spiritualism to sophisticated global religions, each of which adopts its own interpretive frame through which it sees the entire world. This one just happens to be about a

peculiar view of power and its ability to create inequality and oppression.[44]

Further, and here it becomes confusing, "racism" is not just prejudice against race but any position, view, or statement that goes outside of the acceptable postmodern narrative.[45]

Let's review: the Cathedral, those who control our societal narrative, are ideologically committed to the postmodern critique of our society as harbouring systemic racism. That racism is a carryover of our colonial past when White people were on top of the power pyramid. It matters not today if White people are rich or poor, educated or uneducated—they are "privileged" by virtue of their skin colour. They need to "awaken" and become "aware" of their racial bias and correct their behaviour and privilege to ensure they're not perpetuating their racism. Remember, "racism" is now a term applied not only to those who are bigoted in the racial context but in any context that goes against the "progressive" ideology.

We all see the world through a particular lens with premises embedded in it, as Professor Bruce Pardy shared with me.[46] If you don't accept the "progressive," "woke" worldview, you don't simply have a difference of opinion—"you are wrong. It has got to be wrong because you do not agree."

This thinking leads to double standards, which Pardy suggests are "all over the place" in our government and laws. If you're from the left, you must be tolerated, encouraged, and supported, even if it includes violence—even physical violence. If you're from the right, "you must be crushed." We are now in an era of "repressive tolerance," where standards for conduct and

---

44 Helen Pluckrose and James Lindsay, *Cynical Theories: How Activist Scholarship Made Everything about Race, Gender, and Identity—and Why This Harms Everybody* (Durham, NC: Pitchstone Publishing, 2020), 15–16.
45 Ibid., at 15, "When they speak of "racism," for example, they are not referring to prejudice on the grounds of race, but rather to, as they define it, a racialized system that permeates all interactions in society yet is largely invisible except to those who experience it or who have been trained in the proper "critical" methods that train them to see it."
46 You can listen to my interview with Professor Pardy at https://rumble.com/v1mixzk-you-must-be-crushed.html. Accessed May 10, 2023.

speech are different depending upon your ideological commitment.[47] "If you are burning churches or you are blocking railways, but you are doing it for a progressive cause then that is OK," Pardy explains. "But if you are the Trucker Convoy protesting vaccine mandates, well, that is beyond acceptable, civilized behaviour and you must be crushed."

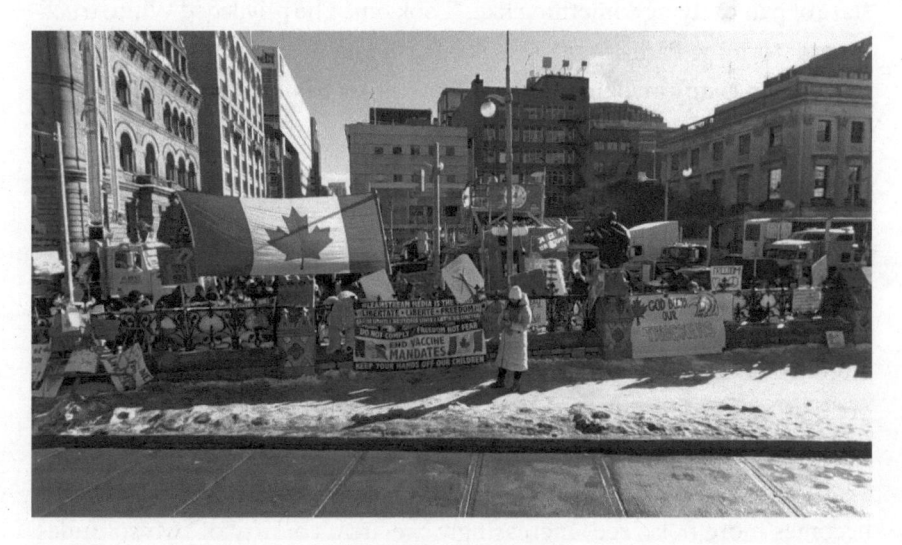

*Patriotism Abounded*

## Time to connect some dots:

I suggest that the prime minister's attack on the truckers was framed in the same way social justice "woke" activists use their version of Critical Race Theory to attack the White colonial aggressors, but these aggressors arrived in semi-trucks in late January into February 2022. They used their "White privilege" to keep everyone up at night by blowing their obnoxious horns just because they wanted the prime minister to step back from authoritarian actions, of which the vaccine mandate was but one example.

---

47  Also see my discussion with Professor David Haskell, "When Will You Stand Up? Feature Freedom Interview with David Haskell," First Freedoms Foundation, accessed May 10, 2023, https://firstfreedoms.ca/when-will-you-stand-up/.

Further, given that Prime Minister Trudeau is the spokesperson for the Cathedral, the trucker opposition wasn't just about the vaccine mandates. It was taken to be against those in the Cathedral and all they stand for in their cynical, critical-race-theory-based opposition to liberal democratic Canada as it was once known. The prime minister and his coterie appeared to be in a state of panic, saying something like, "Look out! The privileged White truckers are storming Parliament! This is our January 6 assault!"[48] Such thinking was used to justify invoking the Emergencies Act to stop the violent rhetoric.

## Two Views of the Same Reality

A common theme throughout this book is that we face two alternative views of the convoy: one positive and one negative. The positive view is based on accounts and impressions from those, like me, who walked the streets of Ottawa during the protest, and many who did not. The "progressive" Cathedral didn't need to walk the streets—they "knew" all they needed to know about "those people."

To be fair, the assumptions and divisions work both ways as our society becomes more polarized. Increasingly, we are a country of two solitudes, and it's not over language but ideology.

Those who walked the Ottawa streets in that cold winter received a very positive vibe from the people who came together to support freedom and each other. The protesters were society's outcasts who were told it was "your choice" to lose jobs and property. Suddenly they got to recognize that they weren't alone. There were tens of thousands of them who yearned to get back to "normal."

The Trucker Freedom Convoy was cooperative with authorities and made sure that emergency lanes remained open. This was made clear in the evidence given at the POEC. The city was not gridlocked. The only street that was blocked was Wellington Street, and that was because of the police barricades. Yet it still had an emergency lane. While there was some inconvenience, the city was able to operate. However, government offices

---

48 "January 6," is a reference to a demonstration that became a riot at the US Capitol Building on January 6, 2021.

closed, and some businesses closed because they didn't want to be seen as "supporting" the truckers.

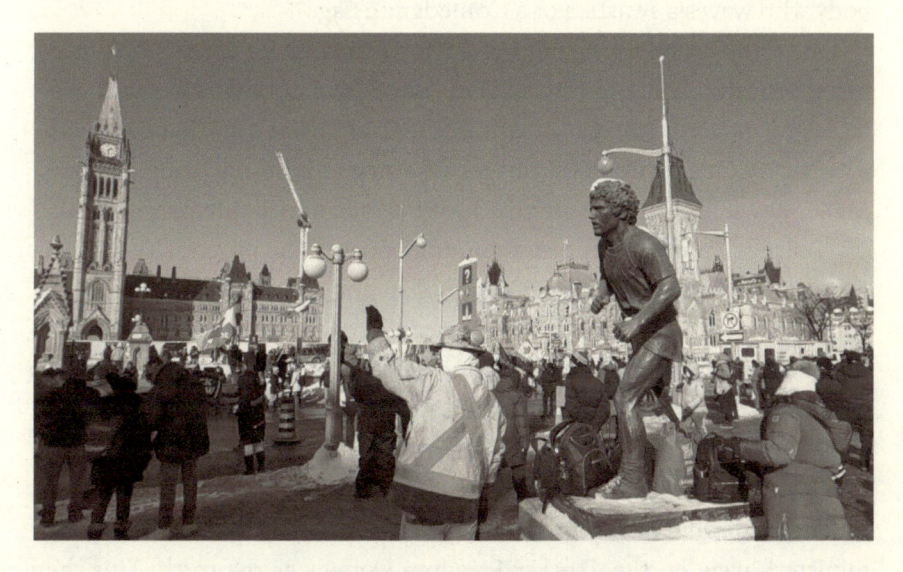

*Terry Fox Monument During Protest*

Many of those who watched from afar have a very negative impression of the protest. Their understanding of the protest comes from Prime Minister Trudeau's cynical reaction and outright lies about it, and from mainstream media's hostile reaction to the protesters and their cause. The prime minister said it was filled with violence, there was harassment, there were Nazi flags and Confederate flags everywhere. As time went on, it became clear to those watching that each of those claims was unsubstantiated.

Reading through the House of Commons debates from February 2022, one is confronted by the profound chasm between the parties. One MP, Christine Normandin, BQ, observed that "We got to the point where some were accusing people of condoning racist, violent acts, and others were saying that anyone against the protest was against freedom of expression, even though that is not what is at issue at all."[49] By exaggerating your opponent's position, it's easier to refute it. Many Conservative MPs urged

---

49 Ms. Christine Normandin (Saint-Jean, BQ), in the Emergency Debate on the COVID-19 Protests, accessed May 10, 2023, https://www.ourcommons.ca/DocumentViewer/en/44-1/house/sitting-25/hansard.

dialogue, while the Liberals repeatedly made blanket comments like that of Mr. Yasir Naqvi, Liberal: "I am not interested in speaking with somebody who waves a swastika or a Confederate flag."[50]

The Ottawa city councillor for Ottawa's downtown denied the protest being peaceful. She said the residents were "seeing the images that we're all seeing, of very right-wing extremist messages: the flags that display the swastika, Confederate flags, images of a prime minister being lynched," McKenney said. "I'm not sure that I would continue to call this peaceful."[51]

As Bruce Pardy points out, the intolerance of the progressive mindset refuses to tolerate anything it deems "beyond the pale." As soon as the convoy was labelled racist, it could be condemned without any attempt to understand or empathize with anyone involved, whatever their views. This was what the prime minister's office wanted as it created the "Truckers are extremist" narrative and sent emissaries to the media with that message.[52] The PMO holds that narrative to this day.

The media and the entire federal government apparatus hold the prime minister's view on the Trucker Freedom Convoy as the truth. This then gets played out in the media coverage and in how people like Tamara Lich, one of the convoy organizers, was unfairly treated by government lawyers, including, it would seem, the Ontario Crown Attorney's office.

---

50  Mr. Yasir Naqvi (Parliamentary Secretary to the President of the Queen's Privy Council for Canada and Minister of Emergency Preparedness, Lib.), in the Emergency Debate on the COVID-19 Protests, accessed May 10, 2023, https://www.ourcommons.ca/DocumentViewer/en/44-1/house/sitting-25/hansard.
51  Adina Bresge, "Calling the Ottawa protests 'peaceful' plays down non-violent dangers, critics say," The Canadian Press, January 31, 2022, accessed September 5, 2023, https://www.theglobeandmail.com/canada/article-calling-the-ottawa-protests-peaceful-downplays-non-violent-dangers/
52  Rachel Aiello, "Convoy organizers had extreme aims, says PM's national security adviser, CTV News,
    March 10, 2022, https://www.ctvnews.ca/politics/convoy-organizers-had-extreme-aims-says-pm-s-national-security-adviser-1.5814097

## Compelled to Write

The Trucker Freedom Convoy was diverse. I was there for three days over two weekends and can attest to the diversity. The convoy didn't represent the language of those in the Cathedral. It was an "earthy" protest in that it represented the common, down-to-earth, hard-working, industrious people whose traditions and way of life are very different from the views espoused by the prime minister. That difference may help explain the disconnect between the prime minister and the truckers.

The 2021 election forced me to take a personal stand against the hatred being advocated by the prime minister toward the unvaccinated. I left my position of ten years and started First Freedoms Foundation to be a voice against the inhumanity being imposed by our own government. It was a bold move. It was the right move. The Trucker Freedom Convoy and the prime minister's brutal crackdown against them only confirmed my suspicion of the totalitarian trajectory on which it seems he is taking the country.

The bravery of the truckers, the moment of freedom their protest represented, the amazing non-violent, peaceful nature of their cry to government to change course will turn out to be a defining moment in Canadian history. As the months have passed since the prime minister's authorization for the brutal takedown of the protesters, I have reflected on what it all meant. I have some thoughts on why Mr. Trudeau and his supporters were so troubled by this protest, which I will share in the coming pages.

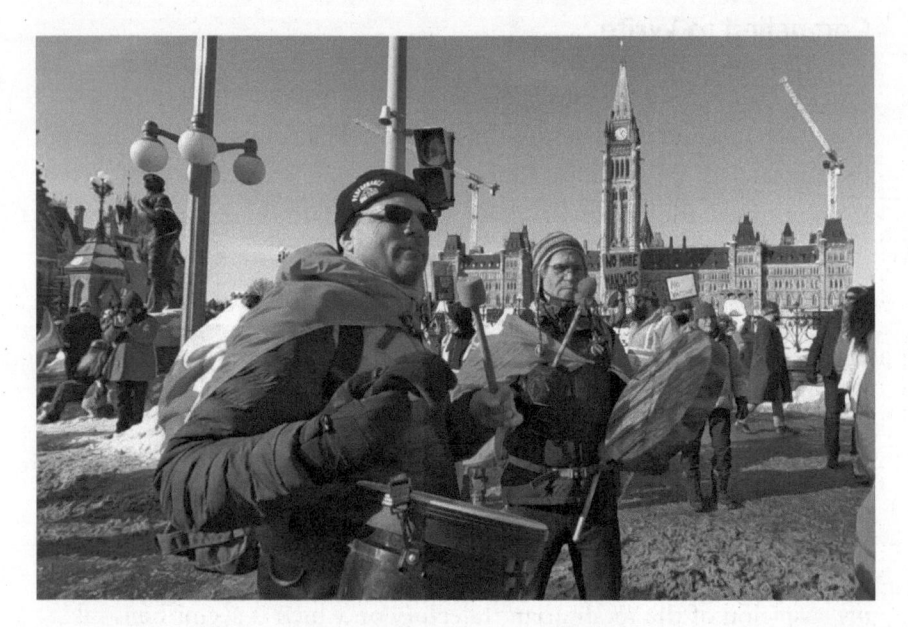

*Drums, Music, Horns Filled The Air*

It's important for average Canadians not to lose hope over the decisions of the prime minister's office against the Trucker Freedom Convoy 2022. Such actions only tell us that those holding power failed to gain the trust and understanding of the people. The brutal takedown is a sign of failure. It reveals a regime with a troubled soul. That realization is important because we now know beyond any doubt what we're up against. And like the crackdowns of non-violent movements in the past, such actions are made by those who recognize they have ultimately lost the war of ideas. Make no mistake the government's crackdown foreshadows their loss of power. It will happen and when it does the pundits will look back to the Freedom Convoy 2022 as the beginning of the end of the Trudeau government.

A wounded regime is prone to hit back hard, and it may yet do worse, but it has already lost the heart and soul of the working people. I decided to be a part of a cause that must ultimately succeed rather than support a cause that must ultimately fail. The Trucker Freedom Convoy 2022 succeeded in causing the Cathedral, the mainstream media, academia, the politicos, and the Ottawa establishment to nervously ask, "What does this all mean?"

My answer: 16 ways the Trucker protest ignited Canadian citizens to stand against any regime that would destroy Diefenbaker's definition of a free Canadian.[53] It is a movement that continues to boil. The Cathedral has every reason to be concerned for soon they will no longer recognize their own place in the new Canada that will be transformed by the renewal of the old virtues of truth, justice, love, humility, prudence, and courage. A place where faith, hope, and charity will be ideals to strive for once again. The Cathedral's failures of the present will be the base upon which to build a better society – a more just society. This was a movement that I had no choice but to write about.

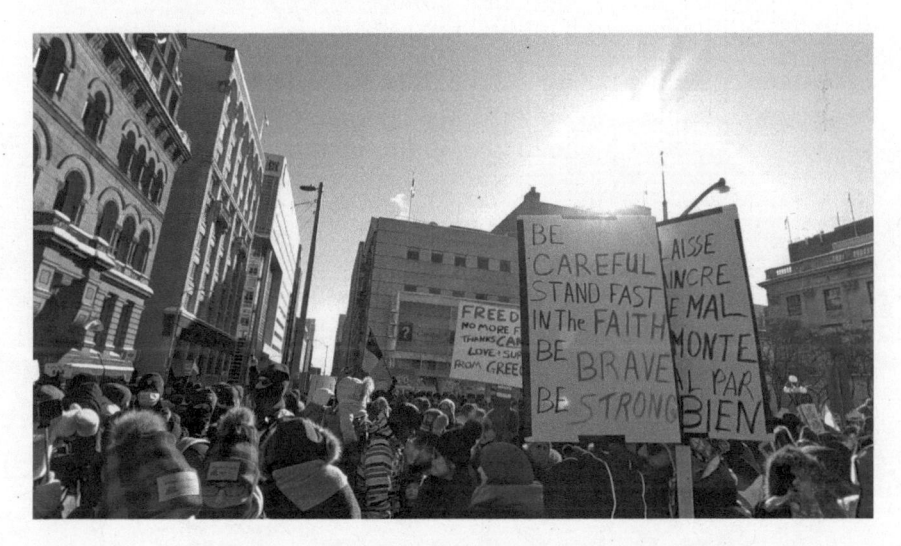

*Canadians Now Willing To Stand Up To Government*

---

53 "I am a Canadian, free to speak without fear, free to worship in my own way, free to stand for what I think right, free to oppose what I believe wrong, or free to choose those who shall govern my country. This heritage of freedom I pledge to uphold for myself and all mankind." Accessed on May 30, 2023, https://www.canada.ca/en/immigration-refugees-citizenship/corporate/publications-manuals/discover-canada/read-online/memorable-quotes.html.

## CHAPTER ONE:

# Setting the Stage

I FIRST BECAME aware of the novel coronavirus in late 2019 and early 2020 when the news carried the story of Dr. Li Wenliang of Wuhan, China. You may remember that he was the young hero physician who warned the world of a virus he thought was like the SARS virus of the early 2000s. His raising of the alarm angered the Chinese authorities, who claimed he was unnecessarily troubling the public order with "rumours." He died from the virus at age thirty-four. His story alone, I think, had a part to play in raising irrational fear for many.

My fascination with those few brave individuals who stand up and speak the truth to a hostile audience has been lifelong. Often, from hindsight, we know that had the people at large listened to and responded positively to the warning expressed by the objectors, the majority would have been better off. It's a basic human characteristic to avoid all that disturbs one's peaceful lifestyle. All is good. Nothing to be gained by worrying. It's like those on the *Titanic* who chose to stay with the warm ship rather than jump into a cold lifeboat.

Of course, we can't be running hither and yon because we're frightened by every negative news story of some disease. Perhaps that explains our collective shrugging of shoulders when we first heard of the novel coronavirus in late 2019. It was far away. Diseases break out consistently around the world, as happened with Africa's Ebola outbreak in 2014, which lasted two years. Ebola didn't affect us here in Canada, so I didn't worry about it.

My first inclination that something might be different with what would be COVID-19 occurred in late January 2020, when we travelled to Michigan to meet up with one of our sons and his family. Coming to meet us there was our other son, who lived in Ohio. My wife and I brought his fiancée with us. At the US border, the agent was wearing latex gloves. I thought that odd. He wouldn't take our passports until we confirmed that we hadn't visited China in the previous two weeks. Again, I thought it odd. Did the American authorities know something about this disease that the rest of us didn't?

We went to Michigan and had a great time of fellowship.

Our son and his fiancée had planned their wedding shower for early March and their wedding for mid-July. It was to be a huge wedding—350 guests. The shower went well, but the wedding turned out to have a grand total of eighteen people, including the photographer, and it was held on our front lawn. COVID-19 suddenly and unexpectedly affected our family tree. The winds of strife that blew throughout the pandemic affected us all.

With each passing day in 2020, the news was saturated with stories of the virus. Some wanted to stop all flights from China. That was considered racist—especially because it was President Trump who closed the American border to travellers from China. The disease spread like wildfire in much more remote places like my home of Newfoundland. No place was safe.

At first, Canada's chief public health officer, Dr. Theresa Tam, said to reporters, "I don't think there's any reason for us to panic or be overly concerned."[54] Indeed, that was the generally accepted pre-COVID-19 protocol around the world. Governments were to do all they could to ensure there was no panic. Yet, as we experienced, they did the exact opposite.

Soon I saw video from China of what looked like hundreds of excavators digging ground for a massive hospital building for the anticipated COVID patients. The Chinese authorities were intent on controlling the virus. However, the medical practitioners I knew, or had access to, informed

---

54 Graham Slaughter, "Canadian health chief: 'I don't think there's any reason for us to panic' over coronavirus," CTV News, January 21, 2020, accessed May10,2023,https://www.ctvnews.ca/health/canadian-health-chief-i-don-t-think-there-s-any-reason-for-us-to-panic-over-coronavirus-1.4775957.

me that there is no human possibility of containing a respiratory virus. Lockdowns and masks were, I was told, ineffective. A virus will eventually sweep through everyone. It was basic textbook understanding and historical knowledge of human experience.

Initially, the headlines agreed with that basic science: "Mass quarantines like in China won't happen in Canada."[55] In fact, one infectious disease specialist told CTV in January 2020 that Chinese efforts to contain the virus amounted to little more than "political theatre," which would cause more harm than good.[56] Studies cited in the news showed that travel restrictions were historically "ineffective, impractical, costly, harmful and ... discriminatory." Other sources made similar arguments, commenting on the many problems associated with mass quarantines.[57]

Looking back, the narrative shifted so gradually but so completely that it's hard to identify the point at which these seemingly rational voices became "COVID deniers" peddling "misinformation" that was said to endanger the health and safety of millions. When did we start "cancelling" doctors who criticized the dictatorial brutality of a communist regime? When did we decide that "science" meant one unanimous and indisputable

---

55  Colin Perkel, "Mass quarantines like in China won't happen in Canada, say authorities," CTV News, January 24, 2020, accessed May 10, 2023, https://www.ctvnews.ca/health/mass-quarantines-like-in-china-won-t-happen-in-canada-say-authorities-1.4781509.
56  Cillian O'Brien, "Can putting a city under lockdown stop the spread of a coronavirus?" CTV News, January 23, 2020, accessed May 10, 2023, https://www.ctvnews.ca/health/can-putting-a-city-under-lockdown-stop-the-spread-of-a-coronavirus-1.4781057. At that point, it was still permissible to observe that "This particular coronavirus does seem nastier than most, but preliminary data shows it's not quite as bad as MERS or the SARS coronavirus"(https://www.ctvnews.ca/health/don-t-panic-a-medical-expert-weighs-in-on-the-coronavirus-1.4777973). It was also permissible to remind people that "the common cold comes from the same family as the latest coronavirus and that the influenza virus kills thousands of Canadians every year." Within weeks, however, comparing COVID-19 to the flu would be enough to get prominent doctors cancelled.
57  Dakin Andone, "China's unprecedented quarantines could have wider consequences, experts say," CNN Health, January 26, 2020, accessed May 10, 2023, https://www.cnn.com/2020/01/26/health/quarantine-china-coronavirus/index.html.

course of action instead of a process or method of inquiry? And why did moderation give way to the very panic we were told to avoid?

Was it fear?

It's natural to be afraid of the unknown, and we knew very little about the virus. We didn't have any personal experience with this new disease, and most of us didn't have the epidemiological training to make sense of the limited data ourselves.[58] We had to rely on whatever we were told by the apparent experts. And most of us, at that point, assumed that the experts could be trusted. We knew that politicians could be self-serving or even corrupt. We knew that journalists could be biased. We knew that doctors could make the occasional mistake. We had faith in the checks and balances that were meant to keep our institutions free and fair. We believed that our leaders were well-informed, and that they were making policies in our best interests. Together, we would navigate the unknown as safely and securely as possible.

We couldn't see the currents of opportunism and greed that swirled under the surface of political and corporate decision-making. Those who did see, or suspected, were accused of being conspiracy theorists. Any discussion that was outside the soon official narrative was considered dangerous.

After all, Canadians aren't generally known for rebellious individualism. We pride ourselves on being polite, apologetic, deferential. We have a habit of coming together during a crisis. We help each other shelter from the blistering heat in the summer or the freezing cold in winter.

Many years ago, while I was in law school, a tornado was spotted near where we lived. My wife babysat to earn extra money, and the parents were at our house when we were informed over the radio to hunker down. We all hustled to the basement to take cover until the "all clear" was given. That's how we react to an emergency. We all help each other. No matter where we are, whatever is needed is shared to get through the crisis.

---

58 Skipping ahead in the chronology, I believe this is one reason that contributed to the Trucker Convoy: by winter of 2022, millions of Canadians had been infected and recovered, often with very mild symptoms, which made it clear how disproportionately severe the restrictions were.

So, when we were told that mass quarantines would help protect our neighbours, we listened. Even if we weren't worried for ourselves, we wanted to do the right thing to help others—although, I must admit, I was skeptical. From what my medical friends shared with me, this didn't make any scientific sense. I went along with it—just to be neighbourly—but I remained doubtful. That skepticism only increased with each passing day.

In early March 2020, after our son and his fiancée's wedding shower, my wife and I went to Vancouver, British Columbia to spend spring break with our daughter and grandchildren. Because we were going to be providing childcare, it was a permitted reason to travel. However, Canada changed over that week. On the flight out to Vancouver, no one wore masks on the plane, but coming back seven days later, about fifty per cent wore masks. It was all so confusing. We were told by Dr. Theresa Tam that a mask wasn't helpful, later she said it may provide some benefit. Which was it?

The first couple of days in Vancouver, we played with our grandchildren on the playground in the park at the back of their house. We kicked the ball; we pushed them on their swings; we climbed with them over the monkey bars. Then the city workers arrived and put yellow tape around the entire playground. Everyone was told to stay inside. It was quite the feat for a family with four very rambunctious children. It was simply insane. Looking back, it was cruel to have done that to our children. When exercise, sunshine, and the great outdoors are the very antidote for respiratory viruses we, as a society, shut our children up in our houses! Cabin fever was a real thing. We took the children for a walk at times when there were few people out and about.

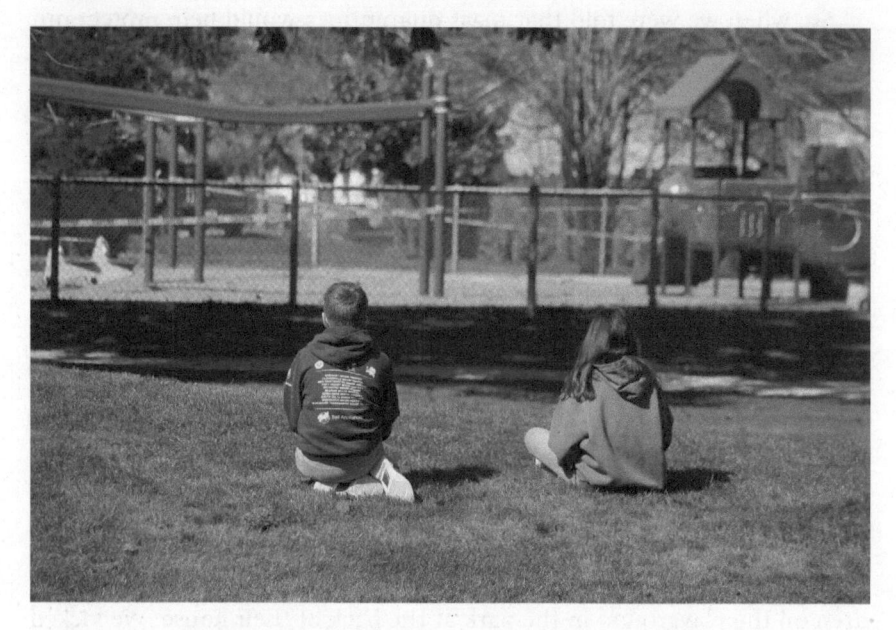

*It Was Cruel To Have Done That to Our Children*

The two-week lockdown, the authorities said, was to slow the exponential rate of transmission long enough to allow hospitals to increase capacity and get the medical equipment, like ventilators, that they needed. The goal was to "flatten the curve." This compassionate appeal certainly struck our caring instinct to do all that we could to ensure that the hospitals weren't overrun with COVID-19 patients, preventing the treatment of other diseases and ailments needing hospital care.

The rapid rate of spread of new COVID-19 variants goes way beyond anyone's control. Lauren Ancel Meyers, director of the COVID-19 Modeling Consortium at The University of Texas at Austin, observed that "[b]y the time we learned about the UK variant in December [2020], it was already silently spreading across the globe."[59] In other words, the original arguments that we all accepted were based upon false assumptions. It was, and remains, a fallacy that we could somehow control a viral disease

---

[59] "Undetected Coronavirus Variant Was in at Least 15 Countries Before its Discovery," *UT News*, April 1, 2021, accessed May 10, 2023, https://news.utexas.edu/2021/04/01/undetected-coronavirus-variant-was-in-at-least-15-countries-before-its-discovery/.

that had already engulfed the world, escaping every measure intended to stop it; that compliance to the lockdown measures was morally good and dissent would be deadly, if not for you, then for your sweet grandmother—thus turning sickness into a moral failing or fault that could somehow be blamed on the noncompliant; that everyone was susceptible and there would be no treatment—no therapeutics; that only COVID-19 posed a risk, and any other cost or loss would pale in comparison; that collective rather than individual decision-making was necessary to prevent the apocalypse.

We were caught up in a moral matrix that refused to look at the competing cost/benefit analysis of the various government-imposed measures. The effects on the economy, on mental health, on personal finances, and on the distribution of goods weren't even considered. Current studies suggest that the aggressive COVID restrictions only exacerbated poor social conditions and should be avoided in the future.[60]

We didn't have the context we needed; no one was talking about daily ICU numbers before the pandemic. No one was publishing running statistics showing the number of deaths from drug overdoses, heart attacks, car accidents. Only later would we come to realize that our healthcare system was already stretched beyond capacity even before COVID-19 entered the scene. So, to blame all the healthcare system issues on COVID was simply wrong. It was manipulative for some other political purposes.

In the meantime, my family had some important issues to deal with. What were we going to do for a wedding in the summer? What about the wedding shower? The March 6, 2020, wedding shower was the last time, until my mother's funeral in July 2021, that our family and friends were able to gather in a large group. And even at the funeral it was limited in accordance with government regulations. It was only in mid-2022 were we on a more normal footing, but until May 2023 family still couldn't travel across the Canadian/US border unless they were fully vaccinated—with a

---

[60] M. Schippers, J. Ioannidis, and A. Joffe, "Aggressive Measures, Rising Inequalities and Mass Formation During the COVID-19 Crisis: An Overview and Proposed Way Forward," May 24, 2022, *Frontiers in Public Health*, Forthcoming, Available at SSRN: https://ssrn.com/abstract=4118910 or http://dx.doi.org/10.2139/ssrn.4118910.

vaccine that doesn't prevent the spread of the virus but has been found to have a huge number of adverse reactions.

Just before my wife and I left for Vancouver, in March 2020, the WHO announced that COVID-19 could "be characterized as a pandemic." Throughout the country, schools and daycares were closed. Businesses and churches were shut. Overnight, our lives changed dramatically. We went to my wife's music studio at the school before our trip out west to pick up a few items in case the school was still closed when we got back. We had no idea that she wouldn't be able to return to her studio until the fall of 2022!

New words and phrases entered our vocabulary: Zoom calls, co-morbidities, social distancing, sheltering at home, vaccine, and mask mandates. Everywhere there were bottles of alcohol-based sanitizer to wipe down everything we touched.

Grocery store shelves were bare. The run-on toilet paper was bizarre. The bare shelves were so unusual that pictures were texted. We'd seen such pictures in the past in communist countries, but to have that in Canada in 2020 was shocking. Items that were always available became rare. We had a rough time getting flour, yeast, eggs, and milk. Basic food items were in short supply.

For the first few weeks, everyone went along with the new reality. We didn't know what we were up against. However, as the two weeks stretched into four, then eight, people began questioning the wisdom of the government authorities. One of the earliest centres to raise objections and get the attention of the press were a few churches who defied the public health orders. Churches throughout the country decided they couldn't remain closed while the government allowed large box stores to remain open. From Pastor Henry Hildebrandt of the Aylmer Church of God in Aylmer, Ontario to Pastor James Coates of the Grace Life Church near Edmonton, Alberta, pastors began to speak out.

Several of my acquaintances called them "rogue pastors." The sentiment was that as church leaders they should be applying the principles of the Christian faith to "love thy neighbour" and not do anything that would put others in harm's way. If the experts said that churches are to be closed, then they must be closed.

Churches got creative, as did Pastor Hildebrandt's, and held worship services with the pastor preaching from a podium in the church parking lot. In Pastor Hildebrandt's case, his congregants remained in their vehicles with their windows up as they listened to his sermon via their radios. For many, this was too much and could not be tolerated.

When in the spring of 2020 Pastor Coates' church was taken over by the government, and hundreds of police officers were placed around it, it seemed to me that as a country we had crossed a line we had never crossed before. It seemed unjustified to allow Costco and Walmart to remain open with hundreds of people in an enclosed area at the same time and not allow churches to hold parking lot services. Further, consider the "Black Lives Matter" protests that swept the country, spilling thousands into public streets with politicians, including the prime minister, joining them in close proximity as they knelt together in protest, many without masks or social distancing.

From those early COVID days, the disparity between how big businesses and churches were treated made no sense. And that disparity extended far beyond churches. Local businesses were also shuttered for a long time, while the big box stores remained open. That crippled the "little guy," with many going bankrupt and some committed suicide because they lost it all.

One could argue that this disparity was due to government incompetence rather than any type of malicious government intent against churches per se. However, it seems to me there is a wider context to be seen. We are currently in an age when the presumption is that churches present a problem. They are viewed as discriminatory, to have been part of the "colonizing force" in our history and no longer a force for good. Religious individuals and communities were given, up until recent times, accommodations to practice their religious beliefs and customs. That presumption of accommodation has now all but been taken away. Religious communities are on the defensive.[61] While government may or may not have been specifically targeting churches, the systemic bias against churches suggests

---

61 Barry Winston Bussey, The Legal Revolution against the Accommodation of Religion: The Secular Age versus the Sexular Age (June 27, 2019). Available at SSRN: https://ssrn.com/abstract=3460346 or http://dx.doi.org/10.2139/ssrn.3460346.

that the government wasn't willing to give them any benefit of the doubt. Churches were seen as a problem if they didn't comply. Any that disagreed with the narrative were not only wrong but had to be crushed into compliance. Therefore, multiple arrests were made.

In 2020-2022 we were dealing with a health pandemic, but the principle of speaking out and challenging the government narrative remained the same. The state was imposing its authority on any group that dared defy their orders, based on the views of those proclaimed to be experts. In the meantime, gaping holes in their dictates allowed for gatherings in box stores and at "approved" public protests. Think also of public transit. I never heard of public transit being the source of an outbreak. It made no sense. There was a yearning within peoples' hearts for answers.

## CHAPTER TWO:

# The Election That Changed Canadians

THE 2021 ELECTION was—like most of this current government's undertakings—a totally unnecessary, multi-million-dollar extravagance.[62] However, it did accomplish one thing: it initiated and reinforced a hateful campaign against unvaccinated Canadians.

Constitutionally, Mr. Trudeau had three years before he had to hold another election. Given his political "bromance" with Mr. Jagmeet Singh, leader of the NDP, Trudeau's minority government wasn't likely to fall.

Apparently, that wasn't good enough for Trudeau. In August, he dissolved Parliament and called a snap election for September. It looked like a smart political move. At the time, he was higher in the polls than the new Conservative leader, Erin O'Toole. If he was successful in obtaining a majority government, he would go unchallenged for at least another four years, with no need to rely on the good graces of Singh. Nor would he have to worry about the opposition asking pesky questions about the We Charity scandal (just one of many scandals infecting his administration).

Despite his political manoeuvring, Trudeau failed to achieve his goals. He ended up in virtually the same position after the election (minus the $600 million wasted). His party gained only three seats compared to

---

62 The $600 million spent was mere chicken feed compared to the $660 billion the self-proclaimed "disnumeric" prime minister has burned through since 2015.

the previous Parliament, emerging with another minority government. Worse, Trudeau actually lost the popular vote by a narrow margin. Of the 17 million Canadians who cast their ballot on September 21, some 5.56 million (32.6%) voted for the Liberals, while 5.74 million (33.7%) voted for the Conservatives. Given that voter turnout was a lacklustre 62.2%, the Liberal Party only earned the active support of a fifth of Canadian adults. The vast majority of Canadians either voted for another party or were too disillusioned to bother participating in an election that was so transparently self-serving and pointless.

In his acceptance speech, Trudeau praised Canadians, insisting that "Some have talked about division, but that's not what I see ... I see Canadians, standing together." He pledged, "If you did not vote for us, I want you to know that we will stand up for you and work for you every single day. Because, no matter how you voted, just like no matter where you come from, what language you speak, the colour of your skin, the way you pray, I hear you."[63]

Nice words! It reminded me of my grandfather saying, "Now there's a nice chicken," as he grabbed the targeted fowl from the rest and promptly executed it in preparation for the morrow's Sunday dinner. Similarly, Trudeau's fine rhetoric rang hollow for anyone who didn't share his enthusiasm for a "progressive plan." The coming months would expose just how unwilling the prime minister was to hear from thousands of Canadians who disagreed with his policies. By January 2022, the fracturing of Canadian society and politics could no longer be ignored. The early cracks were already appearing in the summer and fall of 2021—and they were chiselled by Mr. Trudeau's own hand.

Sometime before the election call, the Liberal Party made a strategic (if short-sighted) decision to use vaccination as a "wedge" issue to secure left-leaning votes. It was a blatant politically tactical move. Campaign promises to segregate society based on vaccination status were not driven

---

[63] CTV News Staff "Full transcript: Justin Trudeau says Canadians have chosen 'a progressive plan' in victory speech," CTV News, September 21, 2021, accessed May 10, 2023, https://www.ctvnews.ca/politics/federal-election-2021/full-transcript-justin-trudeau-says-canadians-have-chosen-a-progressive-plan-in-victory-speech-1.5593795?

by medical data but by selective polling and focus groups with no scientific expertise or training. The purpose, at least in part, was to deflect attention away from the government's ineffective handling of the pandemic. Indeed, we are now finding out just how political the whole vaccine mandate issue was in government offices. Public health did not advise the mandates. It was a total political machination.[64] Power at all costs is the constant drumbeat of this government. Think only of the recent decision to put the Carbon Tax on hold in the Atlantic provinces as a 'temporary measure' due to the declining political support.[65] Mr. Trudeau's 'carve outs' for political purposes continue.

Scapegoating the unvaccinated would prove to be a profoundly destructive idea. Families were divided, friendships broken, livelihoods lost, and businesses destroyed because of the government's decision to pit "one part of the population against another."[66] And, as I discuss below, the firing of conscientious, unvaccinated government employees helps explain the ongoing struggles this government is having in doing its basic administrative tasks, from running the airports to issuing passports.

Mr. Joël Lightbound, a member of Parliament in Trudeau's Liberal Party, later criticized Trudeau's actions during the election. He confirmed what many had suspected all along: that a conscious "decision was made

---

64  See Noé Chartier, "Health Canada Did Not Recommend Travel Vaccine Mandate, Official behind the Policy Testifies," *The Epoch Times*, accessed May 10, 2023, https://www.theepochtimes.com/health-canada-did-not-recommended-travel-vaccine-mandate-official-behind-the-policy-testifies_4637758.html. Also see my interview with Noé, "On Reporting the News in Canada, Interview with Noé Chartier," First Freedoms Foundation, accessed May 10, 2023, https://firstfreedoms.ca/journalism-in-canada-freedom-feature-with-noe-chartier/.

65  Naturally the other premiers not so favoured by the political move are demanding equal treatment. See: Michael MacDonald and Keith Doucette, "Make carbon pricing measures fair to all Canadians, premiers tell Trudeau government," The Canadian Press November 6, 2023, https://nationalpost.com/news/politics/premiers-meeting-carbon-tax

66  National Post Staff, "Liberal MP Joël Lightbound's full remarks: 'It's time to choose positive, not coercive methods,'" *National Post*, February 8, 2022, accessed on May 10, 2023, https://nationalpost.com/news/politics/joel-lightbound-full-transcript.

to wedge, to divide and to stigmatize." The nastiness that followed was not an accident; it was deliberately inflamed.

"I can't help but notice with regret," Lightbound lamented, "that both the tone and the policies of my government changed drastically on the eve and during the last election campaign." He went on, "I fear that this politicization [of] the pandemic risks undermining the public's trust in public-health institutions. This is not a risk we ought to be taking lightly."[67]

Yet by the time Mr. Lightbound shared his concerns in February 2022, the damage had already been done. The government had made it clear that it cared more about scoring political points than meeting the needs of struggling Canadians. Power is an opiate of those in control.

Indeed, the process of division and exclusion began not with imposition of the vaccine mandates, but with campaign rhetoric that explicitly "othered" a minority of Canadians. In a now-infamous appearance on a French-language talk show, Trudeau used derogatory language to stereotype the unvaccinated. According to the prime minister, the unvaccinated "don't believe in science and are often misogynistic and racist as well." He claimed, "It's a small group of people, but they take up some space. And there we must make a choice, as a leader and as a country: do we tolerate these people?"[68] Re-read his words and let them sink in. They were spoken by the prime minister of a G7 country!

---

67  Mr. Lightbound also pointed out that lockdowns affected people differently: "not everyone can earn a living on a Macbook at the cottage." He observed that Canadians were rightly "worried that measures which ought to be exceptional and limited in time are being normalized with no end in sight, like vaccine passports, mandates, and requirements for travellers. They're worried because they feel it is becoming harder and harder to know where public health stops and where politics begins." To counter this, he recommended that the government establish clear benchmarks for ending restrictions, and "should systematically publish the epidemiological projections and the scientific analysis underpinning the measures it imposes going forward." See *National Post* Staff, "Liberal MP Joël Lightbound's full remarks: 'It's time to choose positive, not coercive methods,'" *National Post*, February 8, 2022, accessed May 10, 2023, https://nationalpost.com/news/politics/joel-lightbound-full-transcript.

68  Julie Snyder. "Le chef du parti ..." Facebook, September 17, 2021, https://m.facebook.com/watch/?v=965926357318548&_rdr at 3:22 to 4:30.

It didn't matter that these labels had no basis in truth. Statistics Canada's own data showed that "far from the unvaccinated being racists and misogynists ... groups most likely to be vaccine resistant included Blacks, Metis, Latinos and Arabs—all with valid historical reasons to be wary of authoritarian initiatives by governments." Editorialist Lorrie Goldstein noted that based on polls, "the typical vaccine-resistant individual is a 42-year-old Ontario woman who votes Liberal."[69] So the point of Trudeau's comments was not to reflect reality but to create a sense of group superiority by dehumanizing the "other." "[D]o we tolerate these people?"

Remember, "racist" doesn't mean, in Mr. Trudeau's environment, simply holding disparaging views against another person based on race, but it has become the choice word to describe anyone who doesn't agree with the progressive Cathedral. One is "racist" under this view if you don't accept the vaccine.

Deepening the "us" versus "them" mentality, Trudeau promised that once re-elected, he would mandate the COVID-19 vaccine for all federal public servants, including the RCMP, and would prevent the unvaccinated from travelling by plane, train, or ferry. He didn't want them to put anyone else at risk. It was their "choice" to refuse the shot, but they couldn't choose to sit next to a vaccinated Canadian. He insisted, "No one is safe until everyone is safe."[70]

It was apparently lost on Mr. Trudeau (and the press) that if the vaccine worked, there would be no need to segregate society. A vaccinated person wouldn't have to worry about encountering an unvaccinated person, since she would be "safe" from infection. On the flip side, if the vaccine did *not*

---

[69] Lorrie Goldstein, "GOLDSTEIN: Even Trudeau knows targeting unvaccinated un-Canadian," *Toronto Sun*, January 8, 2022, accessed May 10, 2023, https://torontosun.com/opinion/columnists/goldstein-even-trudeau-knows-targeting-unvaccinated-un-canadian.

[70] Prime Minister of Canada Press Release, "Prime Minister announces mandatory vaccination for the federal workforce and federally regulated transportation sectors," October 6, 2021, accessed May 10, 2023, https://pm.gc.ca/en/news/news-releases/2021/10/06/prime-minister-announces-mandatory-vaccination-federal-workforce-and.

protect people from the virus, then there would be no scientific rationale for mandates, either, since they wouldn't stop the spread of disease.[71]

One possible argument is that unvaccinated individuals have a higher likelihood of severe symptoms,[72] necessitating hospital care at a time when the hospitals are already overly strained. However, it remains an open question whether an otherwise healthy unvaccinated individual is at a huge risk of hospitalization compared to the immunocompromised unvaccinated or vaccinated individuals. Is it worth the risk of shutting down huge swaths of the economy by the vaccine mandates? That we were not told. Nor do we have any indication that the government sought clarity on that point. Also forgotten was Canada's long history of respect for individual freedom and personal responsibility. In labelling the unvaccinated as bigoted conspiracy theorists, Trudeau left no room for conscientious objections or even valid medical exemptions.

---

71  Later arguments—for instance, that vaccines were necessary on prophylactic or therapeutic grounds, because they would reduce the seriousness of infection, or serve as an "added layer of protection"—were only offered as it became obvious that the shots did not work as initially promised.

72  The Mayo Clinic noted, "People with vaccine breakthrough infections may spread COVID-19 to others. However, fully vaccinated people with a breakthrough infection are less likely to have serious illness with COVID-19 than those who are unvaccinated. Even when vaccinated people develop symptoms, they tend to be less severe than those experienced by unvaccinated people," Mayo Clinic Staff, "Fully vaccinated? Get the facts," August 25, 2022, accessed May 10, 2023, https://www.mayoclinic.org/coronavirus-COVID-19/fully-vaccinated.

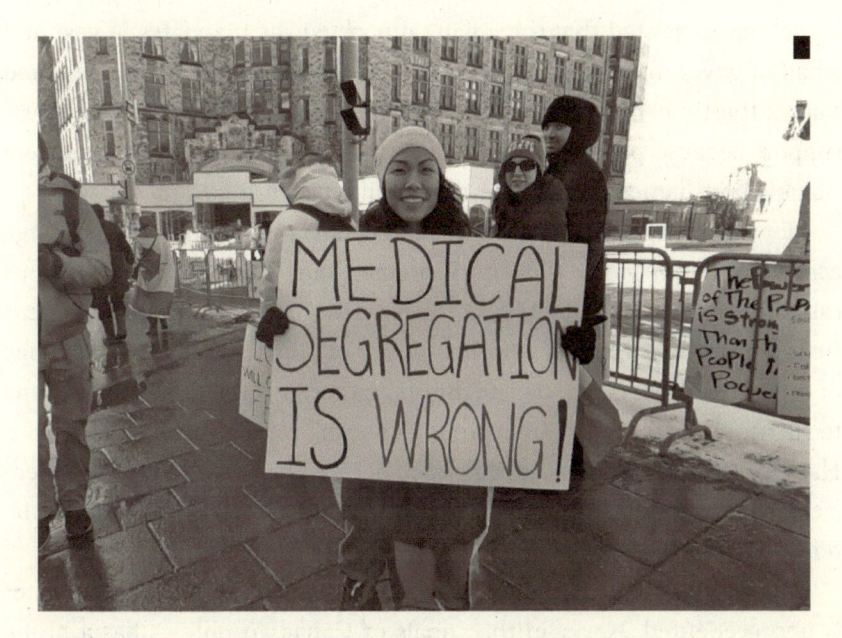

*Medical Segregation Is Always Wrong*

This failure wasn't some kind of careless oversight or inadvertent mistake. It was a deliberate and complete about-face from his comments in May 2021, when Trudeau questioned, "What do you do with someone with an allergy? What do you do with someone who's immunocompromised, or someone who for religious reasons or … deep convictions, decides that no, they're not going to get a vaccine? *We're not a country that makes vaccination mandatory.*"[73] Three months later, the same prime minister promised to introduce some of the strictest mandates in the world while declaring that anyone who refused the vaccine for any reason was simply "wrong."[74] Progressives have a difficult time with people with opposing views.

---

73  Lorrie Goldstein, "GOLDSTEIN: Even Trudeau knows targeting unvaccinated un-Canadian," *Toronto Sun,* January 8, 2022, accessed May 10, 2023, https://torontosun.com/opinion/columnists/goldstein-even-trudeau-knows-targeting-unvaccinated-un-canadian, italics added.

74  "Trudeau calls out 'anti-vaxxers' for putting kids at risk as campaign event is disrupted by protesters," CBC News, August 31, 2021, accessed May 10, 2023, https://www.cbc.ca/news/canada/sudbury/trudeau-sudbury-laurentian-election-stop-1.6159866.

Polling suggested that Canadians supported the mandates. A year and a half of government messaging had its effect. But it should also be noted that at the time, opposing voices were silenced. It seemed like there was support because people couldn't hear critics, and those they heard were ridiculed or shamed by the government and its subsidized media.

Not surprisingly, the prime minister's harsh language provoked outrage across the country. In 2013, the Supreme Court of Canada, in a famous case known as the Whatcott case,[75] explained that hate speech is different from political speech. In the normal course of politics there is an exchange of opposing ideas, as in a debate. But hate speech is the opposite. It wants to silence the voice of its target group. It doesn't want an exchange of ideas. Hate speech is derogatory, it vilifies and detests the group, not giving them a chance to respond. That, in my view, was exactly what the prime minister was doing.

Such vilification of a group of Canadians by a Canadian prime minister is unprecedented. Never in the annals of Canadian politics has a prime minister reached across the line of hate against an identifiable group of citizens. It made for a troublesome campaign.

As the campaign continued, Mr. Trudeau was accosted by many angry people. At one point, handfuls of gravel were thrown at him by protestors who "appeared angry about COVID-19 health measures and vaccination requirements."[76] When asked about the incident, Trudeau responded, "Nobody should be doing their jobs under the threats of violence or acts to put them in danger."

---

75 "Saskatchewan (Human Rights Commission) v. Whatcott, 2013 SCC 11 (CanLII), [2013] 1 SCR 467," CanLII, accessed May 12, 2023, https://canlii.ca/t/fw8x4.

76 Aaron D'Andrea, "Trudeau says he was hit by gravel, condemns rock throwing as 'unacceptable'," Global News, September 7, 2021, accessed May 10, 2023, https://globalnews.ca/news/8171619/trudeau-hit-by-gravel-rocks-condemns-unacceptable/.

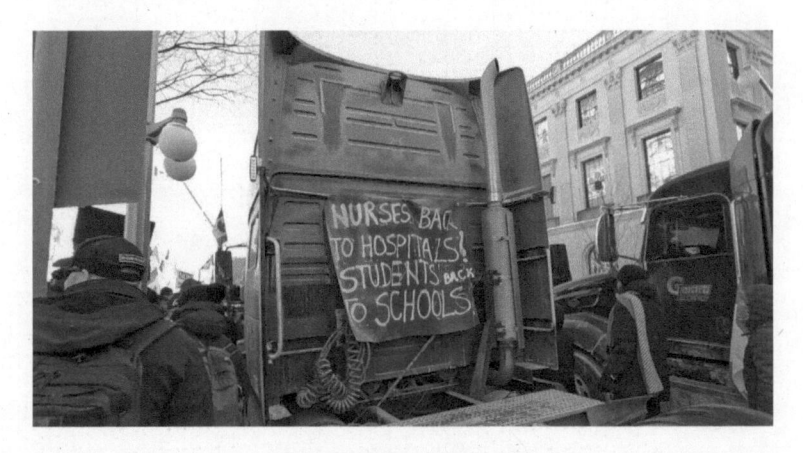

*No One Deserves Coercion*

Violence is never justified. That includes the violence of forcibly preventing people from continuing their employment or schooling because of a personal medical decision. Apparently, that kind of aggression didn't worry Trudeau. Instead, expressly upping the ante against the unvaccinated, he continued, "That's not how we do things in Canada." He condemned his opponents as extremist, "anti-vaxxer mobs, who are not respecting the basic science, and the basic decency that Canadians have rightly come to expect from each other."[77] His use of the term "basic science" is now so ironic as we are finding out just how he imposed those mandates based on politics and not science, as we discuss below.

Gone was the prime minister who proclaimed in 2015 that "a Canadian is a Canadian is a Canadian."[78] Gone too was the basic decency that Canadians once expected from their leaders. Fear of COVID-19 had been amplified and then politicized to benefit the Liberal Party. Little thought was given to the breakdown of unity or trust that would result from these tactics. Nor did the country foresee that Trudeau's policies would lead to the most dramatic, non-violent protest in Canadian history: the Trucker Freedom Convoy 2022.

---

77  Ibid.
78  "'A Canadian Is a Canadian': Liberal Leader Says Terrorists Should Keep Their Citizenship," *Vice News*, September 28, 2015, accessed May 10, 2023, https://www.vice.com/en/article/7xaxby/a-canadian-is-a-canadian-liberal-leader-says-terrorists-should-keep-their-citizenship.

## CHAPTER THREE:

# The Tribal Attack against Unvaccinated Canadians

BEFORE I GO much further, I want to make it very clear that I am not against vaccines on principle. Indeed, nor were the truckers. Two centuries ago, I'm told, 25% of the population never reached the age of one. Some 50% never reached the age of 20. Since then, death from chicken pox, mumps, polio, and the like has been rare, if not eliminated altogether. Much of the credit for this modern-day miracle is the development of vaccinations. Of course, the adoption of basic hygiene, regular exercise, and healthful eating have also contributed to our quality and length of life. We are indeed blessed to be living in this day and age.

When the vaccine for COVID-19 was announced mere months after onset of the virus in the general population, I immediately became suspicious. It made no sense that a "vaccine," as defined by Webster's in 1963, could possibly be created to deal with COVID-19 in such a short time.[79] Dr. Gerhard Sundborn, an epidemiologist at the University of Aukland, pointed out that "the best-case scenario" for a vaccine to be developed is

---

[79] *Webster's Seventh New Collegiate Dictionary* (Springfield, Massachusetts: G. & C. Merriam Company, 1963), 979. Specifically, it states that a vaccine is:
"1. Matter or a preparation containing the virus of cowpox in a form used for vaccination.
2. a preparation of killed microorganisms, living attenuated organisms, or living fully virulent organisms that is administered to produce or artificially increase immunity to a particular disease."

four years; the average is up to ten years—and there are many viruses that have no vaccine, such as HIV."[80]

However, as the COVID-19 crisis swept the world, we were told to erase from our minds the "science" of the past and accept the new "science" and new definitions. "Vaccine" now defined by Webster is "a preparation that is administered (as by injection) to stimulate the body's immune response against a specific infectious agent or disease."[81] So just like that, the old is cast out in favour of the new. The term "vaccine" has magically been redefined to meet the official narrative. As long as "a preparation" is made and injected in the body "to stimulate the body's immune response," it is now a "vaccine." Gone is the requirement that it contain the virus. That's all good if what we call a "vaccine" today does at least what the "vaccine" of the past did.

It's true that work on the mRNA technology had been ongoing for some time.[82] The immediate advantage is clear: rather than having to take ten years to develop a regular vaccine, this new technology promises that a vaccine can be created in months. However, all previous attempts to use this technology were abandoned due to its instability: "RNA in general had a reputation for unbelievable instability," says Paul Krieg, University of Arizona in Tucson. "Everything around RNA was cloaked in caution."[83]

The technology has origins going back to the 1960s, but its use for vaccines dates back only to around 2010. We're dealing with very new vaccine technology. The COVID-19 crisis was used to override efficacy and safety

---

80 Gerhard Sundborn, "COVID is not as dangerous as the fear instilled in community," on Kerre McIvor Mornings (August 13, 2020) iHeartRadio podcast, accessed May 10, 2023, https://www.iheart.com/podcast/1049-kerre-mcivor-mornings-pod-46787367/episode/gerhard-sundborn-COVID-is-not-as-70204639/.
81 *Merriam-Webster Dictionary*, s.v., "vaccine," accessed May 10, 2023, https://www.merriam-webster.com/dictionary/vaccine?utm_campaign=sd&utm_medium=serp&utm_source=jsonld.
82 "The Long History of mRNA Vaccines," Johns Hopkins, accessed May 10, 2023, https://publichealth.jhu.edu/2021/the-long-history-of-mrna-vaccines.
83 Elie Dolgin, "The tangled history of mRNA vaccines: Hundreds of scientists had worked on mRNA vaccines for decades before the coronavirus pandemic brought a breakthrough," *Nature*, September 14, 2021, accessed May 10, 2023, https://www.nature.com/articles/d41586-021-02483-w.

concerns. Therefore, we are amid the largest human pharmaceutical experiment of all time. Right now, all we have is a lot of promises.

The promoters of this technology see the COVID-19 vaccine as a great success and to be emulated in creating vaccines for other diseases, such as the seasonal flu. Others maintain that the cost in adverse reactions and lack of effectiveness of the technology outweigh any benefits, and its use on human beings should be abandoned until further advancements are made.

The COVID-19 pandemic was seen as an opportunity to enhance the technology, serving not only the current situation but also the future. No doubt many scientists were motivated by the desire to do something good for humanity. However, the politics over the debate of this new technology requires that opposition and/or questioning be labelled as "disinformation." This cantankerous attitude has led to restrictions on free speech and coercive measures, and it has quickly spiralled into a full-blown loss of confidence in the vaccine for a significant minority of people—people whose concerns were given voice by the Trucker Freedom Convoy.

Justin Trudeau's campaign rhetoric in the fall of 2021 opened the door to a nationwide attack on the unvaccinated. With few exceptions, both the public and private sectors embraced vaccine mandates to "encourage" vaccine uptake. The unvaccinated were systematically barred from full participation in Canadian society, while simultaneously being blamed (and shamed) for the latest wave of COVID-19 infections.

Even before Trudeau won his second minority government, airlines announced that they would require travellers to be vaccinated. They took their cue from the government. On August 13, 2021, before the election was called, Transport Minister Omar Alghabra said the vaccine mandate for travellers would be in place "by no later than the end of October."[84]

Porter Airlines and WestJet supported the government's proposal. They swiftly implemented policies mandating COVID-19 vaccines for

---

84 Marieke Walsh and Laura Stone, "Trudeau says people who are not fully vaccinated won't be able to travel on domestic planes or trains," *The Globe and Mail*, August 18, 2021, accessed May 10, 2023, https://www.theglobeandmail.com/politics/article-trudeau-says-people-who-are-not-fully-vaccinated-will-not-be-able-to/.

their employees and passengers. Air Canada followed suit "in line with federal rules."[85] This corporate support helped legitimize the government's position. It showed people that these institutions agreed with Trudeau's proposals and solidified the view that the unvaccinated were unreasonable. If some "racist anti-vaxxer" chose not to get the shot out of ignorant selfishness, then they would have to live with the consequences, even if that meant being unable to fly to a loved one's deathbed or attend a child's wedding.

The airlines proved to be as political as the politicians in trying to follow the crowd. Once the federal government eventually reversed their policy on the vaccines, Porter Airlines came out saying that "this is something we've been asking for,"[86] and Air Canada said the "measures were not justified by science"![87]

"That is why I am so frustrated with these airlines," said Greg Hill, co-founder of Free to Fly Canada.[88] "They come out now and made these statements as if they realized this all along. Where were ya? Where were you the last year or two? If you knew the science was not solid ... they could have spoken up." But as Hill notes, they didn't, and that was their choice.[89]

While many countries limited unvaccinated international travellers, there were few, if any, that refused the unvaccinated the right to travel within their borders. Canada's vaccine requirements for travel within the country took matters to a whole other level. On September 3, 2021, Prime

---

85 "Air Canada suspends more than 800 unvaccinated workers under new federal rules," CBC News, November 3, 2021, accessed May 10, 2023, https://www.cbc.ca/news/business/air-canada-vaccine-suspensions-1.6235222.
86 Tom Yun, "Travel, aviation industry leaders applaud lifting of vaccine mandates," CTV News, June 15, 2022, accessed May 10, 2023, https://www.ctvnews.ca/health/coronavirus/travel-aviation-industry-leaders-applaud-lifting-of-vaccine-mandates-1.5946596.
87 "Air Canada Welcomes Government of Canada Decision to Lift Mask, Testing and ArriveCan Requirements," Air Canada, September 26, 2022, accessed May 10, 2023, https://media.aircanada.com/2022-09-26-Air-Canada-Welcomes-Government-of-Canada-Decision-to-Lift-Mask,-Testing-and-ArriveCan-Requirements.
88 https://www.freetofly.ca.
89 "Calling Out the Airlines—Interview With Greg Hill," First Freedoms Foundation, accessed May 10, 2023, https://firstfreedoms.ca/calling-out-the-airlines-interview-with-greg-hill/.

Minister Trudeau tweeted: "When you board a plane, you want to know that the people sitting around you are fully vaccinated. We'll move forward with mandatory vaccines on planes, trains, and cruise ships to make sure you stay safe while you travel."[90]

Since when do we want to know the personal medical history of those next to us on an airplane? "Excuse me, sir, but are you vaccinated? If not, get off the plane!" is not how we normally would start a conversation with our seatmates enroute to our destination. It is difficult to comprehend but there actually were people who wanted to know everybody's medical status. This "busybody" mindset reminded my Eastern European friends of their time under communism. Today we know, as we did in the fall of 2021, that the vaccine doesn't prevent spread of the virus. The prime minister's position was pointless, and it damaged our civic peace.

His sentiments and others only fuelled the animosity against the unvaccinated, as evidenced by one of Trudeau's followers, @KaathyLa: "The whole world should do this, the unvaccinated can just stay home."[91] Such bigotry against the unvaccinated was a direct result of the egging on by the prime minister. Vilification of the minority was in full swing. A Trudeau critic, @djlange, tweeted to him, "The vaccinated can still transmit the virus and you know this. So why is your entire campaign based on demonizing the unvaxxed?"[92] Good question.

In my role at the First Freedoms Foundation, I heard firsthand the stories of many hurting people who lost jobs, houses, education, and security for "their decision." They would not be coerced by government and employer vaccine mandates, despite the terrible costs. Based on Trudeau's logic, they got what they deserved. That view came out in spades in the average person who took up Trudeau's hateful rhetoric.

---

90  Justin Trudeau (@JustinTrudeau), "When you board a plane, you want to know that the people sitting around you are fully vaccinated," Twitter, September 3, 2021, 8:31 PM, https://twitter.com/JustinTrudeau/status/1433950810296172544?t=FuN2VOG0SYNE4hnHypHDMA&s=19.
91  @KaathyLa. Twitter reply, September 2021, https://twitter.com/JustinTrudeau/status/1433950810296172544?lang=en.
92  @djlange. Twitter reply, September 2021, https://twitter.com/JustinTrudeau/status/1433950810296172544?lang=en.

The mistreatment of the unvaccinated was so widespread and normalized by politicians and journalists that it extended well beyond federal mandates or corporate policies.[93] I heard chilling stories of people angrily calling for the unvaccinated "to be lined up and shot" for not following Trudeau's dictates. Others refused to allow the unvaccinated into their homes. Teenage athletes couldn't play sports unless they got the vaccine. Even some churches—traditionally places of refuge from oppression—insisted that their congregants show proof of vaccine status before entering the sanctuary.

I became very unsettled by the animosity I saw developing day after day. I listened to the struggles of six university students who came to our house for help in writing their religious exemption applications. Their pastors refused to help them. They felt alone.

Hannah Arendt, who suffered during WWII, told us that totalitarian domination becomes possible when people suffer from a deep and damaging loneliness. Not mere solitude, the loneliness she describes is characterized by fear and mistrust: it is "the experience of being abandoned by everything and everybody."[94]

Those young people were abandoned by their universities, their professors, for some their families, and for most, their own Christian communities. They were alone and trusted no one. It was difficult to hear. Even worse, I found it hard to comprehend how our society had come to reject those who simply wanted to follow their conscience on a personal medical issue that had absolutely no impact on others. In some circles, the bigotry against the unvaccinated continues to this day. Fear, based on lies and half-truths, has ripped our social fabric.

None of this was based on scientific evidence (or even logic).[95]

---

[93] A fascinating perspective of an immigrant to Canada is found at "COVID in Canada Was Worse Than Communism—Interview with Dr. Emanuel Baston," First Freedoms Foundation, accessed May 10, 2023, https://firstfreedoms.ca/covid-in-canada-was-worse-than-communism/.

[94] Hannah Arendt, *The Origins of Totalitarianism* (New York: Harcourt, 1968), 476.

[95] See the previous chapter for more on the politicization of the vaccine and the pandemic response as a whole.

The attack on the unvaccinated was tribal in the worst sense. If you were vaccinated, you were "one of us." If you were unvaccinated, you were "one of those people." Your unique beliefs, experiences, skills, and needs were irrelevant. Your vaccine status mattered more than your personal dignity or individual worth. You could be labelled, excluded, threatened, and abused because you were a threat to "basic decency," as the prime minister warned.

For Trudeau and his supporters, it was a "win-win" scenario. Those on "the inside" could rest secure in their moral superiority, even gaining virtue points by posting photos on social media to prove they had rolled up their sleeves for the obligatory shot(s). Meanwhile, those on the "outside" became a convenient scapegoat for every failed policy of the pandemic and beyond. Hospitals understaffed, ICUs overflowing, surgeries delayed? Blame the unvaccinated. Airports congested, luggage lost? Blame the unvaccinated. Shelves empty and parcels delayed? Blame the unvaccinated. It might seem like I'm taking the case too far, but not by much. Consider the prime minister's statements:

> People are seeing cancer treatments and elective surgeries put off because beds are filled with people who chose not to get vaccinated; they're frustrated. When people see that we're in lockdowns, or serious public health restrictions right now because [of] the risk posed to all of us by unvaccinated people, people get angry.[96]

And,

> If you make a choice a personal choice to not get vaccinated then I will have no sympathy for you when you come to me and say, '...I can't go out to a restaurant with my friends,' or 'I'm not being allowed to go to the gym,' or 'my employer is telling me I have to continue to work from home.' You don't have a right to endanger others. You have a right to make choices about ... your own status

---

[96] Rachel Aiello, "Canadians are 'angry' with the unvaccinated: Trudeau," CTV News, January 5, 2022, accessed May 10, 2023, https://www.ctvnews.ca/politics/canadians-are-angry-with-the-unvaccinated-trudeau-1.5728855.

and your own health decisions, but you can't impose those decisions at risking everyone else. So, no, I won't apologize for being extremely unequivocal and standing up for the vast majority of Canadians who've done exactly that.[97]

No need for pesky questions pointed in the wrong direction. Like a magician's sleight-of-hand, blaming the unvaccinated kept the scrutiny away from bloated bureaucracies, corporate monopolies, or political incompetence (not to mention outright lies about "the science"). It was also far simpler to focus on a defenceless minority than to deal with broken supply chains, skyrocketing inflation, government inefficiencies, or staffing shortages caused by the very mandates that created such divisions. Not to mention the outrageous overspending and refusal of the government to allow industries, such as oil and gas, to access the natural resources we have in this country that would have helped lower the costs.

The manipulation and misdirection became especially obvious when the prime minister began pushing the false narrative that the unvaccinated were delaying the "return to normal." If nothing else, a return to normal would mean cutting back on government powers gained over the last two years. That's as unlikely as the concept of ever getting back to "normal." What is "normal" has changed.

As Lord Sumption, former Supreme Court Justice in Great Britain, said recently, when we allow governments to "keep us safe" from a wider and wider range of issues, we become increasingly dependent on the state. We grow less resilient and less capable of solving our own problems. That means we also grow more compliant. Our personal lives become less and less private as the government gains more control over our day-to-day decisions. And just as we lose the habit of thinking or acting independently, the government develops a habit of authoritarian rule.[98]

---

97   Toronto Star, "Althia Raj challenges Justin Trudeau over his handling of anti-vaxxers," accessed August 30, 2023, https://www.youtube.com/watch?v=eXQblsa7Lzs

98   Roger Scruton Memorial Lectures, "Roger Scruton Memorial Lectures 2021—Jonathan Sumption," YouTube, November 3, 2021, 1:29:48, accessed May 10, 2023 https://youtu.be/oZHMTrSZyZE.

To those who say that pandemic restrictions were only temporary and necessary to save lives, let's not forget the kinds of orders that were put in place by both federal and provincial governments. The authorities took it upon themselves to dictate exactly where Canadians could or could not go, what they could or could not do, and what they could or could not buy, down to an absurd level of detail that had no scientific rationale. In Manitoba in the fall of 2020, winter jackets and snow pants were on the "essential" list, blue jeans were not. Snowmobiling was allowed, but toboggan hills were closed.[99]

Most of these restrictions have now been lifted, but the underlying assumptions are still active: Canadians cannot be trusted to assess the risks for themselves. They must rely on the government to keep them safe. And even if one threat has passed, there will always be a new emergency that justifies repeating the same—or harsher—measures. Just look at the cycle of invasive mandates that have been imposed, then lifted, and then re-imposed in the last two and a half years of the pandemic. Once we give the government the power to decide when and how our freedoms can be exercised, we are no longer truly free. We are at the mercy of the state.

The unvaccinated know this truth all too well.

Not only were they banned from work, school, and travel, they were subjected to once-unthinkable arguments made by Canadian politicians and journalists. In Quebec, Premier François Legault threatened to tax anyone who still refused the shot. Like the prime minister, he referred to the unvaccinated as "these people" who "put a very important burden on our health-care network."[100] Yet the health-care network was already overburdened. The unvaccinated were unfairly shouldered with the blame.

---

[99] Joyanne Pursaga, "City rinks, toboggan runs can open, with pandemic restrictions, *Winnipeg Free Press*, December 11, 2020, https://www.winnipegfreepress.com/local/2020/12/11/city-rinks-toboggan-runs-can-open-with-pandemic-restrictions, See also the letter of Cameron Friesen, Minister responsible for administration of The Public Health Act, https://www.gov.mb.ca/asset_library/en/proactive/2020_2021/orders-soe-11222020.pdf.

[100] Verity Stevenson and Isaac Olson, "Unvaccinated Quebecers will have to pay a health tax, Legault says," CBC News, January 11, 2022, accessed May 30, 2023, https://www.cbc.ca/news/canada/montreal/unvaccinated-health-contribution-quebec-1.6311054.

Others went even further than Premier Legault, calling for the unvaccinated to pay for their own medical care.[101] Can you imagine such an argument being made in normal times? But then, we aren't living through "normal" times.

There was no appreciation for the personal loss the unvaccinated faced when the prime minister verbally attacked them. His Liberal and NDP supporters pushed a false narrative that the pandemic had now become a "pandemic of the unvaccinated." By the way, there was not much succor from the Conservatives. Mr. O'Toole was part of the official chorus calling for everyone to be vaccinated and rather ambiguous about standing up to Mr. Trudeau's extreme rhetoric. Official opposition was uncharacteristically muted.

Prime Minister Trudeau's statement bears repeating, "When people see that we're in lockdowns or serious public health restrictions right now because of the risk posed to all of us by unvaccinated people, people get angry."[102]

---

101 Diane Francis, "Make the unvaccinated pay for their own health care: Public health measures should not be confused with freedom of choice or rights," *Financial Post*, December 22, 2021 https://financialpost.com/diane-francis/diane-francis-make-the-unvaccinated-pay-for-their-own-health-care.

102 Amanda Wawryk, "Prime Minister Trudeau says Canadians are 'angry' with the unvaccinated," *Daily Hive*, January 5, 2022, https://dailyhive.com/vancouver/canadians-angry-unvaccinated-prime-minister-trudeau. Also note this quote from Lord Sumption, former Supreme Court Justice in Great Britain said recently,

"The more routine the perils from which we demand protection, the more frequently will those demands arise. If we confer despotic powers on government to deal with perils, which are an ordinary feature of human existence, we will end up doing it most or all of the time. It is because the perils against which we now demand protection from the state are so much more numerous than they were that they are likely to lead to a more fundamental and durable change in our attitudes to the state. This is a more serious problem for the future of democracy than war."

Freddie Sayers, "Lord Sumption: Civil disobedience has begun, The retired Supreme Court justice believes we have no moral obligation to obey the law,"UnHerdMarch4,2021,https://unherd.com/2021/03/lord-sumption-civil-disobedience-has-begun/?=refinnar

As I write this, I can't get over the above quote. How, with what we now know he knew,[103] could Mr. Trudeau say that with a straight face and not care about the hatred he was stoking against the unvaccinated? It is truly unbelievable and scary that a Canadian leader would ever do such a thing.

The government's insatiable desire for more power demanded a scapegoat to legitimize the totalitarian tendency, as have the governments of many other countries. The government of Canada found one in the unvaccinated. This was evident in the systematic denial of the unvaccinated to work, attend classes, or travel. But there was more. Diane Francis, a columnist for the *Financial Post*, argued that Canada should follow Singapore: "If you don't want to be vaccinated and don't protect yourself, then fall ill, nobody else should have to pay for your personal negligence and irresponsibility."[104]

Setting aside the fact that all of us in Canada pay for universal healthcare through our taxes, let's pause to think about this argument. While it's assumed that the vaccine helps reduce severe symptoms of COVID, can we use that to say that every person not vaccinated who requires hospitalization is to be personally responsible for health care expenses?[105] If so, are we also going to tell alcoholics they must pay for healthcare related to their alcohol consumption? What of those who "negligently" eat sugar and develop diabetes? Must they pay for dialysis treatment? What about lifetime smokers who irresponsibly put their own health and the health of others at risk with their second-hand smoke? Do we force them to pay for their lung transplant or chemotherapy drugs?

---

[103] Consider: Blacklock's Reporter, "Wanted 'Winning Messages' On Vax Injury: Secret Memo," June 6, 2023, https://www.blacklocks.ca/wanted-winning-messages-on-vax-injury-secret-memo/, accessed August 8, 2023, "The Privy Council Office in a secret memo said Covid vaccine injuries and deaths 'have the potential to shake public confidence' and must be carefully managed with 'winning communication strategies.'"

[104] Diane Francis, "Make the unvaccinated pay for their own health care: Public health measures should not be confused with freedom of choice or rights," *Financial Post*, December 22, 2021, https://financialpost.com/diane-francis/diane-francis-make-the-unvaccinated-pay-for-their-own-health-care.

[105] That is assuming we can accurately determine for each case that the refusal of the vaccine led to hospitalization.

If this is our approach to medical care, how do we decide who deserves treatment and who does not? If someone who is vaccinated gets COVID, should they be punished with a pile of medical bills? After all, they're burdening our healthcare system, too. If they're deemed worthy of care when an unvaccinated COVID patient is not, then we have a system where access to public services is based on whether or not someone agrees with the government in power: a very dangerous precedent indeed.

When it comes to public health, there's a tricky balance to be found between personal autonomy and public welfare. This debate has been going on for centuries. Public officials must weigh the risks and decide what they deem to be in the public interest. It's no easy task, to be sure.[106] There's something terribly amiss in this country when people call for the exclusion of certain citizens from health care based on their conscientious beliefs. If you get sick in Canada, whatever the circumstances and whatever the disease, you should be treated with respect and compassion. Period.

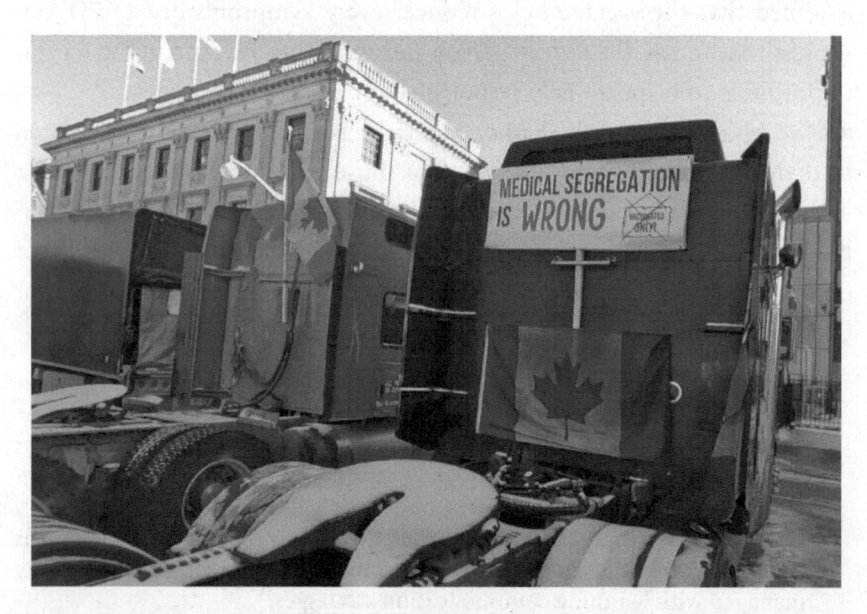

*The Truckers Resonated The Same Sentiment Of The People*

---

[106] As Jason Kenney found out, see John Ivison, "The downfall of Jason Kenney will reverberate beyond Alberta," *National Post*, October 6, 2022, accessed May10,2023, https://nationalpost.com/news/politics/john-ivison-the-downfall-of-jason-kenney-will-reverberate-beyond-alberta.

It's worth emphasizing that the minority who refused the vaccine did not make that choice lightly. Many of those I met decided not to get the vaccine because of their conscientious beliefs. Some took a religious stand. They wouldn't accept an injection that was developed or tested using aborted babies, for example. Others, seeing their body as the temple of God, refused to get a shot that could possibly harm their physical health and interfere with their spiritual journey.

Others objected to the COVID-19 jab as a matter of truth. They couldn't take a vaccine that was subject to so much conflicting information. Many had legitimate questions about the safety of the vaccines. At the time, these concerns were ridiculed as conspiracy theories. Now we know that many adverse effects have been linked to the vaccines, from Guillain-Barré Syndrome to myocarditis.[107]

Still others were determined not to comply because they were troubled by the government's coercive tactics. They witnessed the damage done by lockdowns and other measures and chose to refuse the vaccine as a way to show their opposition to government overreach.

"It was an intrusion into my personal life, and my personal choices into what I needed to do to be healthy and not be healthy," said James Topp, who commenced his own walk across Canada in the summer of 2022. He continued, "It's not anybody's business what my vaccination status is, okay? Like ... what's next? [Are] we going to start walking around with a collar?"[108]

I overheard one man giving an interview on the Ottawa streets that expresses the views of many. "My life is gone because of these people," he said. "I am no one now because I do not want to take something they are forcing me to take. How is that fair? It's not fair!" Then he emphatically stated, "I don't want it. It has nothing to do with it being a conspiracy theory. I don't believe any of that. I don't want it. I had an allergic reaction

---

[107] "Reported side effects following COVID-19 vaccination in Canada," Government of Canada, March 3, 2023, accessed May 10, 2023, https://health-infobase.canada.ca/COVID-19/vaccine-safety/.
[108] "Freedom Marches On—Interview with James Topp," First Freedoms Foundation, accessed May 10, 2023, https://firstfreedoms.ca/freedom-marches-on-interview-with-james-topp/.

to the flu shot and now I have to take this shot? And I can't get a medical exemption? How is that fair? I don't want it."

In normal times not wanting to be jabbed was not a career-ending move. Today it is. As the man said, "How is that fair? It's not fair!" Nor, I say, is it moral. Is this the kind of society we want?

It's true that suspicion of nonconformists is nothing new. Conscientious objectors have been harassed in our society for a long time. Years ago, the young men who refused to bear arms during the World Wars were sent to labour camps around the country. The boring hard work in these camps was seen as an opportunity to recruit the men. The hope was they would break down from the boredom and join the war effort "voluntarily." In some cases, it "worked," as the recruitment officers made their rounds to see if the inmates had had enough. Many, however, remained steadfast despite the hardships they faced.

Nevertheless, the government made allowances for conscientious objectors. Even under the *War Measures Act*, which was used to violate the rights of many Canadians who were labelled as "enemy aliens" and unjustly interned, the government was willing to accommodate nonconformists by providing alternatives to military service on the front lines.[109] After service in the work camps, the conscientious objectors of WWII re-entered regular society and carried on their lives as would any conscript who was discharged upon completion of their term of service.

Pacifists certainly faced societal pressure to compromise their beliefs and enlist, but there was no widespread campaign of coercion led by the prime minister himself. Indeed, during a parliamentary debate on conscription in 1940, William Lyon Mackenzie King promised, "the government has no desire and no intention to disturb the existing rights of exemption from the bearing of arms which are enjoyed by the members of certain religious groups in Canada, as for instance the Mennonites. We are determined *to respect these rights to the full.*"[110]

---

[109] "Defense of Canada Regulations," Archive.org, accessed May 10, 2023, https://archive.org/details/defenceofcanadar1939cana/page/n3/mode/2up?view=theater&q=alien.

[110] Debates (H.C.), 1940, Vol. 1, p. 904, as quoted in J.A. Toews, *Alternative Service in Canada During World War II* (Winnipeg: Canadian Conference of

Six decades later, the government took a very different approach. Instead of respecting the rights of a small minority, federal and provincial leaders trampled over the fundamental freedoms of Canadians. Under government rules—and rhetoric—there was no room for conscientious objectors on campus, in the workplace, or at an airport. Even medical exemptions were denied, as doctors who dared to provide exemptions to mask or vaccine mandates were severely punished.[111] Indeed, whether they fell under federal jurisdiction or not, the institutions and corporations that refused to accommodate conscientious beliefs were acting in line with federal objectives.

According to court documents revealed in the summer of 2022, the lack of accommodation was intentional.[112] When it came to the travel restrictions, the Liberals took pride in designing "one of the strongest vaccination requirements for travelers in the world."[113] Although airline carriers were permitted to issue waivers on medical or religious grounds, few were granted, and accommodation for other reasons (such as compassionate exemptions) was specifically excluded. The goal was not simply to push more people to get vaccinated. The point was to punish the unvaccinated. As Trudeau exclaimed on January 5, 2022, Canadians were "angry," and the Liberals gave citizens a target for their frustration: the unvaccinated.[114]

---

the Mennonite Brethren Church, 1959) 43. Italics added.

111 See e.g., "Ontario doctor accused of spreading COVID-19 misinformation barred from providing vaccine, mask exemptions" CBC News, September 28, 2021, accessed May 10, 2023, https://www.cbc.ca/news/canada/toronto/patrick-phillips-COVID-19-misinformation-college-1.6191906.

112 See Affidavit of Jennifer Little, April 22, 2022, filed in Ben Naoum v. Canada (Attorney General), 2022 FC 1463 (CanLII), <https://canlii.ca/t/jsnp4>, retrieved on 2023-09-05; being "Part 3" at, accessed September 5, 2023: https://www.jccf.ca/justice-centre-federal-vaccine-travel-ban-evidence/

113 Noé Chartier, "Compassionate Exemptions Cast Aside by Ottawa's Desire for 'Strong' Travel Vaccine Mandate: Court Documents," *The Epoch Times*, August 5, 2022, accessed May 10, 2023, https://www.theepochtimes.com/compassionate-exemptions-cast-aside-by-ottawas-desire-for-strong-travel-vaccine-mandate-court-documents_4646794.html.

114 Rachel Aiello, "Canadians are 'angry' with the unvaccinated: Trudeau," CTV News, January 5, 2022, accessed May 10, 2023, https://www.ctvnews.ca/politics/canadians-are-angry-with-the-unvaccinated-trudeau-1.5728855.

Tribal allegiances and attacks were promoted at the expense of Canadian unity. It would take a mass protest to start bringing Canadians back together again.

## CHAPTER FOUR:

# The Trucker Reaction: Not on Our Watch!

WE SHOULDN'T BE surprised that it was the Canadian truckers who finally said, "Enough is enough." Look around you, everything is moved by a truck. For the most part, truckers operate behind the scenes. They aren't usually centre stage for policymakers or consumers, yet our economy can't function without them. They ensure that when we go to the store, the shelves are stocked. They're the ones delivering medical supplies to hospitals, building materials to construction sites, food to grocery stores.

When we pick up a package of fresh spinach, for example, we rarely pause to think about how that leafy, green vegetable reached the produce aisle of our local grocery store during a snowy Canadian winter. That single purchase is the culmination of a complex journey involving many people. Their hard work allows the average consumer to enjoy a varied diet year-round, which our great-grandparents could hardly imagine.

At the centre of that story is the truck driver who leaves his home one early morning. Climbing aboard his rig, he heads for the American border. Many solitary kilometres lie ahead of him as he travels to Monterey County, California, where he'll pick up a load of freshly picked spinach bound for the grocery stores of the greater Toronto area.

It's a complicated business: his rig must be clean and at the proper temperature to carry the spinach back during the return journey. Timing and fuel prices are everything. He must make sure he has the right documentation for his trip and the handling of the cargo, along with the proper authorizations necessary to cross the border. There is little to no room for error. He is one of scores of truckers who carry only spinach, but he represents just a small fraction of the many truckers on our roads, all of whom play a vital role in our economy.

It's no exaggeration to say that nearly every aspect of our lives is dependent on the hard work of a truck driver. But when given a choice between applauding or attacking the truckers who deliver everything that we buy or use on a daily basis, Ottawa decided to attack.

And the truckers decided to push back. A cross-border vaccine mandate was the final straw. Trucker opposition to the mandate was only one chapter in a much longer story.

For nearly two years, Canadians witnessed the harm caused by invasive government policies. They grieved as their children developed eating disorders or depression brought on by fear and isolation during school closures. They saw their life savings evaporate and businesses crumble that took generations to build. They were unable to worship at church. If they refused a certain medical treatment, they weren't permitted to travel to see their families because they were denied a seat on a plane, train, or ferry.

Although most Canadians continued to obey the mandates, by late 2021, they were starting to question measures that seemed increasingly arbitrary and unjustified. When they tried reaching out to their elected officials, they were told that the government could only "follow the science." Given how often the "science" seemed to change or contradict itself in service of political goals, one couldn't help but be skeptical.[115]

---

115 See Preston Manning, "Determining the Role of Science in Shaping Public Policy,"
*C2C Journal*, December 10, 2022, accessed May 10, 2023, https://c2cjournal.ca/2022/12/determining-the-role-of-science-in-shaping-public-policy/. I summarize his points:
1. Public and media understanding of "the scientific method" as it actually is needs to be vastly increased, starting in the educational system, reducing the vulnerability of the media and the public to believing that "science is being followed" with respect to a public policy when it is not.
2. The minimal requirements that must be met before the developers and administrators of a public policy can claim it to be truly "science based" must be clearly established, with scientists taking the lead in defining those minimal requirements.

It was even harder to trust in the government's good intentions when orders were issued from behind closed doors. There was no open debate that considered the needs and perspectives of all citizens.

Finally, after a year and half of rule by fiat, the September 2021 election was supposed to give Canadians a chance to "choose how we finish the fight against COVID-19." As fall turned to winter, the end of the fight seemed to be nowhere in sight.

By early 2022, countries around the world were beginning to talk about easing restrictions. Even though case numbers were high, it was clear that the Omicron variant was less severe than previous waves. It was also clear that being vaccinated didn't stop people from getting COVID-19. The rationale for curfews, vaccine passports, and other mandates crumbled. The social capital to continue living in fear had run its course. A sizeable group had a belly full of the government narrative and could take no more.

In Canada, however, the government refused to loosen its grip. The authorities wouldn't even provide an endpoint or benchmark for lifting the restrictions that kept schoolchildren masked, barricaded places of worship, prevented families from socializing, and segregated the unvaccinated from the vaccinated. When pressed, they simply repeated their threadbare talking points about—you guessed it—following the science.

In fact, the government showed no signs of responding to the science that said it was time to shift away from harsh pandemic policies that were doing more harm than good.[116] Instead, they hardened their position by moving ahead with new restrictions. These added regulations included the

---

3. Our scientists must be encouraged and better equipped to directly communicate their science to decisionmakers and the public—including the scope and depth of the relevant science required and the need for the freedom to consider alternative hypotheses—rather than having that science filtered, censored, and misinterpreted by ill-equipped third parties.
4. Our politicians, civil servants, media communicators, and legislative caucuses must be better equipped to more ably and effectively "bring science to bear" on public policy, while also appreciating the limitations of science as an exclusive guide to policy development and implementation.

116 In the words of Liberal MP Joël Lightbound, "there is no appetite from our government to adapt so as to reflect the changing data and the changing reality of the Pandemic of the world," in *National Post* Staff, "Liberal MP Joël Lightbound's full remarks: 'It's time to choose positive, not coercive

vaccine requirement that would apply to all Canadian truckers crossing the American border. The mandate went into effect on January 15, 2022, despite warnings from the industry that the new rules would disrupt already fragile supply chains. There was no clear explanation as to why truckers were suddenly a danger to society after being hailed as heroes for working in the early days of the pandemic. The only justification was the government's mantra that vaccination was "the only way out" of the pandemic.

Likely, the government expected that initial criticism of the mandate would fizzle out once it was implemented. After all, for nearly two years it had imposed its will on Canadians with almost no major public resistance. If there were murmurs of dissent, they were quickly silenced or labelled as "misinformation."

But for the truckers, it wasn't just about the mandate. The government had pushed its authoritarianism too far, and now the truckers were pushing back.

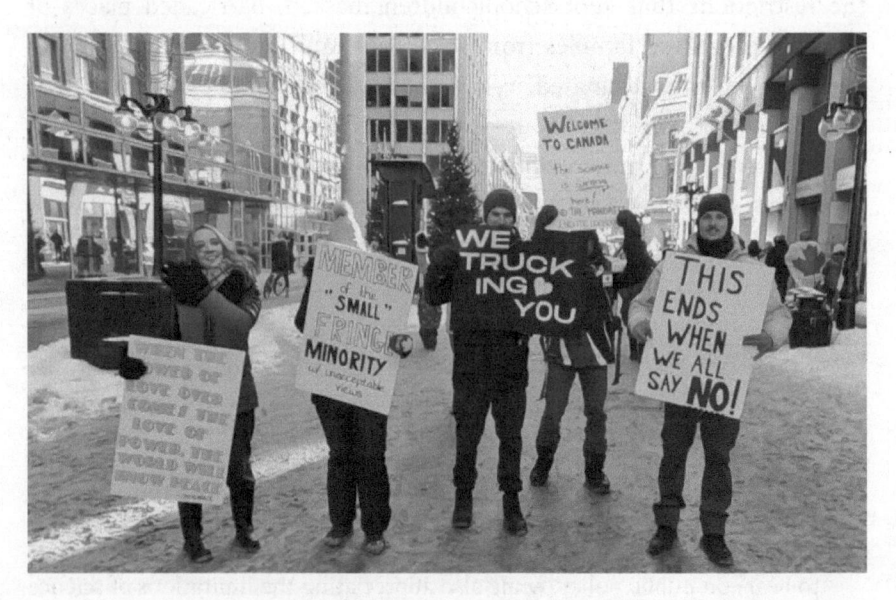

*Members Of The Small Fringe Minority*

methods,'" *National Post*, February 8, 2022, accessed on May 10, 2023, https://nationalpost.com/news/politics/joel-lightbound-full-transcript.

The plan was simple: take their frustration to the prime minister's doorstep. They would make a statement by rolling from coast to coast, converging on the capital. They would force the government—and the wider public—to stop and pay attention. It would be impossible to ignore them camped out on Parliament Hill. And maybe, just maybe, they would be able to make Trudeau hear their side of the story and end the nonsense.

Not surprisingly, there were almost as many different priorities as there were truckers. A few key figures helped to organize routes or raise funds, but the men and women who joined the convoy came independently, with their own goals and intentions. After all, it was their maverick tendencies that motivated them to resist the government in the first place.

In this way, the movement was "grassroots" in the truest sense. And like a prairie grassfire, it gained momentum as it travelled. The vaccine mandates were the proverbial "final straw;" the truckers were the spark that lit a flame of resistance that quickly spread across the country. They broke the seal of the pent-up frustration and anger boiling under the surface of a growing number of citizens.

They knew the costs. They faced slander and abuse from politicians and the mainstream media. The truckers also saw firsthand that Canada was at a tipping point. Canadians would have to choose between defending freedom or accepting a dictatorial regime that demanded control of their very bodies.

They weren't just tired of the pandemic; they were tired of the empty platitudes of the politicians walking the halls of Parliament, tired of the Ottawa and provincial bureaucrats issuing edicts from behind their laptops, tired of the judicial system that was taking way too long to hear their grievances with government. The protestors were tired of the disrespect shown to their rights and freedoms.

Freelance journalist Andy Lee tweeted (prior to being banned from Twitter for her political views):

> This is not just about truckers.
> This is about our parents who died trapped alone in nursing homes. This is about children who have never played with other children. This is about lost lives and livelihoods.

This is for them, and more.
This is for justice.[117]

In a video posted to Facebook on January 15, 2022—the same day the vaccine mandate went into effect—British Columbia trucker and organizer Colin Valentim explained:

> This Convoy is to bring awareness to the mandates and the severe harm that the government of this country is specifically looking to cause against the people. We are truckers organizing this one because we are now the latest to come under fire. It's not specifically for us. This has affected health-care workers, municipal workers, fire, and other emergency, police, ambulance workers as well as hospitality industries. Anyone is welcome for this, any kind of vehicle is welcome to this. The idea behind this Convoy is now to go all the way to Ottawa. It originally started as single cities and it has morphed into a national event and that's great, that's awesome ... We are specifically looking to this Convoy to be as loud and as large as possible ... We do not want to specifically block roads. We just want to continue down in the righthand lane doing our thing, making our miles ... We need to show this government that what they're doing is wrong.[118]

---

117 Her Twitter handle @Hannah_Bananaz—has since been suspended.
118 Valentim, Colin B. "Convoy to end Mandates," Facebook, January 15, 2022, https://www.facebook.com/colin.valentim/videos/1201208053737954/. As of August 2022, the video had been viewed more than 211,000 times and had generated over 4,500 comments.

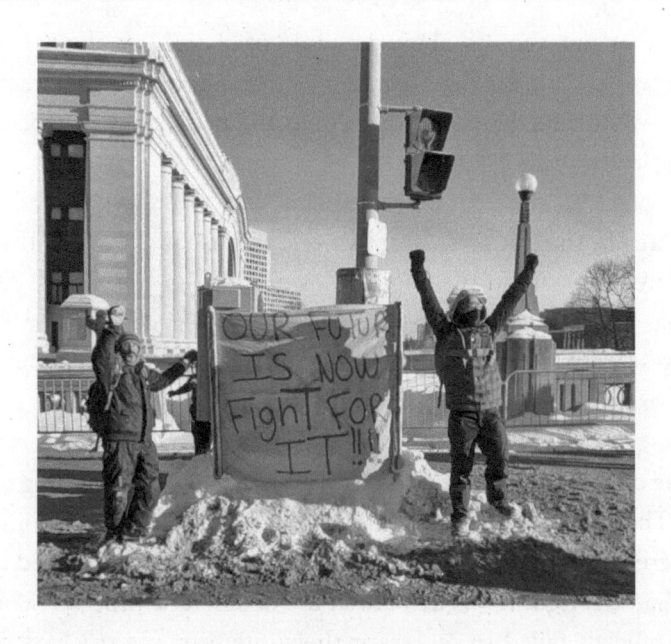

*We Must Fight For Our Future*

Valentim made it refreshingly clear that anyone and everyone was welcome, regardless of their medical status. He was adamant: "I will never, ever, for any kind of service, for any kind of entertainment, or in this case for my job, show segregation papers. I will never do that. That is what we need to fight."[119]

Elliot McDavid, who organized a parallel Slow Roll protest in Grande Prairie in January 2022, echoed a similar position when he explained, "We don't do this because we got nothing to do. We do this because we want what is best for everybody ... Whether you're vaccinated, unvaccinated, it doesn't matter. We are all family in the end. We have just got to unite and get together."[120]

Another trucker, whose social media posts went viral because of their uplifting spirit, shared that "We want people to know this is not about

---

119  Ibid.
120  Curtis Galbraith, "Slow Roll Freedom Convoy to go through Grande Prairie Saturday," *Everything GP*, January 28, 2022, accessed May 10, 2023, https://everythinggp.com/2022/01/28/slow-roll-freedom-Convoy-to-go-through-grande-prairie-saturday/.

being Vac or not Vac. It's about freedom of choice, it's about family, it's about friends. Coming together as a whole and supporting each other, which is what Canada used to be. We as the people have a voice and it's time our leaders heard us!"[121]

This positive attitude helps explain why so many Canadians felt empowered by the truckers. After two years of fear and division, the convoy represented more than the anger of overburdened Canadians. Although there was a strong sense of resentment against Prime Minister Trudeau, the protest wasn't about division or demonization. It wasn't about stirring up rage or fear. It was about hope, unity, and courage.

At long last, Canadians could see that they weren't alone: others shared the same concerns. And the truckers weren't simply complaining on social media. They were doing something constructive about their convictions. They were acting on the belief that Canada was a free nation, and that free people had the right to participate in the democratic process. When their elected officials failed to represent their interests, the truckers took the only course left to them: peaceful protest.

Of course, not everyone was enthusiastic (especially those who saw their power threatened by the protests). As the convoy gathered steam, Prime Minister Trudeau blamed the movement on a Conservative "campaign of disinformation." He accused the truckers of somehow "risking the lives of our frontline workers" and told reporters that:

> The small fringe minority of people who are on their way to Ottawa, who are holding unacceptable views that they're expressing, do not represent the views of Canadians who have been there for each other, who know that following the science and stepping up to protect each other, is the best way to continue to ensure our freedoms, our rights, our values as a country.[122]

---

121 Luke Kendze, Jan. 24, 2022, Facebook.com.
122 "PM Trudeau on Expanded Military Support to Ukraine, Trucker Convoy Protests," CPAC, Wednesday, January 26, 2022, accessed May 10, 2022, https://www.cpac.ca/episode?id=b23f9bf5-008e-4c79-8a3a-7cf82b3e9a65.

Government-funded journalists fell in line with the prime minister's position. The truckers were accused of being foreign-funded extremists bent on overthrowing a democratically elected government.[123] As the protests continued, they would be falsely painted as "most aggressive citizens," with "giddy inchoate rage,"[124] racists,[125] Nazis,[126] arsonists,[127] and behind it all were Russian actors.[128]

However, the Cathedral's front was beginning to crumble. The authorities no longer had control of the narrative. In a defiant twist, many Canadians proudly embraced the label of "fringe minority," eagerly printing bumper stickers, hats, and t-shirts proclaiming their sympathy for the "unacceptable views" of the truckers. It was this groundswell of support that turned a truckers' convoy into such a powerful movement. Across the country, people lined up on the highways and the overpasses, prepared sandwiches, and waved flags as the Trucker Convoy grew longer and longer. It was a far cry from the threatening "mob" being described by mainstream media.[129] The government's seal on the lockdown imprisonment of the people burst open.

There's hardly a better way to refute the lies and distortions than to share the firsthand accounts of the men and women who participated in the convoy.

---

123 https://www.ctvnews.ca/politics/convoy-organizers-had-extreme-aims-says-pm-s-national-security-adviser-1.5814097

124 https://www.thestar.com/opinion/star-columnists/2022/01/27/we-have-to-live-with-the-dangerous-freedom-convoy-fringe-but-politicians-dont-have-to-lend-them-support.html

125 https://globalnews.ca/news/8635223/harassment-threats-journalists-freedom-convoy-protests/

126 https://www.thestar.com/news/canada/2022/02/07/nazi-flag-at-freedom-convoy-sparks-bill-to-ban-hateful-symbols-but-enforcement-is-seen-as-tricky.html

127 https://thepostmillennial.com/freedom-convoy-arson-hoax-spread-canadian-media-debunked

128 https://www.onenewspage.com/video/20220129/14244638/CBC-TV-Suggests-Russian-Actors-Are-Behind-Freedom.htm

129 Gary Mason, "Trucker convoy has evolved into something far more dangerous," *The Globe and Mail* January 27, 2022, https://www.theglobeandmail.com/opinion/article-trucker-convoy-has-evolved-into-something-far-more-dangerous/

Starting his drive from Alberta, mechanic Luke Kendze described his first impressions rolling eastward on January 25, 2022:[130]

> So today was something unreal pretty much had goose bumps all day with the unity and love people have for each other. This convoy keeps growing and growing. Listening to truckers on the radio shows just how much they care about people, their hearts are very big.
>
> The support for this is unbelievable. Going through Alberta and Sask. There are people packing overpasses. For miles in and out of towns trucks and people lined up with signs dancing jumping SMILING (yes we can see their smiles) I have had people come up to the truck and say thank you and they start to cry, it is overwhelming. On cross roads in the middle of nowhere there are packs of 50 + people with augers lifted high and signs attached. Crane trucks, fire trucks, everything you can imagine in support. There are people with camp fires in the ditches with fire works.
>
> The police and RCMP have been very helpful and kind. It is amazing when people come together. In Medicine Hat there was over 500 meals prepared and given to us through our windows. It truly makes me proud to be Canadian! We need to remember that this is not about being Vac or unVac it is about freedom of choice and unity! Being Canadian! Please be loud and share everything possible, very important to stay peaceful! We are not here to cause pain we want to be heard and we want change!!!!

---

130 The quotes that follow can be found at https://www.facebook.com/justyn.kendze. Some posts may no longer be available. These quotes are used with permission.

Two days later, Kendze posted on Facebook:

> The convoy is 100 kms long and growing all the time. The support people have is overwhelming. Coming into Winnipeg yesterday was pretty emotional. The com radios went pretty quiet because no one could find words to express what we felt.
>
> There were people packed on the shoulders of the streets. Cars parked and people for miles and miles on the ring road around the city. The horns never stopped honking on the four lanes going out of Winnipeg. We thought it was hammer down time but ended up driving 5 to 20 km/hr for hours and hours. People had camp fires going in the ditches, fire works, a sprayer with booms out with big Thank you! signs on the booms. Crane trucks with the booms up with signs, lights flashing, and flags. The shoulders of the four lanes were packed with people and cars. Overpasses packed with people. Tons of families with little kids all bundled up. Everyone was jumping, dancing, waving signs, flags, and flash lights. All in minus 30 degrees. Seeing how happy kids are, their smiles make you a little emotional at times. *This is how Canada is supposed to be.* [italics added]
>
> This morning going into Ontario, the support is amazing ...—When we came to Thunder Bay, they had a big area plowed off. Tents put up, big fires and an insane amount of food. Beef on the bun, spaghetti, sandwiches, coffee, donuts and you name it. They brought pallets of windshield washer fluid for everyone. Very humbling how kind everyone is. This is what freedom feels like. I felt normal for once—not alone like the last two years. Thanks for all the support it is much appreciated!!

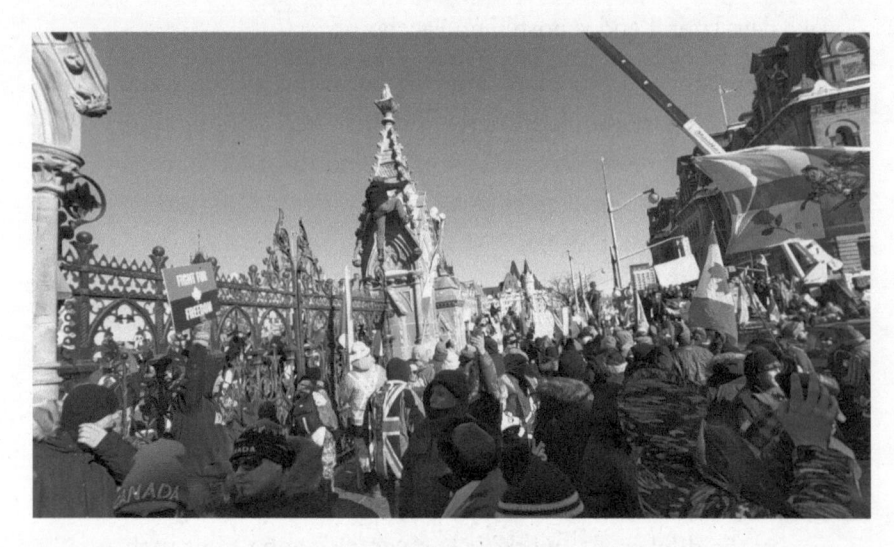

*Overwhelming Support*

On reaching Ontario, Kendze continued to urge kindness and positivity. His personal experience and attitude contrasts with media stories of belligerent truckers accosting business owners or refusing to wear masks. He emphasized that his approach was not unique—it was emblematic of the respect, empathy, and optimism that most of the truckers displayed.

> Hey everyone, today has been such a high for me. The people we meet and the truckers in the convoy have such compassion for everyone! I did not run with the convoy most of the day today. One driver's truck broke down, so we got parts and got him all fixed up. As we drove, we got to talk a bit on the radio. The people in this convoy are very humble. They are here just as I am for our friends and family. That our kids can grow up in a world like we did! The views we have are so united. There is a lot of fear in the world, and it is very broken. Just like the flags on our trucks as we drive getting tattered and torn.
>
> I would like to encourage people to not judge but be respectful. When we got to the hotel last night, I went in to get our room, I could tell the ladies up front were stressed

about masks. I was asked to put one on, so I did (which is not my view but out of respect for them) after talking with them for awhile. They don't want to be wearing one either and are extremely nice. They have families to support. I explained some of the giving and emotions we are having on the trip, how people are feeding us, housing us, fueling us, and so much more. Then a guy I did not know put his card on the counter and paid for my room. The kindness astonished the ladies.

This is what this is about Unity, peace, love to each other! There is fear in this world, I hope people can look past and not judge each other for being Vac or not Vac, wearing a mask or not wearing a mask. Be kind, and respectful. We don't know their situation.

I tell you this is a trip of a lifetime the highs and lows are exhausting. The encouragement of everyone messaging me is overwhelming. I have been getting messages from people all over the world — Germany Japan Australia Europe. I find myself tearing up as I drive and then be like, "grow up you baby!" Sorry I can't get back to everyone. I get nonstop calls and messages. I do appreciate it. I just get busy trying to keep guys on the road! I pray that this would be peaceful all the time. This is so much bigger than one individual.

As January turned to February, Kendze kept on urging a positive message. He acknowledged, "I know there is a lot of false and misleading information on mainstream media. Don't trust everything you hear and watch." He praised the Ontario Provincial Police (OPP) and Ottawa police officers for being helpful, and continued:

Everyone in the Convoy has been fed and fuelled as needed. I see truckers with garbage bags picking up garbage and shoveling snow on sidewalks. When something happens like a statue gets defaced by some group of people, there are people right after cleaning it up and scrubbing it down. It is truly amazing. To me we have already won, the unity and people knowing they're not alone is amazing.

… Stand up for what is right in your community, protect our kids. This is why we are here. Our friends, family, and our future. Show compassion and love to one another! Even if your views are different. Please give my wife and my kids a hug from me when you see them. I miss them more than anything! Thanks again for all the support. It is amazing. Please pray for peace, unity. I do believe I am here for a reason and have been put in a position that will help make a difference!

Later he added:

I run into people that have fear and anger. Lots of the time we get to talk to them and after they hear stories about what actually happened and is happening, they start to think about it all. Our job, everyone's job, is to get the truth out. Be respectful and talk with people. Start conversation — it is ok to disagree. This is the only way people start to think about stuff and their opinion. It goes a lot farther to be nice with someone who thinks different than to get mad back. Pray for our government, pray for Canadians, pray for the innocent in Ukraine. Thanks for all the support!

The desire for truth, positivity, and respectful dialogue that Kendze expressed (as did thousands like him) stands in stark contrast to the federal government's response. As the protests unfolded, Trudeau twisted the truth while refusing to talk with the truckers. The prime minister who told Canadians "I hear you" after the September 2021 election would not listen to the protestors calling for his compassion.

When Trudeau and the City of Ottawa sent in the riot police and the mounted police to break up the peaceful protest and freeze their bank accounts the eyes of many Canadians were opened. Tensions mounted as the protests stretched into the middle of a bitterly cold February. The aggressiveness of the mounted police, the pepper spray, and the violent arrests resulted in a growing admiration and respect among a substantial number of Canadians for those truckers and protesters who were willing to peacefully speak truth to power. Unlike the protests favoured by the government, there were no smashed cars or burnt buildings there were no broken windows, save for what the police did to the truckers' windows on the day they cleared Wellington Street. Now those truckers are remembered for saying, "Not on our watch." The fallout from the protests continues to impact Canada today. While the federal government may seek to control the narrative, and certainly it has greater tools to do so with the passage of the online regulation Bill C-11, the reality on the ground is that Canadians are no longer fooled. The Trucker Freedom Convoy 2022 burst the dam.

Now, let's discuss the 16 Ways the Truckers Ignited Canada for the Long Haul.

# PART TWO

## 16 Ways the Truckers Ignited Canada for the Long Haul

# 1. Gave People Hope

OUT OF THE rising mist came a foreboding yet majestic sight. At over 43,000 tons, the *HMS Prince of Wales*, escorted by two destroyers, made its way into Argentia, Placentia Bay, Newfoundland on August 9, 1941. Aboard was Prime Minister Winston Churchill. Two days before, US President Franklin D. Roosevelt had arrived on board the much smaller 9,000-ton *USS Augusta*. The harbour was a beehive of activity as the American military continued their construction of the air and naval base while the two men and their respective delegations discussed the pressing issues of WWII. The Atlantic Charter was the result, stating the war aims of the ongoing conflict. This document gave hope to war-torn Europe that the great powers were looking beyond the end of the war to a time of prosperity and freedom for all colonial subjects.

Some 120 kilometres away in the hamlet of Foxtrap, Conception Bay, a young couple, subsistence farmers, were pregnant with their fourth child, who was born the next spring. It's little wonder that his name was Winston, my father. Twenty-three years later, I was christened with the same as my middle name.

Having the name of a famous person causes one to wonder who that person was and what they stood for. I gained much inspiration in life for being named after a man who didn't give up, despite the darkest of circumstances.

Winston Churchill was courageous; he gave people hope of deliverance from the arduous journey of war. London and multiple areas in Britain had been bombed by Nazi Germany. Everything was rationed. Food was in short supply. Times were difficult. It took someone who understood the folly of human nature and the importance of history to lead the nation through such dark times. "All the great things are simple," Churchill said, "and many can be expressed in a single word: freedom, justice, honour, duty, mercy, hope."

Freedom, justice, honour, duty, mercy, and hope—such words will not be remembered as part of Trudeau's oratory during the COVID crisis. Rather, what will be forever remembered is his vilification of the unvaccinated.

What the Trucker Convoy did was bring people hope! Not only in Canada but around the world. Listen to these words spoken by Christine Anderson, a member of the European Parliament:

> ... and out of all of these movements it is the Canadian truckers that stand out and shine brightest. Because it was the Canadian truckers, their boldness, their courage, their determination to stand up to their governments. And it was they who inspired so many others all over the world to finally come together and be determined to put a stop to governments tearing down the very foundation of our democracies.
>
> And the reason I'm telling you all of this is [that] while I might have given hope to people like I said, it's only half the story because the other part of the story is this, I too needed hope. I too needed to know that I am not the only one fighting this fight.
>
> We all needed this help. We all did. And this is what you have given us—hope. Hope. That not all is lost. Yet hope that freedom and democracy can still be restored. And it is that hope that nurtures my strength and my determination to keep up fighting on my end of the bargain because it is not enough for a handful of MEPs to stand up and tackle this fight. It is not enough.
>
> We need you—the people—because you are so infinitely more powerful when it comes to convincing governments that they are not doing the right thing. So please, first of all, thank you for doing all of this. For paying us the

strength we need to do our job here but please stand up to your governments and follow the brave Canadian truckers' lead. They did exactly the right thing.[131]

I spent three days at the trucker protest, in Ottawa, over two different weekends—January 28, 29, and February 13. It was a thrilling experience to walk among the people. As I stood at the intersection of Wellington and Metcalfe streets in the throng of people listening to the speakers on the flatbed/staging area, I realized that this was an historic moment not only for me but for the entire country. *When will I ever be here again in the middle of this intersection with so many people supporting the cause of freedom in Canada?* I remember thinking. It was no ordinary protest. It was a celebratory moment of being with like-minded people who wanted hope, peace, and deliverance from the last two years of government overreach.

A truck mechanic from London, Ontario told me why he was there: "One of the biggest things is everybody is together right now," he said. "I have not seen so many people with smiling faces and just happy as all can be in the last two years as I have in the last two days, the last two hours even." He continued, "It's about being part of something that has got to be a change for the better. You can only stay suppressed for so long."

Indeed, he was right. Suppression had to end, and the truckers were the catalyst to break open the suppression. We simply couldn't go on without that hope much longer.

"I'm just a burger flipper," one speaker declared on a makeshift stage that was set up on Wellington Street in front of Centre Block of Parliament Hill. "I'm just a guy who owns a restaurant and who stood up for himself." He went on about the use of "social distancing" by government during the pandemic: "When you're socially distanced you are separated from your friends and neighbours. You're isolated. You're made to feel alone. When you speak out and you're made to feel alone it's scary because you wonder, 'Am I crazy? Does anybody else feel this way? Am I all by myself over here in this little isolated bubble thinking something's wrong?'

---

131   Christine Anderson member of European Parliament, "Emotional tribute to the Canadian truckers," February 18, 2022, https://www.youtube.com/watch?v=7rl8jg4yqLI.

"My message to you today," he said, "is if you're feeling like that, I'm sure none of you are here, but for those who're watching and aren't here, if that's how you're feeling—you're not alone! And what we've seen over the last couple of weeks here are men and women from all walks of life, right from the average business owners to the medical adviser to the White House standing with the truckers."

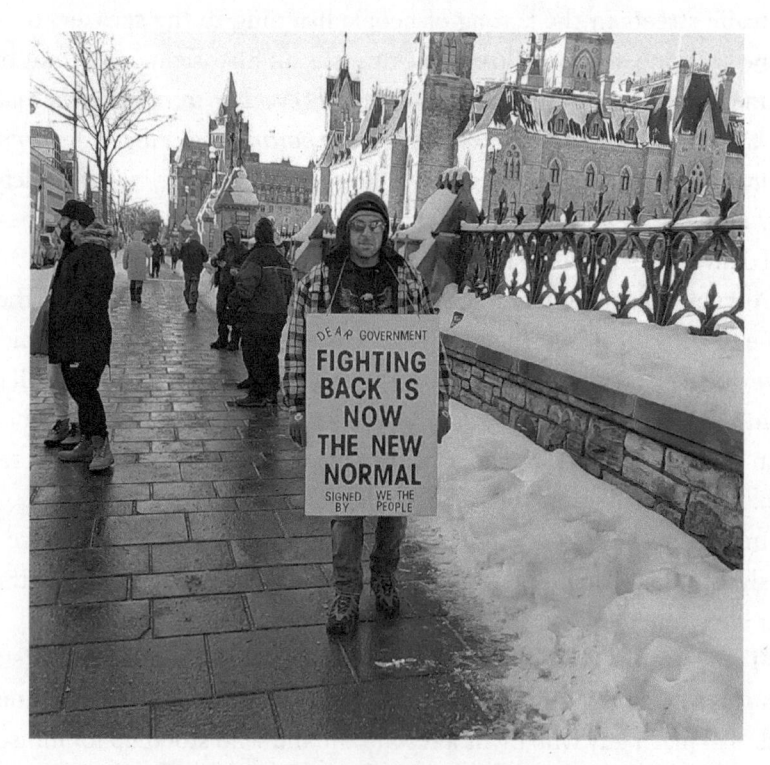

*The New Normal Just Before The Trucks Arrived*

For two years, he pointed out, the pressure had been building. "I've been thinking for the last year, after I stood up, man we really need something that's going to unite and ignite Canadians and get them to stand up together." He continued,

> I thought it might be the restaurants, then it might be the gyms, then it might be healthcare workers who're getting fired. Then it might be the police and the military. And, it never happened. In drives the trucks! ... That's what

we needed to get Canadians out of their homes onto the streets looking around and seeing they're not alone! We're not crazy! We're not crazy as Canadians to think that we should be free! Now we have this monumental occasion where people from all over the world are coming together. Brave men and women are sticking their necks out and they're speaking up and they're potentially losing their jobs, or appointments, or their income to speak up for you and I.

After listening for a while, I left the staging area and walked among the crowd around Parliament Hill, I came across a couple who both worked for the federal government. They'd refused to be vaccinated, and both lost their jobs. The lady held a sign with the words, "Free Will is the Foundation of a Just Society."

"I am here because my grandparents escaped persecution from dictatorship," she told me. "They worked their asses off to come here and I had a great stable life, and I will not take my freedom for granted."

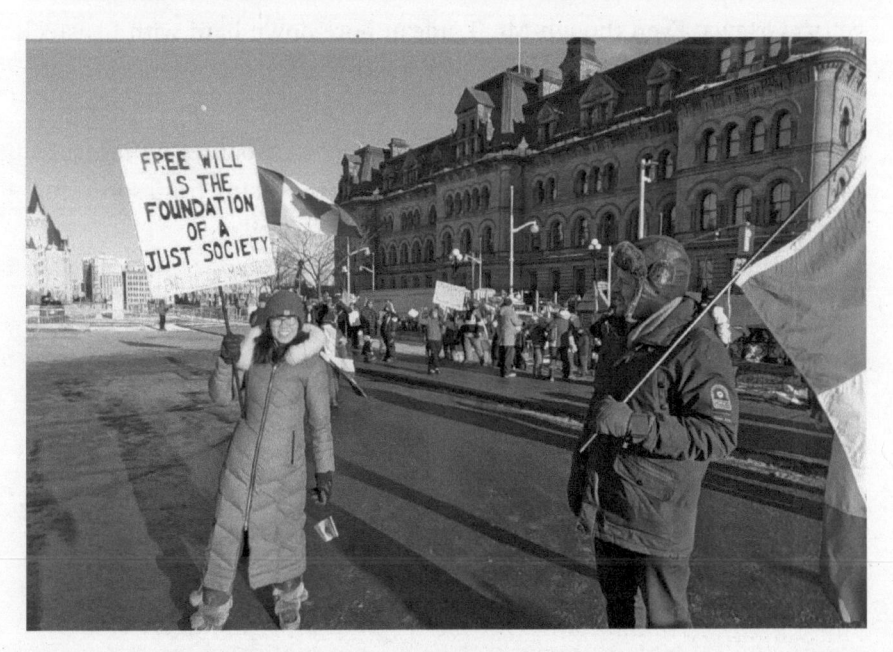

*My Grandparents Escaped Persecution From Dictatorship*

With conviction she stated, "This is the first time in my life where the theory of freedom and the reality is actually coming to a head. I had a decision to make, and I decided to stand for this freedom that I've been talking about for forty years."

Her husband, carrying a Canadian flag, summed up why he came: "Those truckers have brought so much hope when they came to town three weeks ago. I was crying. We were very desperate, and we were really questioning and trying to figure out a way to leave the country, you know, to escape this."

Their son hadn't been able to do any sports for two years. "He still can't do anything. It's horrible. It's horrible. And those truckers, of everybody in society ... we have been on so many walks for freedom and stuff, but there has never been anything that has so much impact. We really feel we're going somewhere with these guys. Finally, we're seeing, we're feeling, we're seeing results. It brings a lot of hope."

When Churchill and Roosevelt met in Newfoundland, the tide of World War II had not yet turned. But their message brought hope. So too did those massive semi-trucks as they pushed through the wind and snow to get to Ottawa. Even though Mr. Trudeau bore down hard with his steel fist and continued his arbitrariness for months after, this protest brought hope for deliverance from a government that had lost its way in an orgy of irresponsible spending, surveillance, and unnecessary oppressive measures to fight a virus that no human agency could possibly stop from spreading. The hope the truckers generated continues with us still.

## 2. Broke Trudeau's Monopoly over the COVID Narrative

FEBRUARY 13, 2022, was my third day on the Hill wading through the joyous crowd. How could I forget it? The very next day, Valentine's Day, Trudeau would send his "love" to the truckers with invocation of the Emergencies Act: the first time this legislation was ever invoked.

He grabbed the most draconian power possible under Canadian law to bear down on a peaceful protest of the working class—for the most part, the class without a university education or a multimillion-dollar trust fund, or an iconic name upon which to ride to power in the highest office of the land without the necessary competence. The working class dared to challenge the prime minister's COVID narrative. He wanted retribution. His grab for emergency power was a doubling down on his narrative.

But there was no emergency.

I marvelled at the carnival atmosphere of the Truckers' Convoy. The children, along with adults, were playing street hockey. There were other games for the kids, games you would normally see on a lawn in the summer, like lawn bowling. Music flooded Wellington Street from various sources.

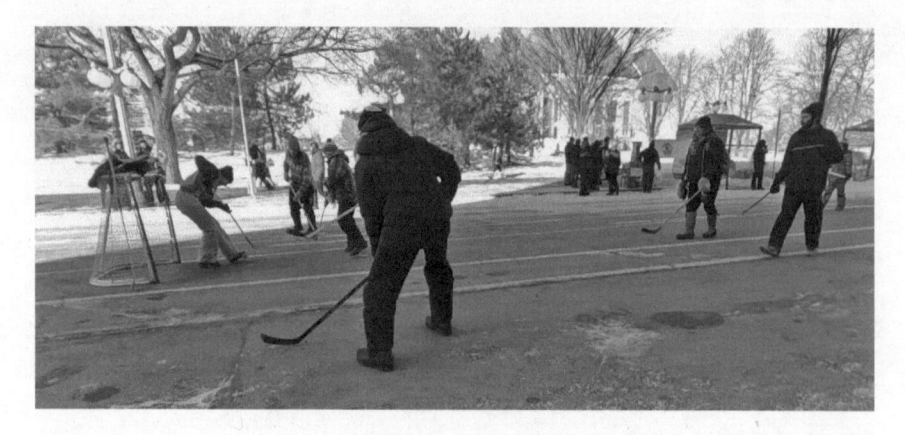

*Street Hockey At The Trucker Protest*

I attended the convoy on the first weekend and the third weekend. There was a dramatic difference between the first and third. At the first there was a lot more energy and, quite frankly, anger at the government. "F*ck Trudeau" flags and banners were everywhere. People were frustrated. Personally, I find such flags offensive, and they take away from the message and spirit of the protest. However, on the third weekend it was much more subdued. Hardly any "F*ck Trudeau" banners and flags. There was a more relaxed atmosphere.

Two young ladies from Quebec went up to random people: "Hi! Can I give you a hug?" they asked in their beautiful French accents. "Why of course!"

As I walked toward the stage at Wellington and Metcalfe streets, I heard a familiar voice. I could just barely hear it. The crowd was applauding to some comments and was deathly quiet on others. I wanted to get closer to hear more. I stood by the Centennial Flame to be in the sunshine. I needed warmth. The government authorities turned the flame off when the truckers came to town. I'm sure it was in the public interest. After all, why should those protesters benefit from the heat? It was cold. A beautiful day but deceptively freezing. One couldn't be out for long.

As I tend to do wherever I go, I took pictures. Lots of them. The posters along the fence line caught my attention: "Mainstream Media Is The Virus," "End Vaccine Mandates," "Keep Your Hands Off Our Children," "Freedom Not Fear." These were but few of the hundreds I saw.

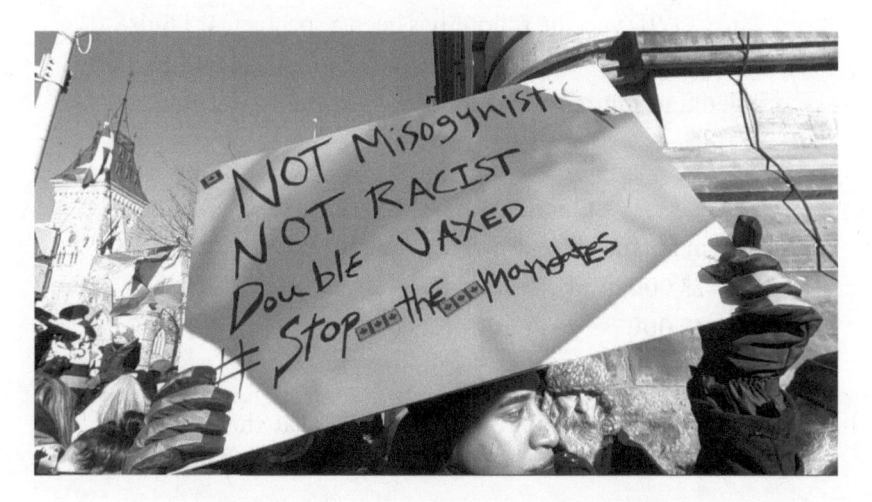

*People Are Tired of Government Misinformation*

The voice on the stage continued:

> When the government demands to inject an experimental substance into your body that you do not want, they are claiming ownership of your body. We have to say no. This is slavery.

The crowd was shouting and cheering, so I quickly made my way east of the Centennial Flame toward the stage. The area was packed full. The voice continued,

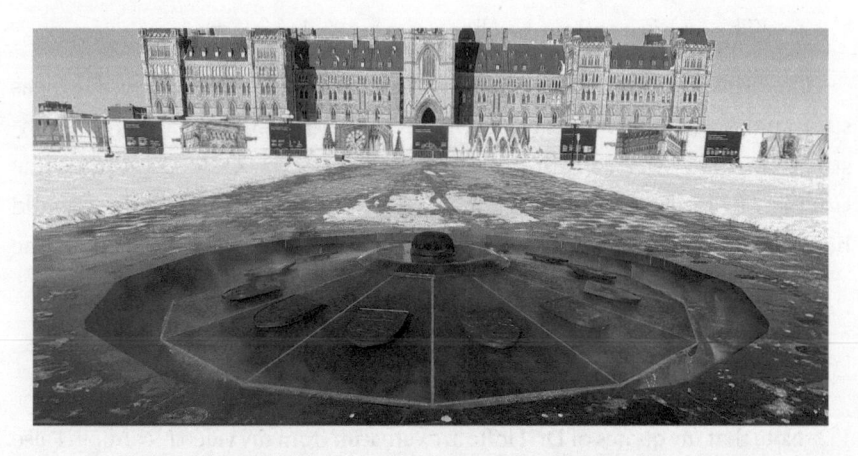

*Centennial Flame Extinguished Soon After The Truckers Came*

The COVID vaccine rollout has been a spectacular failure. Never before in human history has any medical treatment killed and injured so many people in such a short space of time.

A brief look at Open VAERS, the vaccine injury reporting system for the USA, will show you;
- 23,000 dead
- 42,000 permanently disabled
- And 1.1 million vaccine injuries

These were all people who were told that this injection would keep them safe.

Meanwhile in Canada, almost 90% of the population over the age of 12 are fully vaccinated, yet we have more COVID than ever before!

So, it is not hard to see that none of the mandates, restrictions, or injections imposed upon us has done anything to stop the spread of COVID, or to change the course of this pandemic.

Seventy-five per cent of those hospitalized with COVID in Canada now are fully vaccinated.

The vaccine rollout has been a spectacular failure.

The crowd voiced its support. I made my way so I could see who was speaking. It was Dr. Charles Hoffe of Lytton, British Columbia.[132] The mainstream media criticized him for his opposition to the COVID vaccine. The College of Physicians and Surgeons of BC stated at that point they would hold a disciplinary committee into Dr. Hoffe's public statements about the

---

132 Note that my quotes of Dr. Hoffe are verbatim from my video recording. I also verified these with a copy of his written speech which he provided me a copy.

COVID-19 vaccine.[133] Hoffe's opposition came from his personal experience of seeing a number of his patients suffer adverse reactions from the vaccine.

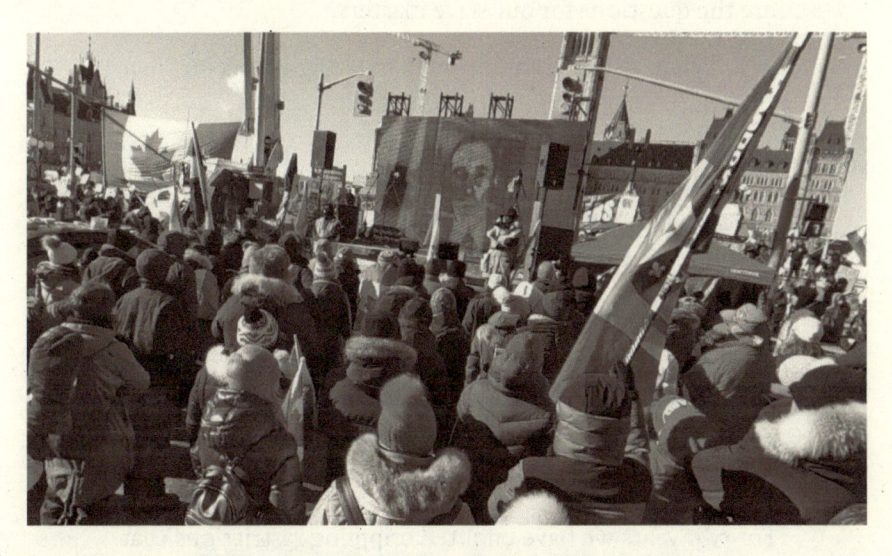

*Dr. Charles Hoffe Speaking To Protesters Via Video*

I stood among the crowd, spellbound by what he had to say. It was totally against the Trudeau narrative. The crowd were enthralled to hear from someone who expressed what they had experienced. Hoffe continued:

> The effectiveness of the COVID shots against omicron is almost ZERO. Omicron has 30 mutations and is so different from the original virus that the shots are near useless.
>
> So there is no logical reason why anyone should be vaccinated. The shots are useless.
>
> In fact, the shots are worse than useless—because they permanently damage your immune system. Triple-jabbed people are four times more likely to die from COVID than unvaxxed people because of the damage to their immune system through pathogenic priming.

---

[133] "Citation Re: Dr. Charles Douglas Hoffe," CPSBC, accessed May 10, 2023, https://www.cpsbc.ca/news/citation-re-dr-charles-douglas-hoffe.

None of the mandates or restrictions make any sense scientifically or logically. They have only caused harm. These are the questions for our slave masters:

1. What is the purpose of mandating a vaccine that does not stop the spread of disease?

The crowd shouted, "Control!"

It has no community benefit whatsoever! You can't keep anyone else safe by being vaccinated.

2. What is the purpose of restricting travel, to stop the spread of a virus that is already everywhere? The same virus is on both sides of the fence. So mandating a useless vaccine to stop the spread of a virus that is already everywhere, defies all reason and logic.

For two years we have endured crippling restrictions that were supposed to keep us "SAFE." Yet they have done nothing to stop the spread of COVID, or to change the course of this pandemic. Instead, they have ruined our lives, our businesses, and our nation.

An eerie silence fell upon the crowd.

Yet the determination of the authorities to continue these destructive and devastating restrictions that have utterly failed in their purpose shows that this is not about science, nor about health or safety. It is only about power, oppression, and control. This is slavery.

And the fact they now want to vaccinate our healthy children with the most dangerous vaccine in history—

"I won't have it!" shouted someone.

>—to protect them against a disease that poses almost no risk to them, shows that this is not about science, health or safety. It is profoundly evil.[134]

Silence followed as the crowd was enthralled with Dr. Hoffe's presentation.

> For two years we have endured this madness. But now more and more people are waking up to the evil, deceit, and control of our governing authorities.

Sporadic shouts of approval.

> The truckers of Canada have united this nation like nothing ever before.

The audience was now getting louder, and clapping almost drowned out Hoffe.

> Your bravery, your sacrifice, and your initiative have inspired and encouraged us all. You have made us proud to be Canadians again.

The roar grew louder and then quieted down.

> You have set an example to us all. You have tossed a snowball down a hill that has become an avalanche, that is reaching right across our nation, and across the world. You are changing Canada. You are changing history and you are changing our world. Well done!

Shouts rose again along with applause and flag waving. Then quiet.

> We are so grateful for the stand that you have taken. You have shown love for your fellow man and for your nation,

---

[134] Virginia Stoner wrote on May 4, 2021, "There has been a massive increase in deaths reported to the Vaccine Adverse Event Reporting System (VAERS) this year. That's not a 'conspiracy theory', that's an indisputable fact. You can try to explain it or justify it, or even argue it doesn't matter, but you can't deny it" in https://www.virginiastoner.com/writing/2021/5/4/the-deadly-covid-19-vaccine-coverup

by standing up for all of our freedoms. This is a war of good against evil, and our weapon is love.

Again shouts, applause, and flag waving.

You have changed our nation, and you are changing the world. Thank you for your sacrifices and your courage. Stand firm. You have filled us with hope and joy. We love you and appreciate you. Thank you.

Shouts of approval continued.

Dr. Charles Hoffe grew up during the Apartheid era in South Africa, and after immigrating to Canada, he practised medicine for 31 years. He knows prejudice. His family rebelled against it in South Africa, and when he saw the prejudice against the unvaccinated in Canada, he rebelled against that too.[135]

No matter what the Trudeau government and its media backers say, the government spell on the COVID-19 vaccine narrative was broken by the Trucker Convoy. No wonder Mr. Trudeau was angry. Court cases winding their way through the judicial system are slowly dripping out knowledge of how the vaccine mandates were based as much as, or more, on politics than science.[136]

Professor Bruce Pardy observes, "The Trudeau government has claimed to follow the science[137] on COVID, but that science is strangely different

---

[135] See, "Don't Give In To Fear: Interview with Dr. Charles Hoffe," Freedom Feature, https://firstfreedoms.ca/dont-give-in-to-fear-interview-with-dr-charles-hoffe/ accessed June 21, 2023.

[136] Rupa Subramanya, "Court Documents Reveal Canada's Travel Ban Had No Scientific Basis: In the days leading up to the mandate, transportation officials were frantically looking for a rationale for it. They came up short," *The Free Press*, August 2, 2022, accessed May 10, 2023, https://www.commonsense.news/p/court-documents-reveal-canadas-travel.

Arjun Walia, "Court Documents Reveal Canada's Travel Ban Had No Scientific Basis," *The Pulse*, August 3, 2022, https://thepulse.one/2022/08/03/court-documents-reveal-canadas-travel-ban-had-no-scientific-basis/.

[137] See also, "What Did the Government Know? And When Did They Know it? Interview with Dr. Joseph Hickey," First Freedoms Foundation, accessed May10,2023,https://firstfreedoms.ca/what-did-the-government-know-and-when-did-they-know-it-freedom-feature-with-dr-joseph-hickey/.

than it is everywhere else. Instead, its policies are based on spite, divisiveness, and pure politics. COVID now serves as an excuse to punish the government's ideological enemies."[138]

Can it be that Mr. Trudeau's anger against the truckers' insubordination was due to a deep-seated fear that the truth would be revealed through their protests? I think so. That explains why he had to double down.

Now think about this: How many people across this country have been denied the opportunity to travel to see their dying loved ones one last time? How many were unable to visit their newborn family member, or attend a long-anticipated wedding, or visit an aging parent, or attend a funeral, or suffered the loss of a government job or a job in a federally regulated industry, because of Mr. Trudeau's politically inspired vaccine mandates?

Consider that Mr. Trudeau was able to travel the world at our expense and not have to worry about such measures as mask mandates like us common people. No, Mr. Trudeau did not miss out on anything of importance to himself. He just decided to subject everyone else to his political whim and legitimated a campaign of harassment with his COVID narrative.

"I don't believe that he ever says a word that's true from what I've been able to observe," Jordan Peterson declared after seeing a video clip of Mr. Trudeau condemning the Trucker Convoy. Peterson's analysis of Trudeau continued. "It's all stage acting. He's crafted a persona. He has a particular instrumental goal in mind, and everything is subordinated to serve that."[139]

When Peterson said that he was in an interview with Peter Robinson, of Uncommon Knowledge, Robinson asked Peterson what Trudeau's motivation could be.

"The same motivation that's generally typical of people who are narcissistic," said Peterson, "which is to be accredited with moral virtue in the absence of the work necessary to actually attain it."

---

138 Subramanya, 2022.
139 Hoover Institution, "The Importance of Being Ethical, with Jordan Peterson," YouTube, April 29, 2022, 1:02:52, https://www.youtube.com/watch?v=DcA5TotAkhs&t=0s.

We can be thankful that the truckers put into motion the process of breaking through Mr. Trudeau's disinformation campaign of his politically inspired COVID narrative. We can never accept what any politician speaks as "truth" again without the strictest of reviews. And even then, I would question it still.

# 3. Gave the Average Canadian a Voice

THERE'S NOTHING MORE frustrating than not being given an opportunity to speak. In my practice of law, I've seen cases settle just because clients were given the opportunity to tell the world how poorly they were treated by the defendant. The money didn't matter as much as having the ability to air their grievances.

As parents having to arbitrate sibling rivalry, we experience something similar when the aggrieved child gets to tell her story. It seems that as soon as she's given that opportunity to speak, a way to settle the dispute is found.

We have a basic need to tell our story. We want to be heard. We must be heard, especially when we've been wronged. Our physical health depends on it.

The success of any civilization necessitates the freedom of its citizens to express themselves. We flourish when we can dialogue and exchange ideas. The ongoing open and honest conversations in all fields of human endeavour benefit the whole body politic. We learn from each other and can do much to solve the problems of our age, whether they be economic or social.

Recognizing the importance of free speech, section 2(b) of the Charter lists the following right,

> "(b) freedom of thought, belief, opinion and expression, including freedom of the press and other media of communication."

That right is there for a reason. Let's be frank. Wars were fought over the right to speak. King Charles I literally lost his head when he refused to allow Parliament a say in the running of Great Britain in the seventeenth century. Free speech is serious business.

If ever there was a need for freedom of speech it was during the COVID-19 pandemic. Average Canadians woke up every morning to confusing signals from the government and its media supporters about what should or should not be done in dealing with it. It ranks as the most exasperating experience of my life. All around me people were saying that there was something not right about the government narrative. Close friends in the medical profession were sharing with me the absolute breakdown in the medical community's approach: "In all my years of practice I have never seen anything like this. Barry, never have we tried to coerce people against their will this way. Never in modern medicine have we used lockdowns to prevent a virus. A virus runs its course. It will mutate as all viruses do. Any vaccine will take years—at least ten—to be developed." On and on I heard a similar analysis from reputable physicians. The dichotomy between what my medical friends shared and what government and the media were saying was huge. It was like living in two different worlds.

My wife is a piano teacher, and she taught our three children piano. I married up—my music skill is limited to turning on the stereo system! I vividly remember one of our sons practising one day when she and I were in the kitchen. She stopped as I was putting the dishes away in the cupboard. "Barry, please go in there [the studio] and tell him that he's doing it wrong! He must play that section over again! It's driving me nuts!" Not being attuned to dissonant notes as is my wife, I thought our boy was doing a great job on the keyboard. I marched in as one with great musical authority and know-how and informed my son of his need to repeat "that section" over again, as it was being practised incorrectly!

Imagine being taught all the principles of modern medicine and science, including the need to debate and question any new approach in the sincere hope of finding out the truth of the case, but being told that there is only one view of the problem, only one method of treatment, and any evidence to the contrary must be kept quiet on pain of your job! Those medical and scientific minds could hear an audible scream: "You're doing it all wrong! Play that section over again, and please do it right this time!"

Public health officials constantly changed the rules. Masks were not necessary one day but absolutely required the next. Lockdowns like what was happening in China weren't necessary, and then they were. Travel restrictions were racist until they weren't. We could go on with a litany of examples.

"The science has changed," we were told. At the same time, scientists and doctors who weren't part of the government apparatus, or on the mainstream media circuit, were drowned out and criticized for not repeating the accepted public health narrative. And worse—they were "putting people's lives at risk." We all saw the inconsistencies. But interpreting those inconsistencies fell into two camps—one supporting the government narrative, and the other not.

Were the COVID numbers accurate? At least anecdotally something was amiss. My neighbour informed me of their family member dying of heart issues but labelled as a COVID death nonetheless! Something was way off.

Once the vaccine arrived, the press reported hospitalized COVID patients according to their vaccination status. Naturally, at first the unvaccinated outnumbered the vaccinated. The media, public health, and politicians said the pandemic was now because of the unvaccinated. The unvaccinated were causing the increased death rates! Imagine the off-putting of guilt that gave because you weren't vaccinated you were causing the death of others! Such reporting continued until the vaccinated hospitalizations were more than the unvaccinated. Then the reporting stopped. "Let's not let facts get in the way of the narrative!"

The contradictions, the half-truths of politicians and the public health officials were in plain sight. But we were told that what we saw was not what we saw. Such gaslighting was unprecedented. Every attempt to voice opinions contrary to the narrative was immediately shut down. Big tech companies—Twitter, Facebook, YouTube, Google, and the rest—made sure that any mention of COVID on their platforms was compliant with the standard narrative. This is still the fact as Jordan Peterson's interview with Robert F. Kennedy, Jr., was taken down from YouTube![140]

Young medical professionals let us know that their qualifications to speak on everything COVID were unimpeachable. Meanwhile, my physician friends whom I'd known for decades were telling me that there was a mass formation process in the works, where everyone was afraid to speak out for fear of losing their jobs. How crazy is that?

It was bad manners, even in the presence of family, to say anything that wasn't in keeping with the official narrative.

But it was the truckers who said, "No! We're not going to take it anymore!" The rolling of the trucks to Ottawa was an act of defiance that put everything into perspective. It removed the tape of censorship. It smashed the seal of political correctness. When I walked among the protestors on Parliament Hill, I had to admit that at first, I was taken back by the harsh language of the signage and flags. The "F*ck Trudeau" message was the most jarring I saw in Ottawa. I even saw young children—perhaps less than ten years old—carrying the same message. How could this be?

I struggled mightily with the abundance of "F*ck Trudeau" flags, signs, t-shirts, hats, and the like. It took away from the message of the convoy, and it could imply intended violence against our prime minister. I respect Mr. Trudeau as the holder of the office of prime minister. I certainly do not respect his policies or his scapegoating of the unvaccinated. But I'm of the view that he should not be accosted with the "F*ck Trudeau" mantra. I have never seen or heard of a prime minister being talked about like this—so polarizing has he become.

Ken Boessenkool and John von Heyking criticized the convoy's "omnipresent 'F-ck Trudeau'" paraphernalia. "Never has there been a more indolent and more feeble expression of disdain," they said. "This indolent and feeble expression is, to make things worse, politically impotent, which is another way to say it is an empty expression of rage populism." They recognized that such displays were underlying legitimate concern about

---

140 Robert F. Kennedy, Jr. on Twitter, "What do you think ... Should social media platforms censor presidential candidates? My conversation with @JordanBPeterson was deleted by @YouTube," https://twitter.com/RobertKennedyJr/status/1670445104564252674?, accessed June 21, 2023.

"government overreach and abuse of power, [but] doing so is just political theatre that makes the waver feel good. No amount of waving obscenity-laced flags will change the government ..." The authors were warning Pierre Poilievre not to be seen supporting such flags, as it won't attract "swing voters to swing their vote to the Conservative side."[141]

Professor Bruce Pardy observes that "in any free country the citizen has got to be able to insult the leader of the country. You can't go around advocating actual violence. You can't stand on the soapbox and say, 'Alright, you people get your torches, we are going to go down to the prime minister's residence and do the following thing.'" As Pardy notes, "That's not on!" However, it is part of living in a free country to be able to express extreme disapproval of the leader. "Any free person in any free country is allowed to say that very thing ["F*ck Trudeau"] and worse about whoever it is that leads the country at that particular moment." In Pardy's view "to not allow that means we are being far too sensitive, and we are giving reality to this 'words are violence' idea which is not true."[142]

I recognize that the Charter, when not suspended by the prime minister, allows us to speak our minds as long as we don't engage in hate speech—meaning something that vilifies and marginalizes people based on their identity or group membership. In other words, we can't delegitimize people, "reducing their social standing and acceptance within society."[143] So hate speech means we're out to ostracize, segregate, deport, and ultimately be violent to the victim. I consider "F*ck Trudeau" to be offensive language. I wouldn't want to use it—although I have to admit that I have used similar language myself.

Even in "polite Canada," there is no right not to be offended. Unfortunately, many people can't handle opinions different from theirs. In

---

141 Ken Boessenkool and John von Heyking, "Getting to government is one thing, but how you govern is just as important: Three ways of understanding the conservative disposition," *The Hub*, September 9, 2022, accessed May 10, 2023, https://thehub.ca/2022-09-09/opinion-getting-to-government-is-one-thing-but-how-you-govern-is-just-as-important/.
142 Barry W. Bussey and Bruce Pardy, October 13, 2022.
143 "Saskatchewan (Human Rights Commission) v. Whatcott, 2013 SCC 11, at para. 71," CanLII, [2013] 1 SCR 467, accessed on May 11, 2023, https://canlii.ca/t/fw8x4.

extreme cases, a perpetrator justifies violence because they were offended by the speech. That is, unfortunately, where we seem to be headed in this country.

The truckers had every right to offend the prime minister and his supporters. They had every right to offend my own sensibilities with their use of "F*ck Trudeau." The populist urge to use such language, in my view, was a mistake. I was pleased to see that by the third weekend of the protest, the visibility of such paraphernalia was drastically reduced. As the protest continued, things calmed down amongst the truckers. They settled in for the (pardon the pun!) long haul.

The value of the truckers speaking their mind was the fact that they allowed the average Canadian a voice. In many ways, the protest acted as a Canadian safety valve that let off pent-up societal pressure that resulted from the government and its supportive media deeming only one narrative as "acceptable." Not only were other views suppressed, but those "fringe" people with "unacceptable views" lost their jobs, their houses, and/or placements in educational institutions because they dared to not comply.

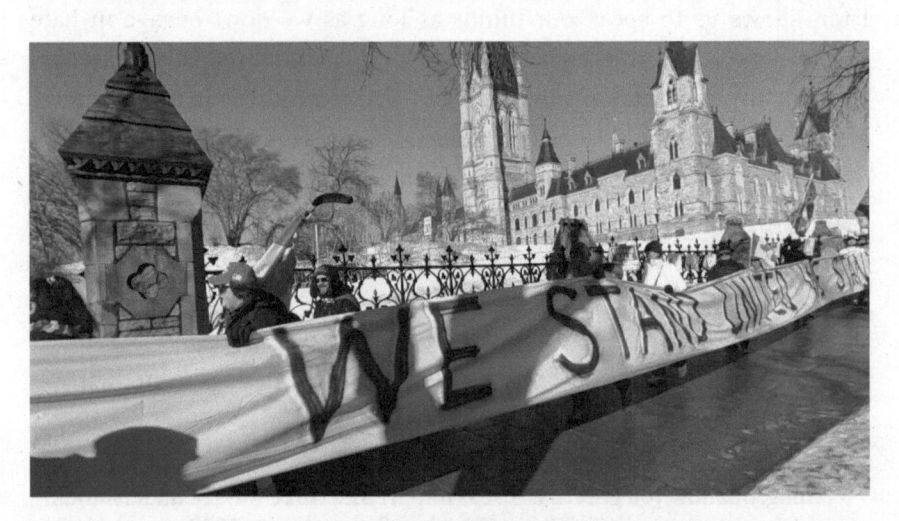

*We Stand United As Never Before*

## 4. Showed That Elites Can Push Only So Far

DAVOS, SWITZERLAND. JUST the mere mention of the town has taken on a conspiratorial ambiance that excites the imagination. In some spheres it's seen as the modern-day Dante's ninth circle of hell—the place of treachery. For others, it's the pinnacle of all that is good. It is, after all, on top of the Swiss Alps, with an awe-inspiring view and where only the richest and self-declared best and their wisdom come to roost.

Here, Mr. Trudeau and the world's up-and-coming leaders and influencers gathered under the auspices of eighty-five-year-old Professor Klaus Schwab.[144] He is the executive chairman of the World Economic Forum (WEF). Under Schwab's leadership, "social entrepreneurship" became a buzzword as his organization sought to bring the most promising youth of the world to his Forum of Young Global Leaders[145] to learn how to save the world in the "Schwabian way."

Basically, the WEF and its related entities is a glorified gabfest where billionaires meet up with other billionaires, political leaders meet other leaders, promising youth meet other promising youth. Connections and friendships are made. There's a certain camaraderie that develops, and opportunities for future projects and undertakings occur. Those who obtain an invitation to attend are awestruck to be so privileged to be among the world's elite.

---

[144] "About Klaus Schwab," World Economic Forum, accessed May 11, 2023, https://www.weforum.org/about/klaus-schwab.
[145] The Forum of Young Global Leaders, accessed May 11, 2023, http://www.weforum.org/young-global-leaders.

Up until recently, it was a mark of some significance to reference one's attendance at such an august gathering. I say "until recently" because it has now become a liability, especially for conservative-leaning politicians, to be associated with the WEF.[146] The newly appointed leader of the Opposition in Ottawa, Pierre Poilievre, made it clear that he will not allow any of his cabinet to attend the WEF. Various conspiracy theories are gathering steam in the conservative digital universe, warning of anyone even slightly associated with Schwab.

To say that Schwab "runs the world" is too simple and not true, although he "certainly pretends to run" it.[147] Any current world leader has probably been to Schwab's gabfest—Emmanuel Macron, Jacinda Ardern, Justin Trudeau, and the like. And, surprise, surprise, they use Schwab's jargon to virtue signal that they're on the cutting edge. It's part of letting each other know "I'm in the club," like the way a Harvard grad tells a group, "Yeah, when I was up in Cambridge ..." Everyone is to take note.

"[W]hat we are very proud of now," said Schwab, "is the young generation like Prime Minister [Justin] Trudeau ... We penetrate the cabinet. So yesterday I was at a reception for Prime Minister Trudeau and I know that half of his cabinet, or even more than half of his cabinet, are actually Young Global Leaders."[148] And yet, according to the longest-serving president of the Liberal Party of Canada, Stephen LeDrew, today's Liberal Party is nothing like the Liberal Party of the past, and there's absolutely no one in cabinet who knows what's going on in public life or in the machinery of government to enable them to solve problems in the government.[149]

---

146 Michelle Rempel Garner, "I went to Davos. The World Economic Forum is not running Canada," *The Line*, February 24, 2022, accessed May 11, 2023, https://theline.substack.com/p/michelle-rempel-garner-i-went-to.

147 Paul Frijters, Gigi Foster, and Michael Baker, "Is the WEF the Headquarters of Evil?" Brownstone Institute, June 15, 2022, accessed May 11, 2023, https://brownstone.org/articles/is-the-wef-the-headquarters-of-evil/.

148 Terence Corcoran, "In Canada, follow the money + the ideas," *Financial Post*, February 18, 2022, accessed May 11, 2023, https://financialpost.com/opinion/terence-corcoran-in-canada-follow-the-money-the-ideas.

149 These words were spoken in August 2022 at a First Freedoms meet-and-greet, see First Freedoms Foundation. "We used to have records..." Facebook, August 10, 2022, https://www.facebook.com/firstfreedomscanada/videos/619742206169805 at 6:50 minutes.

When Schwab's *COVID-19: The Great Reset*[150] was published in July 2020, Justin Trudeau wanted to show that he was with the "in crowd" as he addressed the United Nations in September 2020. "This pandemic has provided an opportunity for a reset," Trudeau airbrushed the room with Schwab's choice words of the moment, letting everyone who is anyone in the WEF world know that he, Justin Trudeau, was up on Schwab's latest dictation on the tablets from the mountaintop released to the public a mere two months before.

"This is our chance," said Trudeau in what has become his much-mimicked diction,[151] "to accelerate our pre-pandemic efforts to reimagine economic systems that actually address global challenges like extreme poverty, inequality and climate change."[152]

"Never let a good crisis go to waste" has become the adage of so many elitists who have already planned what must be done to make the world into their utopian vision. As Ronald Reagan once said, "The nine most terrifying words in the English language are: I'm from the Government, and I'm here to help."[153]

The problem with government and the high and mighty within the progressive intellectual class is that they feel they have all the answers to the world's problems. Very few have ever gotten their hands dirty in the tilling of the earth's soil or in the grease of a mechanic working on a tractor, but they sure have all the answers. It's rather rich for a trust-funded scion of Pierre Elliot Trudeau, whose only experience in life has been as a snowboarding instructor and a drama teacher, to opine on "efforts to reimagine

---

150 Klaus Schwab and Thierry Mallert, *COVID-19: The Great Reset* (Zurich, ISBN-Agentur Schweiz, July 9, 2020).

151 Canada Proud (@WeAreCanadaProud), "Is this the best impression of him you've ever seen?" Twitter, July 17, 2022, 4:48 PM, https://twitter.com/i/status/1548771582629257223

152 https://www.cbc.ca/news/politics/great-reset-trudeau-poilievre-otoole-pandemic-covid-1.5817973

153 "Reagan Quotes & Speeches," Ronald Reagan Presidential Foundation & Institute, accessed May 11, 2023, https://www.reaganfoundation.org/ronald-reagan/reagan-quotes-speeches/news-conference-1/.

economic systems," when he later admitted, "You'll forgive me if I don't think about monetary policy."[154]

Indeed.

He said this before doubling the national debt, leading in no small part to our skyrocketing inflation levels not seen in decades. Under Mr. Trudeau's watch, the federal per-person debt increased by a whopping 35.3% to $47,070, according to the Fraser Institute.[155] The Canadian Taxpayers Association says it's more like $56,000![156] Can we forgive him for not thinking about monetary policy? He would have served us better if he had. But then again, that wasn't in his script. Our grandchildren and their children are going to pay heavily for the obscene monetary failures of Mr. Trudeau.

Part of Schwab's reset is to redistribute wealth from capital to labour. Mr. Trudeau is doing his darnedest to destroy small businesses in Canada with his ideologically-driven policies that make no business sense while supposedly helping the "middle class." His oft-stated point of raising taxes on the wealthiest one percent so he could lower taxes on the middle class is simply rubbish. A recent report on the Trudeau tax changes have meant that sixty per cent of families who are in the bottom twenty per cent of earners are now paying $233 more on average in taxes.[157] What a waste.

---

154 CTV News, "Trudeau: You'll forgive me if I don't think about monetary policy," August 19, 2021, 1:25, https://www.youtube.com/watch?v=G7VOLChLKG4.

155 Jake Fuss and Evin Ryan, "Examining Federal Debt in Canada by Prime Ministers Since Confederation, 2022," *Fraser Research Bulletin*, accessed May 11, 2023, https://www.fraserinstitute.org/sites/default/files/examining-federal-debt-in-canada-by-prime-ministers-since-confederation-2022.pdf.

156 Franco Terrazzano, "Each Canadian is on the hook for $56,000 in government debt," Canadian Taxpayers Federation, June 30, 2022, accessed May 11, 2023, https://www.taxpayer.com/newsroom/each-canadian-is-on-the-hook-for-56,000-in-government-debt

157 Milagros Palacios, Nathaniel Li, Jason Clemens, and Jake Fuss, "Impact of Federal Income Tax Changes on Canadian Families in the Bottom 20 Percent of Earners, 2022," Fraser Institute, February 2022, accessed May 11, 2023, https://www.fraserinstitute.org/studies/impact-of-federal-income-tax-changes-on-canadian-families-in-the-bottom-20-percent-of-earners-2022 for full report, see: https://www.fraserinstitute.org/sites/

On the WEF website Mr. Trudeau's biography includes, "His team is focused on creating good middle-class jobs, making life more affordable, keeping Canada's communities safe, fighting climate change, and moving forward on reconciliation with Indigenous Peoples. A proud feminist, Justin appointed Canada's first gender balanced cabinet."[158]

Consider his record: middle class life has actually gotten harder not easier,[159] Canada's communities are in fear as his policies of releasing violent criminals is devastating;[160] climate change by virtue of carbon tax is showing little results[161] but it is all a matter of politics;[162] Indigenous Canadians are anything but happy with his flippancy and virtue signaling and empty promises;[163] and his feminist mystique is anything but polished after his treatment of Jody Wilson-Raybould.

The WEF club, despite Klaus Schwab holding Mr. Trudeau up as one of his poster boys, does not deliver what is advertised. The world is not a better place because these billionaires "fix" the world's problems through their gabfests.

The WEF's promotion of green policies for the developing countries is dubious at best. Take for example the recent disaster that unfolded in Sri Lanka. In August 2018, the Sri Lankan prime minister was front and centre on WEF's website on how he was going to make Sri Lanka rich by 2025.[164] Western elites were delighted that Sri Lanka followed its green climate change initiatives, including organic farming eliminating synthetic

---

default/files/impact-of-federal-income-tax-changes-families-in-bottom-20-percent-of-earners-2022.pdf.
158 https://www.weforum.org/people/justin-trudeau, accessed June 20, 2023
159 https://nationalpost.com/opinion/np-view-middle-class-life-keeps-getting-harder-under-trudeau-liberals
160 https://nationalpost.com/opinion/trudeau-liberals-criminal-friendly-bail-reforms-helped-spur-wave-of-violence
161 https://globalnews.ca/news/7646946/canada-carbon-tax-experts/
162 https://www.nature.com/articles/s41558-021-01268-3
163 https://vancouver.citynews.ca/2021/10/04/trudeau-tofino-indigenous-relationship/
164 Ranil Wickremesinghe, "Sri Lanka PM: This is how I will make my country rich by 2025," Wayback Machine, August 29, 2018, accessed May 11, 2023, https://web.archive.org/web/20190122012624/https://www.weforum.org/agenda/2018/08/this-is-how-we-will-make-sri-lanka-rich-by-2025/.

fertilizers.[165] But rice production dropped 50%. In July 2022, the Sri Lankan economy collapsed. The president fled the country. Hungry people stormed the government buildings.[166] The WEF, in an Orwellian act, took the August 2018 article off its website.[167]

Of course, the Sri Lankan story is more complicated than the climate change policies alone. Things are always more complex. The COVID-19 pandemic meant that many foreign nationals came home from working overseas. These people were a source of income for the country, as they sent money home to their families. Plus, the tourism industry came to a halt. More people needing more food with less money to pay for it combined with a crop failure is a complex mix.

According to some observers, "Klaus Schwab is a glorified and very talented conference planner selling flattery."[168] The WEF is a four-day networking conference where the elites ignore Schwab's own "words of wisdom" to do what they have always done—network to make more money and virtue signal.

Mr. Trudeau has followed the same WEF schtick in Canada: virtue signaling that he is in line with all the latest progressive fads of the day but in reality, doing what is necessary to maintain power. He is a fake feminist, creating a gender-equal cabinet, only to get rid of two women

---

165 I have the utmost regard for organic farming. I doubt that there was little training and ownership in organic farming in Sri Lanka that would have avoided this crisis. In other words, organic farming may well have been great for Sri Lanka if it were properly implemented. The fact is, the way it was implemented failed miserably.
166 Philip Wen, "Sri Lanka Imposes State of Emergency After President Flees Country," *Wall Street Journal*, July 13, 2022, accessed May 11, 2023, https://www.wsj.com/articles/sri-lanka-imposes-state-of-emergency-after-president-flees-country-11657711655.
167 Helen Raleigh, "Sri Lanka Crisis Shows the Damning Consequences of Western Elites' Green Revolution," *The Federalist*, July 15, 2022, accessed May 11, 2023, https://thefederalist.com/2022/07/15/sri-lanka-crisis-shows-the-damning-consequences-of-western-elites-green-revolution/.
168 Paul Frijters, Gigi Foster, Michael Baker, "Is the WEF the Headquarters of Evil?" Brownstone Institute, June 15, 2022, accessed May 11, 2023, https://brownstone.org/articles/is-the-wef-the-headquarters-of-evil/.

cabinet ministers for challenging his unethical behaviour.[169] He uses the green climate change mantra and then buys a pipeline. He says he is for jobs but eliminates two pipeline projects. He makes it near impossible to get mining projects started because of his ideological commitments that have nothing to do with mining.

The truckers were aware of Trudeau's virtue-signaling tactics. The trucker vaccine mandate had nothing to do with the "science" of COVID safety! It was Trudeau's project to get all Canadians vaccinated. Every trucker is quarantined all day on the road. A vaccine that was dubious to begin with wasn't going to change the reality that the truckers were already safe and harmless. It was show. It was imposition of a rule of the most unsavory kind.

According to Trudeau on March 31, 2020, truckers were heroes who work "day and night to make sure our shelves are stocked,"[170] but in January and February 2022, the truckers who went to Ottawa were the "fringe minority ... with unacceptable views."[171]

To the average Canadian, the Cathedral's musings about climate change, vaccine mandates, and woke ideological positioning means nothing to putting food on the table and providing a roof over their family's heads. Common sense prevails, not some high-minded policy birthed on a mountain top in the eastern end of Switzerland.

When the elites impose their costly, virtue-laden nonsense limiting people's ability to earn a living, there will be pushback. The Canadian truckers did it and woke up the world. The Sri Lankans did it. In the

---

[169] Mario Dion, Conflict of Interest and Ethics Commissioner, after investigating the scandal noted in his *Trudeau II Report 2019*, "The actions [of the prime minister] ... were improper since they were contrary to the Shawcross doctrine and the principles of prosecutorial independence and the rule of law." Accessed August 30, 2023, https://ciec-ccie.parl.gc.ca/en/publications/Documents/InvestigationReports/Trudeau%20II%20Report.pdf,

[170] Justin Trudeau (@JustinTrudeau), "While many of us are working from our homes, there are others who aren't able to do that," Twitter, March 31, 2020, 8:01 PM, https://twitter.com/JustinTrudeau/status/1245139169934016517.

[171] "Trudeau says 'fringe minority' in trucker convoy with 'unacceptable views' don't represent Canadians," Global News, January 27, 2022, accessed May 11, 2023, https://globalnews.ca/video/8542159/trudeau-says-fringe-minority-in-trucker-Convoy-with-unacceptable-views-dont-represent-canadians.

irony of ironies, Trudeau's government claims to side with the Sir Lankan people. Another photo-op.

Imagine the gall of Mélanie Joly, minister of Foreign Affairs on July 12, 2022, tweeting,

> The July 9th protests in Sri Lanka were a clear expression of the desire for a better Sri Lanka. Canada supports a peaceful, constitutional path forward that supports urgent action on economic and political reform. (1/2)
>
> Violence against peaceful protestors and journalists is unacceptable and those responsible must be held accountable. The right to protest peacefully must be upheld.[172] (2/2)

These are the same people who stomped on the Canadian truckers in Ottawa, the same group that encouraged Sri Lanka to adopt the WEF climate change policies that played a significant part in this disastrous result. But never wanting a crisis to go to waste, these same people can virtue signal that they are on the right side!

The little people, the ones for whom the elites have no time on an average day—except when the elites want to do their photo ops—those, average hard-working, good-natured people are getting wise to the elite chicanery.

During the summer of 2022, Prime Minister Trudeau went on a "pop-up tour." He hopped around the country popping up unannounced in the most unlikely places—like at a Christian church service. You can't but recognize that he and his handlers are trying to pretend that he's something he's not. No doubt part of the reason for the unannounced visits is his unpopularity—if known in advance where he will be, surely the anti-Trudeau protesters will show up. I'm not a fan of obnoxious protest tactics, because I wouldn't like to be subjected to harassment everywhere I went. I do still believe, even though I strongly disagree with Mr. Trudeau,

---

172 Melanie Jolie (@melaniejolie), "The July 9th protests in Sri Lanka were a clear expression of the desire for a better Sri Lanka," Twitter, July 12, 2022, 10:24 AM, https://twitter.com/melaniejoly/status/1546863098484740096.

that there must be decorum and respect. His office is worthy of it. Yet for many exasperated citizens, being obnoxious is the only way to draw attention to their cause.

Trudeau revealed his cruel authoritarian streak when he imposed the Emergencies Act against the truckers. No number of church visits will take away the scenes of his aggressive, if not brutal, take-down of the protesters in Ottawa. The same spirit was evident during the Canada Summer Jobs scandal. No Christian church holding traditional beliefs on marriage received any Canada Summer Jobs grant for hiring summer students.

It is truly something to behold.

In Newfoundland, I have often witnessed the "Cod'n In" tradition of making a mainlander an "honorary Newfoundlander." Part of the process is that the mainlander must kiss a codfish. At one program I attended, they put lipstick on the cod! It didn't change the fact that the cod was still a cod. And smelled like it.

It doesn't matter how much Mr. Trudeau shows up at churches or daycares around the country. Until he apologizes to the Canadian people for how he treated the truckers and for unjustifiably invoking the Emergencies Act powers, he is still the same authoritarian Justin Trudeau who would do the same thing again tomorrow if he thought it was politically advantageous.

The truckers showed us that the elites can only push so far before there is pushback.

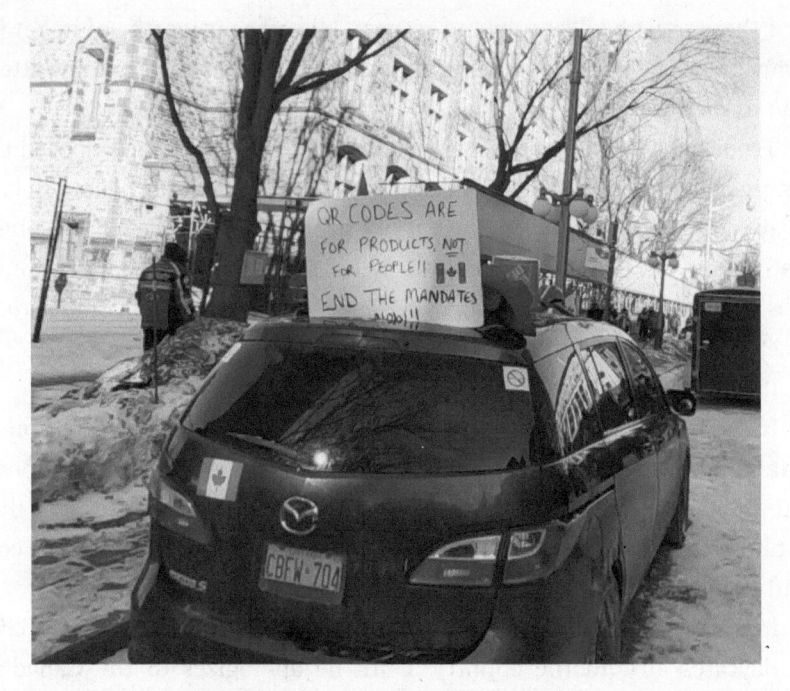

*QR Codes Are For Products Not For People*

# 5. Revealed the Steel Fist in a Tyrant's Velvet Glove

"SOME OF YOU might oppose our grievances," Tamara Lich said as she sat beside the Hon. Brian Peckford in a news conference on February 14, 2022. "However, democratic society will always have non-trivial disagreements and righteous dissidents. There are many reasons for us opposing the mandates. Some of us have ... been mistreated by our government including many of our Indigenous communities who have personally experienced medical malpractice. Some of us simply want bodily autonomy and oppose the mandates on principled grounds. No matter our reasons and opinions it is how the government responds to its citizens that determines the fate of the country. Listen to your hearts Canadians. Is the Emergencies Act the right response to our demonstrations of love and freedom?"[173]

Prime Minister Trudeau's invocation of the Emergencies Act may yet be seen by history as a fatal political mistake.

It seemed he might get away with it. Former Justice Rouleau's decision that the prime minister met the high threshold of the Act to invoke it would again appear to absolve him. It does not. Mr. Rouleau's decision only adds intrigue to the entire affair, for reasons I will elaborate on later. Further, the scandals keep coming. The latest over Beijing's electoral interference in supporting a number of liberal candidates continues what Jody Wilson-Raybould, Jane Philpott, Bill Morneau, and the truckers know: this

---

[173] Bridge City News. "LIVE FROM OTTAWA: Freedom Convoy organizer Tamara Lich, and Charter signatory Hon. Brian Peckford held a press conference Monday afternoon," Facebook, February 14, 2022, https://www.facebook.com/100063516701060/videos/2883409135138326.

too shall pass. With each passing scandal, the evidence of abuse of power gets higher. The power game will soon pass. I am not a prophet or a son of a prophet, but I am certain, as a student of history, that such actions come to haunt those in power, like in a Shakespearean play.

No matter how much our Canadian Macbeth cries, "Will all great Neptune's Ocean wash this blood clean from my hand?" what has been done is done. We can only thank Providence that no one died and little blood was spilled in Mr. Trudeau's trucker crackdown.

Canadian history will come to know February 14, 2022, as a day of national infamy and, for Mr. Trudeau, a personal tragedy. It was yet another example of just how far he was willing to lie and use brute force. His reputation as an authoritarian remains. It was not a proud Canadian moment.

His summer 2022 "pop-up tour" is no doubt an admission by his handlers that his authoritarian reputation threatens his long-term political ambitions.

Consider first the lie of the Emergencies Act[174] invocation. To invoke the Act, there must be a "national emergency." The Act defines it as an "urgent and critical situation of a temporary nature." But there is more. It must seriously endanger the lives, health, or safety of Canadians to such a degree that a province doesn't have the capacity or authority to deal with it. It must also seriously threaten "the ability of the Government of Canada to preserve the sovereignty, security and territorial integrity of Canada and cannot be effectively dealt with under any other law of Canada."

So, a national emergency is urgent, critical, and temporary, and no province has the capacity or authority to deal with it. And it threatens the sovereignty, security, and territorial integrity of Canada. That is a serious situation—one that conjures up images of war or another similar catastrophic event.

Knowing what the Act says, just step back and think about what occurred in Ottawa during the Truckers' Convoy. Did what happened with the truckers in Ottawa even come close to a "national emergency," as noted above? One doesn't have to be a lawyer to answer this. You just need basic common sense.

---

174  https://laws-lois.justice.gc.ca/eng/acts/e-4.5/index.html

Every legal colleague I have spoken to about this (I did not have a chance to speak to Mr. Paul Rouleau!) agrees with me that what happened in Ottawa was *not* a national emergency as defined in the Act. Mr. Rouleau himself expressed that others examining the same evidence that came before him could readily have come to a different conclusion. Invocation of the Emergencies Act was an absolute abuse of the Act and one that must never happen again. It was beyond "over the top." Words are insufficient to describe the inappropriateness.

The Act contains what we call in law "an extremely high bar to meet." There's a reason why the Act was never implemented until February 14, 2022. Its powers are extraordinary. Not only can people be detained without reason, but as we saw, their finances can be seized. It authorizes the state to carry out whatever is necessary to accomplish the government's goal—even war itself. It is not a toy to play with.

How did the events at the Ottawa Freedom Convoy come anywhere close to this level of dire, existential threat required by the Act? The protests in Ottawa were all peaceful. When the court told the truckers to stop honking their horns, the truckers stopped. When the court said, "Get off the bridge," the truckers got off the bridge. Tom Marazzo, a retired Canadian military officer and one of the main organizers of the Freedom Convoy, told me that when someone offered to supply firearms to the truckers protesting in Coutts, the truckers reported it to the RCMP! The truckers then left the border because they were shocked that anyone would even make such an offer! Violence was not what they were about. They hugged the police and sang "O Canada" as they left.[175]

---

[175] See Barry W. Bussey, "Trudeau's Tiananmen Square—Interview with Tom Marazzo," First Freedoms Foundation, accessed May 31, 2023, https://firstfreedoms.ca/trudeaus-tiananmen-square.

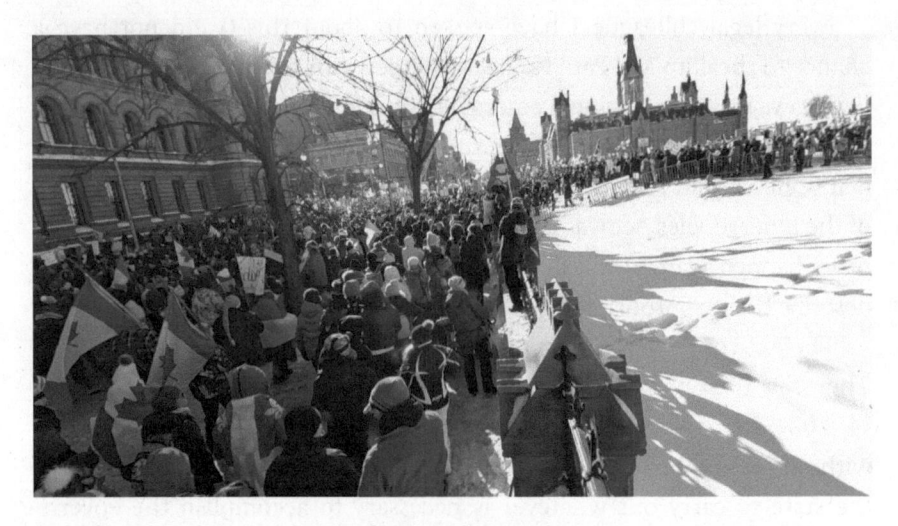

*Peaceful Protest*

The misinformation emanating from the prime minister during this time was incomprehensible. He knew better. He created a spin on a story that he couldn't control. It was obvious that he didn't want the truckers to defy his orders, and he was going to do something about it. His government lied, yet again, and said that the police demanded the extra powers to deal with the protest! We now know that was a complete fabrication.[176]

Not only did the police not request the power, but David Vigneault, director of CSIS, specifically informed the government the day before invocation of the *Emergencies Act* that the protest did not pose a security threat to Canada nor were there signs of international interference.[177] However, he also encouraged Mr. Trudeau to invoke the Act!

---

[176] Ryan Tumilty, "RCMP didn't ask for Emergencies Act to be invoked, commissioner tells Commons committee," *National Post*, May 10, 2022, accessed May 11, 2023, https://nationalpost.com/news/politics/rcmp-didnt-ask-for-emergencies-act-to-be-invoked-commissioner-tells-mps; Sarah Ritchie, "Emergency Preparedness Minister: police did not ask for Emergencies Act," CTV News, June 15, 2022, accessed May 11, 2023, https://www.ctvnews.ca/politics/emergency-preparedness-minister-police-did-not-ask-for-emergencies-act-1.5946705.

[177] Laura Osman and Jim Bronskill, "'Freedom Convoy' did not pose threat to the security of Canada: CSIS director," CTV News, November 14, 2022,

The fact that Prime Minister Trudeau continues to get away with untruths is absolutely shameful to Canada as a whole. Mr. Rouleau's report is now embedded in this narrative, and it will be seen for what it is—a failure to bring accountability. Mr. Rouleau's decision isn't binding on any court. He wasn't in a courtroom but overseeing a statutory commission to explain a political event—the use of the never-used *Emergencies Act*. It was political theatre and again appears to have "worked" to let Mr. Trudeau off. It has not. It has created many questions, and there is fear that his decision has made it easier for another government to use the Act.

There are currently two cases before the federal court that will legally decide whether the government met the Act's threshold. Of course, all bets are off as to how the courts will rule. If we've seen anything during the pandemic, it's that the Canadian courts have shown little sympathy to those who opposed government pandemic measures.[178]

One of these cases has been brought by the Canadian Constitutional Foundation against the federal government for invocation of the *Emergencies Act*. It has revealed to the public that the prime minister was informed twenty-four hours before invocation of the Act that there was about to be a breakthrough between the Trucker Freedom Convoy and the City of Ottawa.

Brian Peckford put Keith Wilson in touch with his contacts, who led a meeting with the City of Ottawa.[179] Wilson noted, "The negotiated agreement between the truckers and City was signed on the Saturday [February 12, 2022]. Logistics mtg was held @ city hall Sunday afternoon. Trucks started moving Monday morning. And then Trudeau invoked *Emergencies Act*. I was there and did the negotiations."[180]

---

accessed May 11, 2023, https://www.ctvnews.ca/politics/freedom-convoy-did-not-pose-threat-to-the-security-of-canada-csis-director-1.6151982.

178 Barry W. Bussey, "Courts Should Uphold Constitutionally Protected Rights Instead of Just Deferring to Governments' Decisions," *Epoch Times*, August 2, 2023, https://www.theepochtimes.com/opinion/courts-should-uphold-constitutionally-protected-rights-instead-of-just-deferring-to-governments-decisions-5438431

179 Email with Hon. Brian Peckford, February 29, 2023.

180 Keith Wilson, K.C. (@ikwilson), "The negotiated agreement between the truckers and the City was signed on the Saturday," August 12, 2022, 1:56 PM, https://twitter.com/ikwilson/status/1558150370366345218.

The *Toronto Star* reported that the "Trudeau government was told of 'potential for a breakthrough' with protesters a day before it used the *Emergencies Act*."[181] So why did the government then invoke the Act the next day? According to journalist Andrew Lawton, Trudeau saw that "his window was closing and there was going to come a time when it wouldn't have been possible to justify it."[182] Everything was winding down with the borders, Ottawa was being freed up and cleaned. "I think they realized it's now or never. We'll never be able to do this." The motivation, as Lawton sees it, was that the government wanted to confiscate all of the money the truckers had raised on the crowd funder GiveSendGo.[183] I think he may be on to something there.

Mr. Trudeau was losing popular support, even though the mainstream media were doing all they could to spin the truckers as seditionists. The truckers did not want, nor did they try, to overturn the government. They just wanted the outlandish government overreach put to an end, including the abolishment of vaccine mandates. The fact that there were some truckers who made intemperate statements against the government was not indicative of the whole.

During all this abuse, we witnessed the prime minister's audacity to accuse the opposition[184] of supporting swastika flags. It was an outright

---

181 Alex Ballingall, "Trudeau government was told of 'potential for a breakthrough' with protesters a day before it used Emergencies Act, cabinet documents reveal," *Toronto Star*, August 11, 2022, accessed May 11, 2023, https://www.thestar.com/politics/federal/2022/08/11/trudeau-government-was-told-of-potential-for-a-breakthrough-with-protesters-a-day-before-it-used-emergencies-act-cabinet-documents-reveal.html ; see also, "Morning Update: Trudeau government invoked Emergencies Act despite 'potential for a breakthrough' with Convoy protesters, documents show," *The Globe and Mail*, August 12, 2022, accessed May 11, 2023, https://www.theglobeandmail.com/canada/article-morning-update-trudeau-government-invoked-emergencies-act-despite/?utm_source=dlvr.it&utm_medium=twitter.
182 The LeDrew Three Minute Interview, "The Magnifying Glass on Justin Trudeau's Egregious Use Of Power," YouTube, July 27, 2022, 3:20, https://www.youtube.com/watch?v=NJylyiQN2gQ.
183 Ibid.
184 Catherine Levesque, "'Stand with Swastikas': Emergencies Act debate turns ugly as opposition grows," *National Post*, February 16, 2022, accessed May

lie. Given that it came from the highest office holder in the land who claims the moral authority to determine what constitutes "disinformation" through the internet,[185] it takes on greater significance. Further, the egregious nature of his insult is amplified, as it was made to a Jewish MP. Rather than make amends, Mr. Trudeau doubled down and repeatedly refused to apologize. He stood by his comments, as they served his cynical political purposes. Power, not truth, is the ultimate goal.

History suggests that one extreme leads to an opposite extreme. I think of when Western society was dominated by Church and State ideology that limited freedom of the individual. The Reformation period led to further abuses. The French Revolutionary fervor brought one extreme after another. The Russian tsar crushed all dissent until the communists crushed the tsar and then crushed dissent again. Russia was finally set free in 1989 with the collapse of the Soviet Union, and then only for a short time. Putin's regime is now in another cycle of limiting dissent. On and on it goes.

We are naïve if we think that the same can't happen here. Consider that we never thought that a Canadian prime minister would take the reins of such dictatorial power as Mr. Trudeau did on February 14, 2022. But we lived through it. Thankfully it was only for nine days, but it was perilously close to being a lot longer and much more severe.

When Mr. Trudeau leaves office, as he will sooner or later, a new wind can be expected to blow. An equilibrium will have to be reached. But who is to say that a new government won't use Mr. Trudeau's example and obtain power for power's sake, and even use the previous government as a proxy for further repression. Or perhaps they'll use it to expose all the inner workings of the Trudeau government as the basis for further investigations of the previous regime?

---

11, 2023, https://nationalpost.com/news/politics/stand-with-swastikas-emergencies-act-debate-turns-ugly-as-opposition-grows.

185 See my discussion with Peter Menzies on the government's internet law: "What's Wrong with Bill C-11—Interview with Peter Menzies," First Freedoms Foundation, accessed May 11, 2023, https://firstfreedoms.ca/whats-wrong-with-bill-c-11/.

The point is this: Just as far as the political and social pendulum swung one way, it can swing the other way. That's why the rule of law is crucial to maintaining long-term stability. Therefore, when Mr. Trudeau knocked down constitutional rights and stretched the credulity of the *Emergencies Act* to punish political opponents, he made it exceedingly difficult to bring about civil peace. He crossed the democratic Rubicon.

Although the prime minister no longer holds the emergency powers, we must recognize that our country was struck a mighty blow. There is still anger in Canada, and if not properly dealt with, it will cause serious problems in the long term.

On February 23, 2022, Ukraine declared a state of emergency after facing several months of Russia building up some 190,000 troops with armoured vehicles and aircraft along its border. *That* is a national emergency that would be beyond the capacity or authority of a provincial government to deal with. By contrast, Canadians coming together to protest government mandates in a carnival atmosphere is not a national emergency. It's the exercise of their constitutionally protected freedom of speech, assembly, and association. Dispelling them with brute force—even strangling their ability to pay for groceries—is a profound failure of leadership.

None of the underlying reasons for the protest were resolved by the use of the Act. In fact, those who felt disenfranchised only had their sense of alienation and mistrust confirmed when the prime minister refused to listen to the pain of Canadians who'd spent weeks in the bitter cold, trying to make their voices heard. Restoring trust will not be easy.

The Public Order Emergency Commission hearings filled the media discussion and political debate about the prime minister's invocation of the emergency powers. The hearings revealed that the government's decision was fraught with more trouble than originally thought.

First, we can't help but observe that it was the prime minister who appointed Rouleau.[186] Rouleau served on the Ontario Court of Appeal,

---

186 "Prime Minister announces Public Order Emergency Commission following invocation of the Emergencies Act," Prime Minister of Canada, April 25, 2022, accessed May 11, 2023, https://pm.gc.ca/en/news/news-releases/2022/04/25/prime-minister-announces-public-order-emergency-commission-following.

and his career included a stint in politics as a member of Liberal Prime Minister John Turner's team.[187] No doubt Mr. Rouleau was recommended by Minister of Justice David Lametti.

The cynic in us can't but remember the way Mr. Trudeau got rid of his former justice minister because she wouldn't violate the rule of law during the SNC-Lavalin Affair. While Justice Rouleau, from all accounts, is a trustworthy arbiter of the law and carried out his duty with the utmost professional care, we can't overlook the shame this government has brought to justice. Therefore, much rode on Mr. Rouleau's shoulders as he weighed the evidence. Now that we have his decision that white-washed Mr. Trudeau's invocation of the emergency powers we are left with more questions.

As former Newfoundland Premier Brian Peckford observes, the inquiry from the beginning was beset with serious problems.[188] The government, in essence, investigated itself. The government determined the terms of reference from which Mr. Rouleau was not to depart. The focus was on the Trucker Freedom Convoy, not on the government's misuse of power. In other words, it assumed right out of the gate that the government did nothing wrong—but the truckers did. That is a serious problem. Mr. Rouleau needed more authority to go beyond those terms, notes Peckford, and do a proper investigation of the government's actions. I agree with Mr. Peckford that there needs to be a commission, independent of government, to investigate what occurred. Otherwise, the government is only feathering its own nest. That is what happened.

Mr. Peckford, the last surviving first minister involved with the creation of the Charter of Rights and Freedoms, was an important voice for Canada during this turbulent time. The voice of an elder statesman who can offer wisdom to the country cannot be overstated.

---

187 Paul Rouleau: Ontario Superior Court Judge interviewed by Carte de visite, unfortunately TFO has taken down the interview. https://www.tfo.org/en/universe/carte-de-visite/100385485/paul-rouleau-ontario-superior-court-judge

188 Brian Peckford, "Canada's Emergencies Act Inquiry (Commission)—It's Outrageous—Government Investigating Itself? And How!" Peckford42, September 6, 2022, accessed May 11, 2023, https://peckford42.wordpress.com/2022/09/06/canadas-emergencies-act-inquiry-commission-its-outrageous-government-investigating-itself-and-how/

Second, now that the hearings of the POEC are over, we're in a better place to provide plausible explanations for why Prime Minister Trudeau invoked the emergency powers. This action was taken even when the police didn't request them, there was no violence during the convoy protest, and CSIS informed him that there was no threat from the protest that would warrant triggering the *Emergencies Act*. The answer lies, in my view, in the fact that the convoy was an ideological threat to the prime minister and his government's narrative. The non-violence didn't matter, the pain suffered by the protestors and those they represented didn't matter, the nonsensical travel mandate didn't matter, and the lack of police and limited CSIS support didn't matter. What mattered was the ideological commitment of the prime minister and those in the Cathedral who demanded total compliance by everyone in Canadian society—including the truckers.

Mr. Trudeau's desire for ideological conformity is eerily like the 1920-30s Soviet Communist Party's demand that the country peasants comply to their dictates, even though it meant countrywide starvation. The communists couldn't have capitalism in the countryside, even though such capitalism provided food to Russian cities. The peasants had to be crushed. Dr. Stephen Kotkin, professor of History and International Affairs at Princeton University, has noted the Marxist-Leninist belief that the "underlying social relations eventually determine the political system."[189] Therefore, "capitalism in the countryside was a permanent threat to the existence of the regime because the underlying social relations threatened the regime at the top." The question for the communists was timing. Ultimately Stalin eradicated the peasant capitalist despite the human cost. The utopian goal removed the significance of human life.

For Prime Minister Trudeau and those in the Cathedral, the trucker "uprising" was a direct challenge to government itself. The non-believing truckers were labelled "violent" merely because they expressed opposition to the government narrative. Their opposition was taken as an existential threat to the regime's legitimacy. They had to be crushed. I suggest that, in

---

189 Hoover Institution, "Interview with Dr. Stephen Kotkin, "Why Does Joseph Stalin Matter?" YouTube, January 25, 2018, 46:19, https://youtu.be/jhi2icRXbHo?t=609.

Prof. Kotkin's words about Soviet Russia, "the underlying social relations" threatened "the regime at the top."

Third, it is now clear from the POEC hearings that the political culture surrounding Mr. Trudeau's inner circle did everything in its power and influence to see that Trudeau's desire to end the protest expeditiously was carried out. In other words, the prime minister's office, the Privy Council, members of the cabinet, CSIS, RCMP, and the government's legal advisers were engaged in an atmosphere of satisfying the prime minister's goals and objectives regarding the convoy.

It is standard procedure that those within a leader's governing team work together to solve the leader's conundrum. Of course, this assumes that the leader's every wish is in the best interest of the organization being led. However, it mustn't be forgotten that those who are close to the leader are in their positions because of their relationship with that leader. Therefore, what's in the best interest of the organization gets foggy when individuals consider their own interest (keeping their job of influence) by ensuring their leader's desires are fulfilled.

For example, at the time of Henry VIII, the "king's problem" of wanting a divorce was everyone's problem within his inner circle. They turned their energies to making sure that the king's problem was resolved. Issues of what was "legal" in fulfilling the desire required his advisors to make the appropriate legal arguments and strategies, all with the goal of reaching the final objective that satisfied the monarch. The law had to be "massaged" to fit the circumstance—that is, the whim of the leader. It's no different today, as is evident with the leadership of Justin Trudeau.

## The Pre-Cursor—The SNC-Lavalin Affair

Consider what happened with Prime Minister Justin Trudeau's inner circle during the SNC-Lavalin affair that saw two women cabinet ministers eventually kicked out of the Liberal caucus because they refused to acquiesce to Trudeau's views. It evinces the same principle of working on "the king's problem." When people get accustomed to having their every whim met by those closest to them, it becomes unbearable to have anyone push back.

Jody Wilson-Raybould was at the centre of the tempest. As the minister of Justice and the attorney general, she refused to interfere with the criminal prosecution of the Quebec company SNC-Lavalin, which her boss, Mr. Trudeau, demanded that she do. She refused to interfere with the arm's-length work of the public prosecutor because it would be against the principles of justice.

In her book, Wilson-Raybould, observes, "The story of the SNC-Lavalin affair ... is one of partisanship and power-seeking over principle. It is a story that highlights a lack of concern with the basic democratic norms that are the bedrock of our systems of government; selfishness and injured pride; and the perils of not being straight and simply speaking the truth to Canadians."[190]

What an indictment of her political boss—selfishness, injured pride, and not speaking the truth. It's an indictment that fits, in my view, with virtually every one of the scandals that has rocked the federal government since 2015. This is especially so with what happened when the prime minister overreached during the Trucker Freedom Convoy.

SNC-Lavalin had been involved in a bribery scheme with the Libyan government that led to the RCMP laying charges against the corporation and two of its subsidiaries. When Mr. Trudeau became prime minister, the company commenced an intense lobbying campaign designed to get the government to implement legislation creating a legal entity known as a "deferred prosecution agreement." This makes room for creative solutions to the criminal charges, basically allowing the criminally charged corporation to obtain a stay of its criminal proceedings. In other words, they wouldn't face a criminal trial, or more importantly risk a criminal conviction that would bar them from government contracts in Canada for a period of ten years under the Financial Administration Act.

In its 2018 budget "omnibus bill," the Trudeau government amended the Criminal Code to allow a deferred prosecution agreement. An "omnibus bill" often has many disparate items thrown into it. You might ask, "Why would the government put so many different items in a budget bill?" Simple answer: politics. It's a common tactic to put into important

---

190 Wilson-Raybould, 2021, 208.

legislation an item that government thinks it couldn't get passed if the item was in its own separate legislation. That would be an issue if the government was in a minority position in the House of Commons.

However, in 2018, the federal government was in the majority position in the House and didn't need to worry about its legislation coming into law. Therefore, it would appear the reason the Criminal Code changes were made in the budget bill was because it was meant to be "hidden" under the shadow of the budget. No doubt the government wanted to avoid the political heat for the inevitable claims it was favouring corporate criminals. There was little opposition.

Everything moved according to plan as the legislation was proclaimed into law. SNC-Lavalin and, no doubt, Mr. Trudeau thought there was little to stand in their way. However, Jody Wilson-Raybould, being both minister of Justice and Canada's attorney general, was "not for turning." She understood the gravity of the need for the independence of justice officials from political interference: "The independence of the Attorney General is so fundamental to the integrity and efficiency of the criminal justice system that it is constitutionally entrenched," said the Supreme Court of Canada. "The principle of independence requires that the Attorney General act independently of political pressures from government and sets the Crown's exercise of prosecutorial discretion beyond the reach of judicial review, subject only to the doctrine of abuse of process."[191]

The Court also noted that, "Prosecutorial discretion refers to the use of those powers that constitute the core of the Attorney General's office and which are protected from the influence of improper political and other vitiating factors by the principle of independence."[192]

From Wilson-Raybould's perspective, the entire SNC-Lavalin affair was "one of partisanship and power-seeking over principle."[193]

---

191 "Miazga v. Kvello Estate, 2009 SCC 51," CanLII, [2009] 3 SCR 339, at para. 46, accessed May 11, 2023, https://canlii.ca/t/26g27.
192 At para. 45.
193 Wilson-Raybould, 2021, 208.

Conflict of Interest and Ethics Commissioner Mario Dion investigated the affair and concluded[194] that the prime minister was in a conflict of interest by using his authority over Wilson-Raybould, trying to change her position on not interfering with the public prosecutions' refusal to enter negotiations with SNC-Lavalin for a "deferred prosecution agreement." However, Mr. Dion faced what has become a familiar pattern of stalling tactics by the government—refusing access to documents due to "cabinet confidentiality," all the while claiming they are open and transparent. This "doublespeak" is rampant.

It must be said that there are legitimate reasons why cabinet documents are not to be released to a public inquiry of government activities. Yet when we're talking about the malfeasance (that is, wrongdoing) of the highest office holder in the land, there must be allowances for an impartial arbiter to have access to all relevant documents. That was not given to Mr. Dion.

In this case, the Privy Council Office decided that it would not "expand the waiver" of confidentiality to allow Mr. Dion access to the material he'd requested. Notice that on the one hand the government said it would waive cabinet confidentiality to allow the investigation, but then on the other hand, when there were documents, the arbiter needed to carry out his review, the waiver could not be "expanded" for those documents! It's a cat-and-mouse game of saying "Go ahead" but then saying "No, not *that* one!"

"Because of the decisions to deny our Office further access to Cabinet confidences," said Dion, "witnesses were constrained in their ability to provide all evidence. I was, therefore, prevented from looking over the entire body of evidence to determine its relevance to my examination."[195]

Mr. Dion noted that when decisions are made that affect his jurisdiction, especially those limiting his ability to receive the evidence he needs to carry out his work, they should be transparent and made "democratically by Parliament" and not by the prime minister whom he is investigating!

---

194 "Trudeau II Report," Office of the Conflict of Interest and Ethics Commissioner, accessed May 11, 2023, https://ciec-ccie.parl.gc.ca/en/investigations-enquetes/Pages/TrudeauIIReport-RapportTrudeauII.aspx.
195 Ibid.

In Dion's view, if his office "is to remain truly independent and fulfill its purpose" then he "must have unfettered access to all information that could be relevant" to his investigation. Otherwise, he can't be sure that there is no conflict of interest in the decisions of "the most senior public office holders."

When Mr. Dion's report was made public, Mr. Trudeau responded in typical fashion: "I'm not going to apologize for standing up for Canadians' jobs because that's my job—to make sure that Canadians, communities and families across the country are supported, and that's what I will always do."[196] No remorse—nothing to see, and as it turned out, nothing politically to worry about. He used the same approach at the POEC, when he said that his job was to "protect Canadians" and that no one got hurt at the Trucker Freedom Convoy because of his decision to invoke the *Emergencies Act*. Whether he will get off politically at the next election is yet to be seen.

The Trudeau government plan of operation, when being investigated, is to give all the appearances of cooperating with the investigations but then pull back when the investigation gets too close to the target. That pullback is justified by "cabinet confidentiality," "state sovereignty," "national interest," and so on. In short, it's a cynical approach to governance, and it was no different at the Public Order Emergency Commission.

As Wilson-Raybould observed, "We may never know the entire backstory to the SNC-Lavalin affair, what people's full motivations or roles or relationships were."[197] She observes a fundamental problem with our system of government in how she was treated. It reveals "the worst and most dangerous aspects of how we are governed."[198] It's not enough to be vigilant and ensure we have the right law and institutions. There needs to be personal integrity more than "representative and partisan 'politics.'"

That integrity is based on "cultural, spiritual, or religious" moral foundations. For her it comes from the teachings of the "Big House" as

---

[196] Catharine Tunney, "Trudeau doubles down on not apologizing for SNC-Lavalin affair," CBC News, August 15, 2019, accessed May 11, 2023, https://www.cbc.ca/news/politics/philpott-snc-report-1.5247792.

[197] Jody Wilson-Raybould, *Indian in the Cabinet: Speaking Truth to Power* (Toronto: HarperCollins, 2021) 209

[198] Jody Wilson-Raybould, 210.

an Indigenous Canadian. This admission is key. I agree with Wilson-Raybould—personal integrity matters. You can have the best law and the best constitution, but if those who administer or interpret the law don't have the integrity to support the underlying spirit or principles of the law, then the law is meaningless. It can be read to mean whatever the office holder wants it to mean.

I am sympathetic to the argument that we need judges who don't make law through their own ideological interpretations. It's fundamentally unjust to interpret or administer the law in a way that is antithetical to the law's plain meaning and purpose. Yet that is increasingly happening in virtually all our public institutions. Unfortunately, there are very few Jody Wilson-Raybould's in our country. Most are willing to violate their consciences for the sake of career advancement.

Our Charter of Rights, our constitution, as well as our statutory or legislative law are meaningless if politicians hold them in contempt and interpret them based on whatever whim catches their fancy. Just by the nature of their official power, while serving in the executive branch of government, politicians can ignore the law in pursuit of their political aims. It takes time and money to hold wayward office holders to account by bringing them in judicial courts or in the courts of public opinion at the ballot box. By then their misapplication of the law will have already made the changes they wanted.

In other words, those politicians without integrity can severely damage average citizens, who are helpless in the face of such assaults on their legal rights. This is why we desperately need men and women of Wilson-Raybould's personal integrity on the judicial benches and in the parliamentary seats. The deep spiritual need in this country for such integrity is particularly acute.

After a fall 2018 meeting with the prime minister, who changed the subject of the meeting to the SNC-Lavalin request for a deferred prosecution agreement, Wilson-Raybould endured a four-month campaign to change her mind. During that time, eleven officials from the PMO, the Privy Council Office, and the Office of the Minister of Finance pressured her. Finally in December, the highest public servant, the Clerk of the Privy Council, Michael Wernick, called her. It was now getting serious.

She had the presence of mind to record the conversation. Not surprisingly, she was threatened when he said, "... it is not a good idea for the prime minister and his attorney general to be at loggerheads ..." and "I am worried about a collision then because he [the prime minister] is pretty firm about this ... I just saw him a few hours ago and this is really important to him."[199]

A few weeks later, she was no longer the minister of Justice and attorney-general of Canada.

Why did she take the stand she did? She answers:

> Simple. Because it was wrong and an affront to the rule of law and prosecutorial independence. And while they tried to pressure me, I did not feel pressured. I was simply doing my job of ensuring the law was followed, and trying to ensure the government did not engage in wrongdoing. [200]

When she was kicked out of the Liberal caucus along with her ally, Dr. Jane Philpot, the prime minister made the announcement surrounded by "a cowardly display of cheering Liberal MPs," and he didn't allow the MPs to have a vote on the expulsion, as required by the Reform Act. [201] That is again true to form. Why bother with following the law when it's inconvenient? A further indication of a lack of integrity in the pursuit of power.

## The Trudeau Way

Wilson-Raybould observed a Trudeau government pattern: access to the prime minister was controlled by his inner circle—at that time Gerry Butts and Katie Telford. That way he could maintain distance and deniability on sensitive files. With the SNC-Lavalin file as with others, "it was the PMO trying to be the government by controlling ministers and what they do."[202] Once the prime minister had made up his mind, it was up to his minions to ensure that his wish was carried out.

---

199 Wilson-Raybould, 2021, 212.
200 Ibid.
201 Ibid.
202 Ibid., 213.

We see this pattern repeated by the prime minister and his inner circle when dealing with the truckers. Trudeau, like Napoleon, uses the same battlefield strategy to win time after time. Like Napoleon at one time, Trudeau's winning streak has yet to be broken. However, there's no telling when a Wellington may come upon the field.

I call it "The Trudeau Way." It consists of the following: decide on a policy, enforce compliance, deny wrongdoing, hide evidence, remove opposition, and ultimately carry on without repercussions. I will address each of them.

**First,** decide on the public policy decision. His public policy decisions tend to be self-serving. The Machiavellian calculus is simple: "What must I do to stay in power?" It matters not what the issue is, whether it is the COVID-19 crisis, the SNC Lavalin Affair, the Chinese Communist Party election interference, or the now four conflict-of-interest violations—what matters is power.

**Second,** use the entire apparatus of the prime minister's inner circle to employ whatever means at their disposal to see that his wishes are fulfilled. Michael Wernick's phone call was but one example of the eleven attempts to seek Wilson-Raybould's compliance.

**Third,** obfuscate—or in other words, muddle about the issue using diction that is often incoherent—when confronted with malfeasance or wrongdoing, to the point that people are baffled as to what to believe. The prime minister's use of "inexactitudes" has become a familiar tactic in his storytelling. For example, at the opening of the SNC affair, he categorically denied pressuring Wilson-Raybould and famously said that *The Globe and Mail* story accusing him of interference was "false." What was false was his denial. As one reporter said upon Mr. Dion's Trudeau II Report, "The allegations in the *Globe* story were true, and the prime minister knew it."[203]

**Fourth,** claim to give open transparency when under investigation but deny it on the key points of access necessary to find out what exactly happened. Mr. Dion's frustration with the prime minister's refusal to waive all cabinet privilege was palpable when studying what happened.

---

[203] John Ibbitson, "Justin Trudeau and things that are not so," *The Globe and Mail*, August 16, 2019, accessed May 11, 2023, https://www.theglobeandmail.com/politics/article-justin-trudeau-and-things-that-are-not-so/.

**Fifth,** once the investigation is over, if not before, remove the noncompliant subordinates from office, since they're no longer helpful in carrying out the necessary goals of staying in power, and put in someone who will do the job without conscientious scruples. Not only was Jody Wilson-Raybould removed but so was Dr. Jane Philpot. In came Mr. David Lametti as the new minister of Justice and the attorney general. Mr. Trudeau seemed to have solved his problem. Although, like the one before him, once Lametti served his usefulness he was let go and replaced with Arif Virani, MP for Parkdale—High Park, who was Mr. Trudeau's trusted vice-chair of the Special Joint Committee on the Declaration of Emergency.[204]

**Sixth,** continue as if everything was properly carried out from the beginning, even when the decision maker (such as a judge or ethics commissioner) determines otherwise. Any lingering objections or criticisms are a "misunderstanding" as a result of the "misinformation" circling about.[205]

To date there have been no long-lasting political consequences to worry about—Mr. Trudeau continues to enjoy the powerful support of the Cathedral.

"Sovereign is he who decides on the exception."[206] It should be clear by now that the current sovereign of Canada is not King Charles III. The

---

204 On July 26, 2023, Mr. Lametti was booted from Mr. Trudeau's Cabinet. See, the Canadian Press, online: The Canadian Press, "Who is in and who is out of Prime Minister Justin Trudeau's cabinet," Jul 26, 2023, https://kitchener.citynews.ca/2023/07/26/canada-prime-minister-cabinet-shuffle/ This even though Lametti carried Mr. Trudeau's "water" a considerable distance from what Wilson-Raybould was prepared to do. Given what we know how Mr. Trudeau sought to control Wilson-Raybould it is reasonable to assume that Lametti's acts, while in office, were ordered from on high. Therefore, his removal cannot be seen as anything but the failure of the prime minister's policies and directives. Lametti's replacement, Arif Virani, MP for Parkdale—High Park, was Mr. Trudeau's trusted vice-chair of the Special Joint Committee on the Declaration of Emergency. https://www.ourcommons.ca/members/en/Arif-Virani(88910)

205 Ian Austen, "What Justin Trudeau Doesn't Regret in the SNC-Lavalin Affair," *The New York Times*, August 16, 2019, accessed May 11, 2023, https://www.nytimes.com/2019/05/17/world/canada/snc-lavalin-justin-trudeau-federal-election.html.

206 Carl Schmitt, *Political Theology* (Chicago: University of Chicago Press, 2005), 5.

monarchical figurehead exercises no ability to decide the exceptions in law on a whim. That role is being fully exercised by Prime Minister Trudeau. He is the one who decides what exceptions from the law are permissible and when and what decisions flow from those exceptions. We have come to a place in Canada when the office holder of prime minister is the sovereign *de facto*. *De facto* is the Latin term meaning "in fact" as opposed to "in law," which in Latin is *de jure*.

This is important to understand because, as Wilson-Raybould observed, "personal integrity matters." The personal moral beliefs and commitments of the office holder will have a direct impact on the efficacy of the law and government institutions in carrying out the work they were meant to do. A prime minister who understands his or her office as one of power, regardless of the law, will be a very different prime minister than the one who exercises caution to keep within the law. The first will see law as a hurdle to jump over to reach a goal in the quickest way possible, while the other will be mindful of the guardrail and follow the legal roads to get to the destination. One will be cynical toward the guardrails as mere conniving powerplays of "privileged" forebears whose "values" are no longer recognized as valid, while the other understands that the guardrails were established for good reason by those in the past who sought to make sense of life and the polity's duty to ensure human flourishing.

Personal integrity matters—it always has, and it always will.

## Prime Minister Justin Trudeau's POEC Testimony

It must be said that Prime Minister Trudeau's testimony at the POEC hearing on November 25, 2022, was, in my estimation, the most articulate presentation he has made since becoming prime minister. He was well prepared for the grand finale of six weeks of grueling and, at times, riveting testimony of some of the key players in the convoy protest.

However, his testimony gives us pause for concern. The same pattern he deployed with the SNC-Lavalin affair he used with the POEC and his involvement with the convoy.

## First, Decide on a Policy

He himself made the decision to invoke the *Emergencies Act* to get rid of the convoy protest. When it was obvious that the truckers weren't leaving after the first weekend, the longer they stayed and the weaker he looked, he demanded action to maintain power. The convoy was seen as an "embarrassment" to the government. Trudeau decided early on that there would be "non-starters" for parliamentary discussion when he spoke of the convoy to Candice Bergen, the interim Conservative Party leader.[207] He admitted that use of emergency powers came into "our minds" "from the very beginning."[208] Trudeau was not going to speak to the protestors because he "worried about setting a precedent that a blockade on Wellington Street can lead to changing public policy." He continued, stating that "using protests to demand changes to public policy is something that I think is worrisome."[209] Of course, he didn't have the same scruples with respect to the blockage of the nation's rail infrastructure two years earlier that demanded changes to public policy.[210] He wanted the convoy protest to end and end quickly, but he was frustrated with the coordination of the three levels of government in getting the police to remove the "occupation."[211] In his view, the "police of jurisdiction had lost control and wasn't able to control the situation."[212] Yet there is evidence in the POEC hearings that the police had established a plan to clear the streets but that the plan was not shared with the prime minister by RCMP Commissioner Brenda Lucki.[213]

---

207 POEC, Volume 31, 20.
208 Ibid., 42.
209 Ibid., 20.
210 John Paul Tasker, "Trudeau asks for patience as rail blockades continue, bars Scheer from leaders' meeting,"
CBC News, February 18, 2020, accessed May 11, 2023 https://www.cbc.ca/news/politics/trudeau-pipeline-protests-house-1.5466878.
211 POEC, Volume 31, 30.
212 Ibid., 36.
213 Ibid., 161. Ms. Rebecca Jones, on cross-examination, suggested that, "Commissioner Lucki didn't brief you [prime minister] and your Cabinet on the fact that there was a complete plan on the 13th [of February]." See POEC, Volume 23, 63, where Commissioner Lucki admits that she was satisfied with the police plan to clear Ottawa. Later on, while being questioned by

## Second, Enforce Compliance

The powerful office of the Canadian prime minister was used to ensure that the decision of the prime minister was implemented. As chair of the Incident Response Group (IRG),[214] a special committee of the PM's inner circle that come together to address national crises, his decisions are implemented. Around the table are representatives of the respective government agencies, cabinet ministers, the bureaucracy, RCMP, and CSIS. They "establish a plan" and "move forward on that."[215] But rest assured, the buck stops with the prime minister. Everyone is expected to carry out his wish—"making sure that everyone is on the same page."[216] This group continues to meet until "the incident is over."

The IRG met about the convoy on February 10, 12, and 13 before announcement of the invocation of the *Emergencies Act* on February 14. On February 10, Mr. Trudeau's question to the IRG was, "What would we do with the *Emergencies Act* if we brought it in that we can't otherwise do?"[217] On top of his mind was to compel the tow truck drivers to tow the trucks from the streets.[218] He also didn't want a "whack-a-mole" situation where the protesters are removed from Ottawa but reappear somewhere else or come back to Ottawa again. In weighing the options, they considered the ability to get legislation passed or write regulations, but in the

---

the Government of Canada lawyer Mr. Brian Gover, the prime minister said he was of the view that the plan Lucki referred to was a plan of engagement, not a plan to clear the area of the trucks. See at 186–187.

214 Incident Response Group (IRG), "Serves as a dedicated emergency committee in the event of a national crisis or during incidents elsewhere that have major implications for Canada. Responsible for coordinating a prompt federal response to an incident, and making fast, effective decisions to keep Canadians safe and secure, at home and abroad." See, https://pm.gc.ca/en/cabinet-committee-mandate-and-membership#incident-response

215 POEC, Volume 31, 40.

216 Ibid., 40.

217 Ibid., 44.

218 Ibid., 44–45. Under cross-examination by Rob Kettredge, Mr. Trudeau denied that the emergency declaration was justified by the need to get tow trucks. However, he subsequently admitted that "Yes, that was one of the barriers they were facing in being able to restore public order" (92). Another example of his "push and pull" during his testimony.

end, Trudeau decided the situation was getting out of control and the government had to act; therefore, *Emergencies Act* powers would get the job done quickly.[219]

The reality was not what Mr. Trudeau described in his testimony. Things were already settling down as the blockades were removed at the border crossings, and there was a deal between Ottawa and the truckers to remove the trucks from the residential areas. The government was aware of the deal and that things were moving in the right direction, but Mr. Trudeau ignored such developments. It would appear that his main issue wasn't so much about Canadians being in danger but that the convoy had no intention of leaving Ottawa until he talked with them. As he had no intention to do so, he wanted them out of Ottawa forthwith. And if that meant emergency powers, so be it.

## Third, Baffle with Inarticulate Nonsense

In his testimony to the POEC, the prime minister came across as articulate with reasoned justifications for his use of the emergency powers.

The argument, no doubt developed by the expansive legal team at his disposal, was that the *Emergencies Act* was a product of the 1980s that came from the *CSIS Act*, which was designed for wire taps for the security of Canada. However, according to Mr. Trudeau and his team, the *Emergencies Act* deals with "reasonable grounds that there are threats to the security of Canada."[220] The two Acts have two different purposes and contexts—says Trudeau and his team. That is true, but that doesn't make the *Emergencies Act* out of touch. I would argue that when read as a whole, the *Emergencies Act* is straightforward and not all that confusing. The prime minister and his team sought to make it confusing because they didn't want to be bound by it.

We must recognise that "reasonable grounds" in the *Emergencies Act* doesn't mean that there is to be a lower threshold of proving that the threat exists. Under cross-examination by Ms. Ewa Krajewska, Mr. Trudeau agreed that the *Emergencies Act* threshold cannot be any lower than that

---

219 POEC, Volume 31, 46-47.
220 Ibid., 49.

in the *CSIS Act*.[221] However, that's certainly what Trudeau implied, and it's the only way he can argue his point. Simply put, there is utter confusion in their approach. There is dissonance in their rationale that does not add up.

In my view, this argument is pure legal fiction crafted for political expediency. The government says it had a legal opinion supporting invocation of the Act, but as of the date of this writing, they haven't released it. Even the mainstream media are demanding its release.[222] That says something. My guess is it will never be released—at least not as long as Mr. Trudeau remains prime minister.

This all represents a misreading of the *Emergencies Act*. Consider that the Act is based on the proposition that there is a threat that existing law can't deal with—that is, a national emergency that challenges the very sovereignty of the country. A peaceful protest in Ottawa did not threaten Canada's existence. No matter how well sounding the prime minister was at the hearing, he was seeking to baffle the public with a huge dose of legal ruminations that sought to justify what was unjustifiable. It was simply attempting to make a square peg fit a round hole. The fact that Mr. Rouleau opined that all is well is simply unconscionable.

What was terribly wrong in this approach was the complete lack of respect for the law over a "political necessity" seen to be of more importance than staying within the legal guardrails.

"[T]he context and the purpose is very different," Mr. Trudeau continues, with his rehearsed lines for his moment upon the public stage. "The people doing the deciding in the case of the CSIS Act ... it's CSIS itself that decides that [the definition of emergency] is met. There's checks and balances afterwards. But for the purpose of the declaration of a public order emergency, it's the ... cabinet, and the prime minister making that determination."[223]

---

221 Ibid., 89–90.
222 The Editorial Board, "Ottawa says it has a legal opinion justifying the use of the Emergencies Act. So make it public," *The Globe and Mail*, December 10, 2022, accessed May 11, 2023, https://www.theglobeandmail.com/opinion/editorials/article-ottawa-says-it-has-a-legal-opinion-justifying-the-use-of-the/.
223 POEC, Volume 31, 49.

Under cross-examination of Mr. Sujit Choudhry, Mr. Trudeau said that the CSIS report, indicating that the convoy did not meet the threshold of a national emergency under the *CSIS Act*, was given to the full cabinet, but that the context for the convoy was different for a public order emergency. According to Trudeau, "the issue was ... the threat of serious violence threshold met in the context of a Public Order Emergency ..."[224]

Therefore, using the logic of the prime minister, he and his cabinet made a political decision for declaring a public emergency under the *Emergencies Act*. Think of the implications of that! The law is to be ignored if there's sufficient political reason to use the immense power of the state to deal with the political reality on the ground. This is beyond anything we have seen in the history of this country.

This interpretation of the *Emergencies Act* will see one protest as a national emergency but another as harmless, depending on the political winds that blow across the country. Prime Minister Trudeau stated that he didn't see any problem with Black Lives Matter protests—no national emergency there—nor was there any national emergency with the country's railway shutting down for weeks. But for the convoy in Ottawa with at least one lane always open for emergencies—that was a national emergency!

If the Supreme Court of Canada accepts this watered down, politically motivated approach to the *Emergencies Act*, then we're in for serious political unrest. Unfortunately, I don't hold out too much hope for the SCC to hold Mr. Trudeau in check. I say that with much regret. In recent years, the SCC has continued to take the side of government actors when assessing whether the Charter has been violated. The precedent of the Trinity Western University Law School cases is the first to come to mind. There, the SCC said, in effect, that if the government actor turns their mind to Charter rights, even though they violate those rights, in the public interest or by claiming "Charter values," then that is okay.[225] The Charter rights are viewed through the "Charter values" lens. The problem, of course, is that

---

224 Ibid., 104.
225 That is the net effect of the Supreme Court of Canada's decision in Law Society of British Columbia v. Trinity Western University, 2018 SCC 32 (CanLII), [2018] 2 SCR 293, <https://canlii.ca/t/hsjpr>

"Charter values" are what the judges say they are—or what the government actor says they are.

I predict—always a dangerous proposition—that the SCC will favour Trudeau's re-interpretation of the *Emergencies Act*. One big clue, of course, is Chief Justice Wagner's statements against the truckers, as I discuss in this book. Another is the tendency to decide with the Trudeau government, as they did with the Carbon Tax decision, even though it reinterpreted the Constitution. The leaning of the court is to support the government where possible, just as it was for Justice Rouleau at the POEC.

Even if the court agrees with the government's use of the *Emergencies Act* against the truckers, it will categorically be the wrong decision. This is a bold position for me to take; however, my reasoning is that it would represent the total capitulation of statutory interpretation as it has been understood to date in order to support a political, not a legal, decision. If, on the other hand, the SCC were to rule against the government, it would be a great victory for Canadians.

In reviewing the *Emergencies Act*, according to Mr. Trudeau, his counsellors centred on the definition of "threats to the security of Canada" in the *CSIS Act*[226] in section 2, subsection (c) that references violence against persons of property for political or ideological objectives. In his view and the view of the IRG, the "threshold" of "reasonable grounds" of threats to Canada's security was met.

Such reasoning disregards the plain reading of the *Emergencies Act* section 3, which requires not only (a) a serious endangerment of the life, health and safety of Canadians that exceeds the capacity or authority of a province to deal with; (b) "seriously threatens" Canadian sovereignty,

---

[226] *Canadian Security Intelligence Service Act* (R.S.C., 1985, c. C-23), s. 2 threats to the security of Canada means ... (c) activities within or relating to Canada directed toward or in support of the threat or use of acts of serious violence against persons or property for the purpose of achieving a political, religious or ideological objective within Canada or a foreign state, and ... in "*Canadian Security Intelligence Service Act*," Justice Laws website, accessed May 11, 2023, https://laws-lois.justice.gc.ca/eng/acts/C-23/page-1.html#h-76161.

security, and territorial integrity; AND there is no other law of Canada to deal with the situation.[227]

We can't lose sight of the fact that with such flimsy legal reasoning, the government and its "inputs" from the RCMP, CSIS, and the Clerk of the Privy Council were able to come to their own conclusions that indeed the "reasonable grounds" threshold was met, and they could advise the prime minister what he already wanted to hear—declare a Public Order Emergency and invoke the *Emergencies Act* accordingly.

Throughout the POEC hearings, not one piece of evidence of serious violence from the protesters that would reach the level required under the *Emergencies Act* was presented. Not one. The only blood spilled, or windows smashed, came from the police enforcing removal of the protesters. Yet the prime minister said there was "weaponization of vehicles."[228] In Ottawa? No, in Coutts! Yet the Coutts protest was over when he invoked the Act!

Trucks in Ottawa, he said, were used as "potential weapons ... with their presence and unknown interiors." Not one gun, not one weapon was found in any truck interior in Ottawa! Yet that was the "serious violence" that no other law could deal with, requiring the Act to be invoked?

---

[227] Emergencies Act (R.S.C., 1985, c. 22 (4th Supp.)), s. 3, in *"Emergencies Act,"* Justice Laws website, accessed May 11, 2023, https://laws-lois.justice.gc.ca/eng/acts/e-4.5/FullText.html.
[228] POEC, Volume 31, 51.

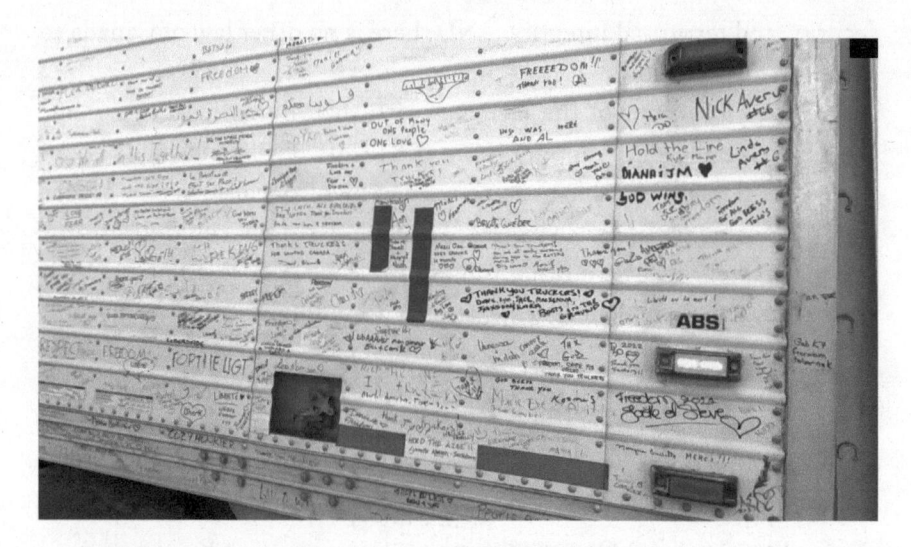

*Rather Than Used As Weapons Trucks Sent A Peaceful Message Of Protest*

Then he said that children were used "as human shields deliberately"![229] As I walked the streets in Ottawa during the protest, I saw many children with their parents. Others were playing street hockey. If Ottawa was a war zone of some sort, then I could see the point of raising the children's presence as a cause of concern.

Then there were claims of "swarming of police" and fears of "lone wolf actors"—all mere speculations of a prime minister who was out to justify the unjustifiable. Where was the violence? There was none. At least not "violence" as rightly understood. The prime minister's definition would include, "unacceptable views."

It is suspicious to say the least. Is it possible that the prime minister's inner circle was called upon to devise a plan and rationale to make the Public Order Emergency palatable to the Canadian public? You be the judge. I have seen the evidence, and it is already clear.

## Fourth, Hide Evidence

Mr. Trudeau felt the police weren't working fast enough in getting the convoy out of Ottawa. "We kept hearing there was a plan," he said. On

---

229 Ibid., 52.

February 13, Ottawa Police Services had a plan, but according to Mr. Trudeau, it "wasn't a plan at all."[230] Under cross-examination by Mr. Sujit Choudhry, Mr. Trudeau was shown that the plan he referred to was in fact redacted to the point that no one could read the plan. Mr. Choudhry then asked Mr. Trudeau to remove the redactions. At that point, Mr. Brian Gover, a government of Canada lawyer, objected, saying it put "the prime minister in an odious position."[231] Unlike Mr. Dion, Commissioner Rouleau agreed that the question was unfair because it would reveal officers from the OPS and OPP and police strategy. That is certainly debatable.

However, the criticism of appearing to be open but not overtly stands clearly in view. Mr. David Lametti, who was still holding the offices after Jody Wilson-Raybould, continuously denied being able to release his department's legal opinion on the emergency declaration,[232] and Mr. Trudeau's counsel continued that position in cross-examination.[233]

## Fifth, Remove Opposition

In the convoy context, no government of Canada official was let go. However, it's noteworthy that Ottawa Police Chief Peter Sloly resigned immediately after the emergency declaration and had his own legal counsel at the POEC hearings to protect his interests. Mr. Trudeau wasn't pleased with the lack of police efficiency in removing the convoy from Ottawa in a timely manner. It wasn't at all surprising to see other police personnel under the prime minister's control on the unemployment line. Brenda Lucki, RCMP commissioner, resigned just before the release of Mr. Rouleau's report.

---

230 Ibid., 54.
231 Ibid., 103–104.
232 POEC, Volume 29, 1–179. https://publicorderemergencycommission.ca/files/documents/Transcripts/POEC-Public-Hearings-Volume-29-November-23-2022.pdf
233 POEC, Volume 31, 107–108. https://publicorderemergencycommission.ca/files/documents/Transcripts/POEC-Public-Hearings-Volume-31-November-25-2022.pdf

## Sixth, Deny All Wrongdoing

The prime minister, true to form, didn't see that he'd done anything wrong. His testimony confirmed his "comfort" that "the system is working as it should," since civil liberty groups are being given the opportunity to oppose his actions. And he noted, "we were able to solve the situation" with invocation of the powers. "There was no loss of life. There was no, you know, serious violence. That we were able to get neighbourhoods back under control, border services opened, and there hasn't been a recurrence of these kinds of illegal occupations since then."

All is well in Canada as a result. Interestingly, he admitted that it was not "the only thing that could have done it, but it did do it." And it is the fact that everything turned out well "that colours the conversations we're having now." And then characteristically he proclaimed, "I am absolutely, absolutely serene and confident that I made the right choice in agreeing with the invocation."[234]

It's worth noting that he "agreed" with the invocation, implying that his inner circle, CSIS, RCMP, Public Service, all recommended that it was the appropriate approach. He intimated that it was from them not him that was behind the decision.

Trudeau refused to take any responsibility for his rhetoric and policies that caused the protest to begin with. Lawyer Eva Chipiuk, counsel for Freedom Corporation, in cross-examination, read several personal accounts of people who suffered from the government policies during the pandemic. One account read, "I am not asking for help; I am begging you to please listen. Hear my heart, feel my pain ..."[235]

"Mr. Prime Minister, you have now heard the statements from some of the many concerned Canadians who felt compelled to support the protesters," Eva said as she faced Mr. Trudeau. "Do you now understand the reason so many Canadians came to Ottawa with such resolve in the midst of a harsh, cold Canadian winter because of the harms caused by your government COVID mandates and they wanted to be heard?"[236]

---

234 Ibid., 68–69.
235 Ibid., 134.
236 Ibid., 135.

Mr. Trudeau responded that he "was moved" and "saw the depth of hurt and anxiety," but his job was to keep Canadians safe, and he did that by relying on the public health officials. He listened to the "experts and science." With eighty per cent of Canadians vaccinated, Canada had fewer deaths, he claimed.[237]

Ms. Chipiuk then went for the core concern as she referenced his comments that the unvaccinated were racists and misogynists, and his officials called the protesters terrorists.[238] She asked if he'd agree that one of his most important roles as prime minister "is to unite Canadians and not divide them by engaging in name-calling?"[239] To which he replied, "I did not call people who were unvaccinated names. I highlighted, there is a difference between people who are hesitant to get vaccinated for any range of reasons, and people who deliberately spread misinformation that puts at risk the life and health of their fellow Canadians."[240]

Of course, a simple review of the transcript[241] of his infamous denunciation of the unvaccinated would clearly establish that his testimony, under his affirmation to speak the truth at the POEC, is an "inexactitude," as Churchill would say. His response was what he would give during Question Period in the House of Commons. Unfortunately, even before the POEC Commissioner it wasn't enough for Mr. Trudeau to admit to what he had said about the unvaccinated. The denunciation of the unvaccinated he gave to the Quebec media made no mention of "those people"

---

237 Ibid., 135–136.
238 Ibid., 136.
239 Ibid., 136–137.
240 POEC, Volume 31, p. 137.
241 Noovo TV program La Semaine des 4 Julie. "Mr. Trudeau arrives," Facebook, September 16, 2021, https://www.facebook.com/watch/?v=965725654005285. Mr. Trudeau stated:
"Yes, we will get out of this pandemic by vaccination. We all know people who are a little bit hesitant. We will continue to try and convince them, but there are also people who are fiercely against vaccination. They are extremists who don't believe in science, they're often misogynists, also often racists. It's a small group that muscles in, and we have to make a choice in terms of leaders, in terms of the country. Do we tolerate these people? Or do we say, hey, most of the Quebecois people—80%—are vaccinated. We want to come back to things we like doing."

spreading "misinformation," as he now claims. Further, the unvaccinated did not put Canadians at risk. Not one iota of evidence exists to give that claim any legitimacy.

Yet he continues to maintain his course, and he does so with such conviction that it is, no doubt, mesmerizing to any who would want nothing more than to believe every word he says. Remember former Liberal MP and cabinet minister Catherine McKenna's assessment that "If you actually say it louder, we've learned in the House of Commons, if you repeat it, if you say it louder, if that is your talking point, people will totally believe it."[242]

## Consequences Are Taking Shape

For a time, it appeared that there were no long-lasting political consequences for Mr. Trudeau to worry about for invoking the *Emergencies Act*. He appeared to be "Canada's Teflon Prime Minister," no matter what the scandal nothing stuck to him. Certainly, the powerful support of the Cathedral and a sizable portion of the Canadian public was behind him.[243] After his testimony to the POEC, some 48% of Canadians supported the use of the *Emergencies Act*, with 18% saying they "somewhat" support.[244] That's an incredible amount of support for an unjustified use of the strongest powers granted government in Canadian legislation.

Prime Minister Justin Trudeau clearly had seasons of enormous popular support—with almost popstar celebrity status for a short season in his early tenure. His ability to obfuscate, cajole, and yet provide a

---

[242] Lorrie Goldstein, "Screeched-in McKenna commits a classic political gaffe," *Toronto Sun*, May 27, 2019, accessed May 11, 2023, https://torontosun.com/opinion/columnists/goldstein-screeched-in-mckenna-commits-a-classic-political-gaffe.

[243] According to a Nanos poll, 46% prefer Trudeau over Poilievre (at 30%): Nik Nanos, "Data Dive with Nik Nanos: Canada has joined the club of angry, polarized countries," *The Globe and Mail*, October 15, 2022, accessed May 11, 2023, https://www.theglobeandmail.com/opinion/article-data-dive-with-nik-nanos-canada-has-joined-the-club-of-angry-polarized/.

[244] Tom Yun, "Most Canadians back invocation of Emergencies Act during 'Freedom Convoy' protests: Nanos," CTV News, December 5, 2022, accessed May 11, 2023, https://www.ctvnews.ca/politics/most-canadians-back-invocation-of-emergencies-act-during-freedom-convoy-protests-nanos-1.6177341.

winsome presence while carrying out the most dreadful policies that have damaged so many people is remarkable. Not even his horrendous spending was enough to dent his electability, despite it leading to an increase of the national debt that eclipses the combined national debt of all previous prime ministers before him. Even former Conservative Prime Minister Brian Mulroney referred to Justin Trudeau as a Biblical visionary figure who will take Canada from "success to success."[245]

Remarkably, not even the May 2023 announcement from the auditor general that the government mismanaged at least $27.4 billion[246] by improperly paying out COVID-19 benefits seemed not to cause much political damage. One could be tempted to think that "it is 2023, after all—things are different now."

I don't think so. As with a wild ride in the stock market – just when you think the prices will only go higher then suddenly the bottom falls out. So, it is with the political capital markets. Every so called politically infallible leader becomes fallible at some point.

---

245 Former Prime Minister "Brian Mulroney offers effusive praise for 'historic' leadership of Justin Trudeau," as noted in Tristin Hopper's write up in the National Post, https://nationalpost.com/opinion/first-reading-brian-mulroney-offers-effusive-praise-for-historic-leadership-of-justin-trudeau (accessed June 22, 2023). Mulroney dismissed all the scandals Trudeau faced as 'trash' and 'rumours' and then gave a stirring analogy of Justin Trudeau as a Biblical visionary figure,
"It's said in the Old Testament that young men have visions and old men dream dreams. Well, great Nations like Canada need a combination of both - visions and great dreams. The object of this conference is to remind us all of the magnificence of Canada and what we can achieve together if we remember the vision and dreams of our forefathers who built this country and now count on us to carry it forward from generation to generation, from success to success from one century to the next. That's what we're here for and that with the prime minister's assistance that is what we're going to do." PM Trudeau delivers remarks to Atlantic Economic Forum in Antigonish, N.S.—June 19, 2023, CPAC at https://youtu.be/HzPBY5KvXYo?t=1610, 26:50-27:37

246 Bill Curry, "Billions in ineligible COVID-19 benefits at risk of going uncollected: Auditor-General report warns," *The Globe and Mail*, December 6, 2022, accessed May 11, 2023, https://www.theglobeandmail.com/politics/article-covid-benefits-auditor-general-report/.

Perhaps, and this is mere conjecture, the secret to Mr. Trudeau's success for so long may have been due to his ability to give most Canadians a sense of security that he is indeed "keeping Canadians safe." His COVID-19 policies hurt the unvaccinated, but they are the minority. They can be forced to pay the price for the "greater good," no matter how "good" or "not good" that turned out to be. Further, and this is key, with a media apparatus supporting him, he had little to fear.

However, if the majority had their bank accounts frozen, then one would suspect that Mr. Trudeau's days as prime minister would be severely limited. Limiting the pain to the vilified minority is a safe bet to remain in power. It's simple, brutal, yet effective, power politics of scapegoating.

All one must do is wait for an incompetent policy that spreads the pain to the wider public and then suddenly it is a whole different political game. The recent Carbon Tax debacle has the makings of a quick rundown of political fortune. You will remember that the Liberal Party won big in the Atlantic provinces in the last number of elections. However, when the Carbon Tax took effect on the heating oil in July 2023, suddenly everyone in those provinces felt the pain. So much so that Trudeau's support plummeted. To rectify the problem Trudeau 'carved out' a special exception for heating oil. Another political ploy to add to his growing list. However, his political strategy meant that everyone else (save for the special provisions for Quebec) still had to pay the Carbon Tax on their heating fuels even though natural gas has a very low 'climate change effect.'

Now everyone is viewed a victim. More victims lead to more political pain. If only Carbon Taxes could be limited to a minority, such as was the scapegoating of the unvaccinated, there wouldn't be such a problem for the government and the majority snug in their comfort would care less at the plight of the minority.

The truckers revealed that what they suffered at the hands of Mr. Trudeau's draconian policy could easily be turned on another group tomorrow. While a huge proportion of the Canadian public has, until recently, been willing to give Mr. Trudeau the benefit of the doubt, that benefit dissipates as soon as personal fear over one's financial security rises because of extreme government measures like we saw in February 2022. Such as the current Carbon Tax firestorm which is but an example.

Canadians must learn not to be deferential to government—no matter the political stripe. Even is this so when we agree with the government. Our survival depends on an informed and vigilant electorate—the truckers showed us how. Gone is the naivete of Canadians with respect to this Liberal government. The truckers' protest showed us to what lengths the current regime can go if its ideological commitments are challenged. That can never be forgotten. However, it is more than that. It is government in general.

It is becoming increasingly evident that the current Liberal government is on its last legs. Indeed, if you take the time to review the data at https://338canada.com/ you will discover that since the Freedom Convoy 2022 the Liberal government has been consistently falling out of favour with the public. At the time of this writing, Mr. Trudeau and his government is in a freefall. But, just as with the stock market nothing is a forever thing – including the government's current woes. However, it is fair to say that the trajectory suggests that, barring no surprises, Mr. Poilievre will be our next prime minister. That for many will be a good day. A very good day.

The lesson from the Truckers Convoy is do not ever, ever, let your guard down. Every political power is subject to hubris and incompetence. Furthermore, the modern state is more than the political leaders. We are saddled with a very powerful public service that has been well entrenched in the thinking of the Cathedral. The managerial state, the power of the bureaucracy must not be overlooked no matter which party is in control over Parliament. Citizens must never relax thinking that government is always their best friend. Far from it. Be constantly on the watch. We have seen what powerful bureaucracies can do as well as political leaders.

"The condition upon which God hath given liberty to man is eternal vigilance, which condition if he break, servitude is at once the consequences of his crime and the punishment of his guilt."[247]

---

247 John Philpot Curran, "Elections of Lord Mayor of Dublin," speech before the Privy Council, July 10, 1790. *The Speeches of the Right Honourable John Philpot Curran*, ed. Thomas Davis, pp. 94-95 (1847).

## 210°CELSIUS

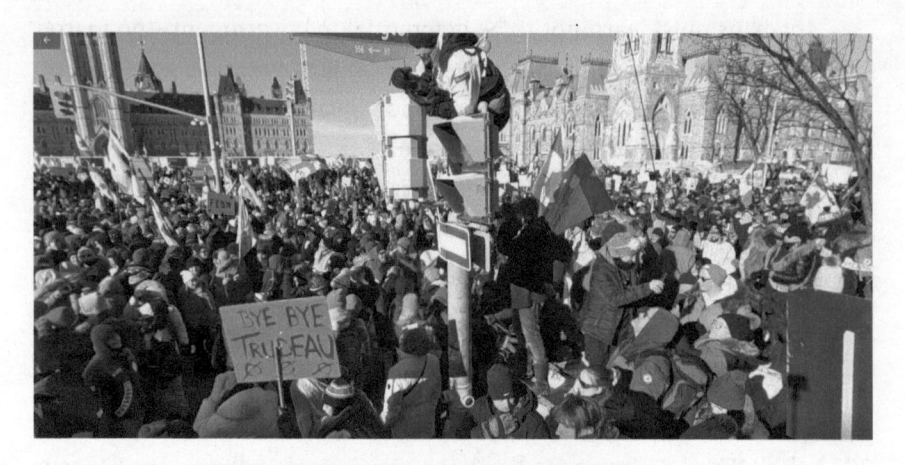

*Canadians Are No Longer Deferential*

# 6. Exposed the Inhumanity of the Administrative State

THE TRUCKERS SPOKE out loud what many of us were thinking: There is something terribly amiss when government agencies, in carrying out the edicts of their political leaders, do so in such a callous manner that affronts basic human dignity.

If we step back and think about what we just went through over the three years of the COVID-19 pandemic, we must give our heads a shake. Can it be real? We allowed our bureaucracy to follow the evil surmising of corrupted politicians to direct employment policy affecting tens of thousands of public servants and employees of government-controlled and/or regulated agencies.

Across Canada, the federal bureaucracy purged the unvaccinated from its ranks. People lost their jobs, their means of earning a living to support their family, because of an ill-conceived rule that their private health decisions could no longer be private and must be disclosed before their entire colleague complement. Every employee was now entitled to know whether their fellow worker in the next cubicle was vaccinated. And, if unvaccinated, it was the new employment culture to shun, ridicule, harass, and ultimately fire those non-compliant types. Their private health decisions were no longer their own to make.

Could there have been a more evil statement to come from many government, health, education, and media circles than that the pandemic was a "pandemic of the unvaccinated"? Think about what that suggested:

- The unvaccinated are causing the death of fellow citizens because of their unvaccinated status.

- The unvaccinated have no human rights but can be discriminated against because of their health status.
- The unvaccinated can no longer have access to government programs such as unemployment insurance because it was "their decision" that led to them to lose their jobs.
- The unvaccinated have rightly lost their houses and property for a "willing" failure to keep their employment.
- The unvaccinated cannot participate in community events.
- The unvaccinated are fair game to be ridiculed by the media and government so that they are now "others" and pariahs to be shunned.

The truckers protesting on Ottawa's streets were literally left in the freezing cold by a government bureaucracy that had lost all heart. The government continued to pay its vaccinated employees, including providing other perks and benefits such as the home office tax break, so these same employees had no incentive to even listen to the concerns of their colleagues who were cut off from unemployment benefits after being fired for not being vaccinated.

Just consider the language of this one bureaucrat who dismissed a nurse whose only misdemeanour was not allowing her employer to force her to get the COVID-19 vaccine, which she felt was akin to experimenting with her health:

> On December 16, 2021, you were provided with a letter advising that you were insubordinate and willfully refusing to comply with the City's COVID-19 Vaccination Policy and that your employment with the City of Toronto would be terminated for cause unless you achieved compliance with the Policy by providing proof of full vaccination to your manager. In the intervening time, you were suspended without pay to provide you with an opportunity to comply with the Policy.
>
> As of January 3, 2022, you were still not in compliance with the City's COVID-19 Vaccination Policy and, as such,

> you have not remedied your insubordination and willful disobedience. Therefore, this letter confirms your termination for just cause effective January 3, 2022.

Notice the language: "*you* have not remedied your insubordination and willful disobedience." Since when have we as a society said that vaccination was necessary for employment? Has this ever been done? Some will say, "But this was a health professional. Surely the employers in the health profession can refuse employment to those who aren't vaccinated. Besides, think of the threat to others!"

First, I'm not aware of any time in Canadian history when vaccinations were a requirement for any health professional. To be certain, I asked a physician friend of mine, and he confirmed my intuition. He said it has never been required—not even a flu vaccine! Indeed, arbitrators ruled in favour of medical freedom for health professionals prior to COVID-19.[248]

Second, even if there were any such requirement, such as in an educational institution, there have always been exemptions for health, conscience, or religious reasons.

Consent once "was a thing." A phrase I hear my children say. Remember when nurses and physicians use to ask, "Do you consent?" before they administered the medication? The pushback during the pandemic—as so often put by the government—well it is up to you—you have a choice! For those who are relying on their jobs to care for their families there is little choice. It is coercion wrapped in the nomenclature of "choice."

Third, there is no evidence that unvaccinated healthcare providers have ever caused any danger to patients. What did cause concern was whether the health professional (vaccinated or unvaccinated) was ill and contagious. And any health professional worth their salt would know to stay home if showing symptoms of a contagion.

---

248 Jennifer Brown, "ONA wins second arbitration against hospitals on 'vaccinate or mask' policy:
For a second time, an arbitrator has ruled in favour of the Ontario Nurses' Association, ordering a major hospital group in Toronto to rescind its 'vaccinate or mask policy.'" Canadian Lawyer, September 13, 2018, https://www.canadianlawyermag.com/practice-areas/privacy-and-data/ona-wins-second-arbitration-against-hospitals-on-vaccinate-or-mask-policy/275455

So, we must ask, "Why was the vaccine mandatory for all government employees and those working in government regulated agencies?"

There is only one answer: politics.

The truckers' common sense recognized that government bureaucrats had no scientific or moral foundation to demand vaccinations. Working long hours day after day, isolated in their semi-trucks, truckers did not pose a contagion risk. For one thing, it was physically near impossible. For another, it was scientifically impossible when they were not contagious. It simply made no sense. Besides, as already noted by far the majority of the truckers were vaccinated—more than the general population.

Yet the administrative state was intent on carrying out whatever COVID-19 policy the public health authorities and their legal teams came up with at the behest of politicians. Just as we noted above, Mr. Trudeau had no scientific basis for the vaccine mandates.

Bureaucrats, being like all the rest of us who simply wanted to keep our jobs during this crisis, faithfully followed the politically inspired vaccine mandate without any concern about how their decisions were going to affect the persons who would lose their jobs. It didn't matter to the bureaucrats. It was more of a paper shuffle. The people represented by that mountain of paper were none of their concern. Getting the job done so that they could carry on with their regular routine was what mattered most.

The dehumanizing effect of the COVID policies implemented by the bureaucrats will, I hope, be systematically studied by curious psychologists in the coming years. What is eerie about our two-plus years of experience is that not only have the bureaucrats been dehumanized by carrying out politically motivated policies, but our entire society has been dehumanized. Our entire society found itself wrapped into a time-warped and dehumanizing cycle that has brutalized thousands of families across this country.

As Tamara Lich observed, "They encouraged us to be suspicious of one another, with snitch lines, and taught us to call each other murderers, and to scapegoat each other. They had tried to turn Canada into an ugly, angry, unforgiving and untrusting nation. They hadn't just dehumanized the unvaccinated. They had dehumanized us all."[249]

Daniel Freiheit, an employment lawyer,[250] notes that if employers had treated their unvaccinated employees with respect and offered them funds to assist in their transition to a new job or provided help with training, it would have been a very different situation, with none of the conflict that was created: "Not only are we going to treat you like crap and fire you without notice we are going to consider it as wilful misconduct for not getting vaccinated. 'Wilful misconduct?' Have you lost your mind? Call it many things, it is not misconduct, my friend!"[251]

Unfortunately, too many people don't care. As long as their own salaries continued to be deposited in the bank pay period after pay period, it mattered not what their cubicle colleague suffered because of their conscientious decision not to receive the vaccine. Nor did it matter that the "science" of the "vaccine" was constantly changing, all while the adverse reactions of many receiving the vaccine were ignored.

Further, it mattered not to the bureaucrats that their respective places of employment were letting go of top-notch workers. Who cares if the office or department is hampered because those conscientious vaccine objectors, with long years of work and life experience, leave huge holes in the operations? The policy was followed. Those non-compliant insubordinates were let go—"as they should be"—for their failure to abide by the COVID policy. At some point an economist will review the loss of productivity of the various government departments, government agencies and other compliant employers of the government COVID policy. What have

---

[249] Marnie Cathcart, "'Hold the Line': Tamara Lich Talks About Her New Book on Freedom Convoy," The *Epoch Times*, April 29, 2023, https://www.theepochtimes.com/hold-the-line-tamara-lich-talks-about-her-new-book-on-freedom-convoy-looks-back-at-protest_5226478.html

[250] Lion Law, accessed May 11, 2023, https://lionlaw.ca/.

[251] "Freedom Feature: Holding Government Accountable," First Freedoms Foundation, accessed May 11, 2023, https://firstfreedoms.ca/holding-government-accountable/.

we lost by going through this totally unnecessary exercise of societally destructive behaviour?[252]

It would have been funny if it weren't tragic when Transport Minister Omar Alghabra opined that the massive airport delays throughout the country were due to "out-of-practice travellers" as they got back into the routine of security measures at the airports.[253] I wonder, could it be that the massive purging of the ranks at the airport were somehow partly to blame for the troubles? What about the other government department breakdowns, such as at the passport office? Or the processing of immigrant applications? Could they not be related to the COVID purging?

Or what about the fact that Canada has, for the first time in eight years, decided that it can't provide any support to NATO fleets in Europe because our military is understaffed and underequipped? But the military is going to continue to make an example of the brave and persistent Warrant Officer James Topp,[254] who will be court martialed for his decision to wear a military uniform while standing against the vaccine mandate.

Some estimates are that the country has lost a billion dollars "in training costs because of vaccine-related discharges"[255]in the military. Even though the military is ending its vaccine mandate, hundreds of members will be let go because they've already gone through the COVID review process. The military bureaucrats were efficient in carrying out the political mandates.

---

252 For a great discussion of the economics of this see, "The Great Covid Panic—Freedom Feature Interview with Authors Paul Frijters, Gigi Foster and Michael Baker," First Freedoms Foundation, accessed May 11, 2023,https://firstfreedoms.ca/the-great-covid-panic-freedom-feature-with-book-authors/

253 Staff, The Canadian Press, "Rusty travellers, not staffing, behind delays at Canada's airports: transport minister," *Global News*, May 11, 2022, accessed May11,2023,https://globalnews.ca/news/8827316/travellers-flight-volumes-airport-delays-alghabra/.

254 His website www.canadamarches.ca is no longer operational but you may see the archive here: https://web.archive.org/web/20220629155240/https://canadamarches.ca/ accessed June 22, 2023.

255 Andrew Duffy, "Canadian military poised to end vaccine mandate," July 21, 2022, *Ottawa Citizen*, accessed May 11, 2023, https://ottawacitizen.com/news/local-news/canadian-military-poised-to-end-vaccine-mandate.

It matters not that we as a country are worse off for the purging of our government, agencies, and military of the vaccine hesitant. What matters most, for these bureaucrats, is that the process was followed.

We can expect that the government will never blame their increased inefficiencies on their disastrous COVID vaccine mandates. No, the problem will be our fault. The citizens are to blame, because our expectations are too high from our pre-COVID memories, when the processing of our passports took only two weeks, or our hospital lineups were undesirable but still within the realm of expected minimums, or we had a functioning military. We must forget what once was and never, ever blame the outrageous public policy of COVID-19 mandates.

Professor Bruce Pardy observes, "The challenge I think is going to be this: Is this just the end of the COVID regime or is this the end of the ideas that led us to this kind of problem? Are we going to have the guts to say, 'No, no, no, at the heart of this problem were a set of bad ideas and one of those ideas is that there are experts within the state whose job it is to direct us in our lives?' That's the idea that has to be buried."[256]

The administrative state has become the all-powerful Leviathan that Thomas Hobbes described.[257] Security was more important to Hobbes than individual freedom. Hobbes saw the monarchy as the ultimate sovereign, but the COVID experience gave us a foretaste of what life under bureaucratic control looks like. Pardy notes, "We have moved away from the rule of law back towards rule by fiat. Control resides not in a monarch but in a professional managerial aristocracy."[258]

"The King's absolute power served him, not his subjects. People who believe that the administrative state is different have been hoodwinked. By

---

256 Interview with Prof. Bruce Pardy on Freedom Feature, "The Experts Don't Own Us," https://firstfreedoms.ca/the-experts-dont-own-us-interview-with-bruce-pardy/
257 Thomas Hobbes, 2008. *Leviathan*. Edited by J. C. A. Gaskin. Oxford World's Classics. London, England: Oxford University Press.
258 Bruce Pardy, "Anatomy of the Administrative State," August 21, 2023, https://brownstone.org/articles/anatomy-of-the-administrative-state/

debating the niceties of policy, we quibble in the margins and surrender the battlefield." [259]

We can no longer keep our heads in the sand. Look around with the truckers' red pill to see what damage our governments and their bureaucracies have wrought and what continues to affect our lives day after day. The absolute power of the bureaucrats during the pandemic served their own kingdom-building interests more than it did the interests of individual freedom.

Pardy is spot on when he notes that "The conceit of our functionaries has become intolerable. Most public policy, good or bad, is illegitimate."[260] The ends do not justify the means.

The Truckers' Convoy exposed the inhumanity of bureaucrats who made decisions without much analysis of how their decisions would impact the daily lives of those affected.

We can no longer surrender the battlefield.

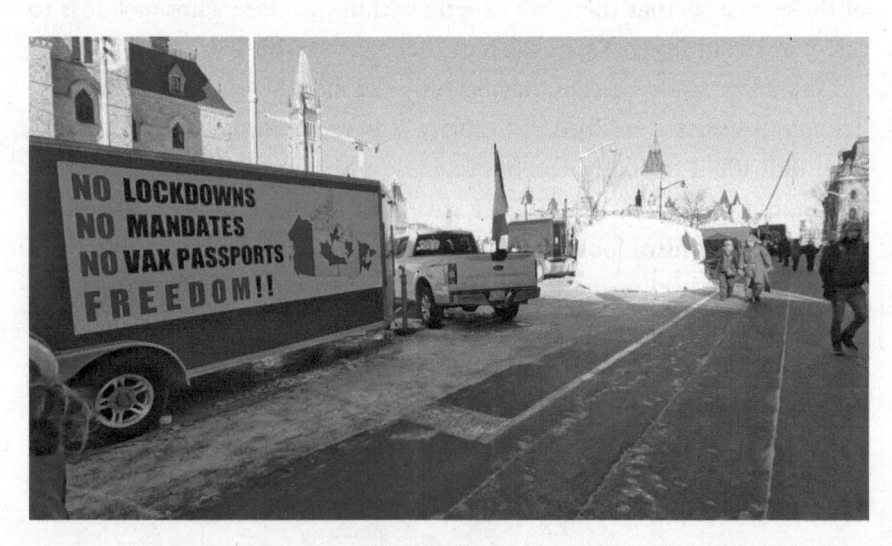

*Wellington Street – Notice The Open Lane For Emergency Use*

---

259 Bruce Pardy, "Anatomy of the Administrative State," August 21, 2023, https://brownstone.org/articles/anatomy-of-the-administrative-state/
260 Bruce Pardy, "Anatomy of the Administrative State," August 21, 2023, https://brownstone.org/articles/anatomy-of-the-administrative-state/

# 7. Revealed the Absolute Necessity of Justice Not Only Being Done but Seen To Be Done

IN THE SMALL village of Foxtrap, Newfoundland, my father, Winston, stood in the lineup at Johnny Butlers' General Store with his father, Peter. It was a busy day. The store's namesake was busy behind the counter serving the customers when he suddenly looked up and stared beyond Pete and Winston.

"Mr. H! Welcome, Mr. H!" He swung around the counter and got a chair for Mr. H to take a seat at the front of the line. "What can I do for you today, Mr. H?"

"Hold on, Johnny!" Peter protested. "Is my money not as good as Mr. H's? Me an' m' b'y were 'ere long before Mr. H. Now how about you serve us!"

"Yes, Pete b'y, what can I do for ya?"

Peter, my grandfather, a subsistence farmer and day labourer, knew what a hard day's work was. He had no education, nor was he part of the shore's money elite. He didn't own businesses like Mr. H. Yet he wasn't willing to be treated differently just because he didn't fit in with the rich. He demanded fairness in all his dealings.

He lost his father at sea in 1914 during the great sealing disaster when he was but four months old. Raised by a single mom in the early 1900s, he understood the importance of impartiality. When he was a teenager, his distant relatives tried to take his father's house and land. The case went before a local justice, who ruled in my grandfather's favour. He kept his father's house and raised, along with my grandmother, eight children.

We expect our economy and our judicial system to be just and fair. We demand it. We must demand it! Our entire civilization is dependent upon it.

The Trucker Convoy took that basic common sense of justice that my grandfather and so many like him relied upon to get through life's challenges to Ottawa. They had endured months of the prime minister's belittling of their concerns during and after the election. The poisoned atmosphere produced by the vaccine mandate made it difficult, if not impossible in some cases, to earn a living. They wanted justice.

Everyone involved in the legal system understands the absolute necessity for the public at large to have faith in the administration of justice. Lawyers, judges, law clerks, police, law professors all recognize that if the public loses faith in the justice system, then the entire societal structure is in danger of collapse. For there to be peace there must be respect for the law. If the public deems justice is "rigged" in favour of some at the expense of others, then look out. It won't be long before there's a free-for-all. True anarchy, no ruler, is the result of people taking justice into their own hands.

The truckers' protest came because they felt their opposition to government overreach, of which the vaccine mandates were a part, wasn't being heard by the prime minister and his government. As we know, the prime minister mocked and "gaslighted" them, which only fuelled the fire of opposition. Not only did they not get justice from the prime minister, but they were also troubled by the comments of the one person who holds the highest judicial office in the land—the Right Honourable Chief Justice Richard Wagner of the Supreme Court of Canada.

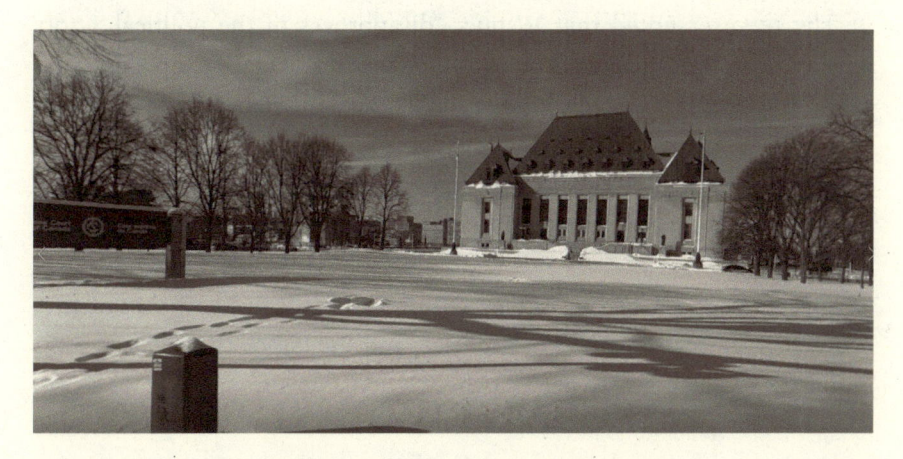

*Supreme Court Of Canada During The Protest*

Never has a person in that office come out before the national press and pronounced such comments against those who exercised their Charter right of free speech and assembly. The fact that Chief Justice Wagner felt so compelled to speak against the truckers in the way he did highlights yet again how effective the Trucker Convoy was in showcasing the fault lines in Canadian society. The elite/commoner divide is stark.

On April 9, 2022, the *Le Devoir* newspaper published an interview[261] with the chief justice about the Trucker Convoy. "What we have seen recently on Wellington Street here is the beginning of anarchy," said Justice Wagner, "where some people have decided to take other citizens hostage, to take the law into their own hands, not to respect the mechanism. [...] I find that worrying."

The article went on to say, "Forced blows against the state, justice and democratic institutions like the one delivered by protesters to the doors of the prime minister's office and the Privy Council, Parliament, the Supreme Court of Canada and the Press Gallery parliamentary between January 28 and February 21 must be denounced with force, and this, by all the figures of power in the country, believes Mr. Wagner."

---

261 Marco Bélair-Cirino, "Le juge en chef du Canada n'a pas oublié l'odeur d'anarchie," *Le Devoir*, April 9, 2022, https://www.ledevoir.com/politique/canada/697566/convoi-de-la-liberte-le-juge-en-chef-du-canada-n-a-pas-oublie-l-odeur-d-anarchie.

The reporter noted that Wagner "disapproves of the political actors who stuck to the Freedom Convoy, which was made up of people of "good faith," but also of "remotely guided" people seeking to bypass the political "system." "It doesn't inspire good feelings in me. I find that disturbing."

The occupation of downtown Ottawa, according to Wagner was fueled by "misunderstanding" and "ignorance" of the basics of Canadian rule of law.

The concept of "the rule of law" requires the different branches of government—the legislature, the executive, and the judiciary to stay in their own lane and by doing so act as a check against any branch that does not. Anytime the government interferes with the judicial role we are not ruled by law but by men and vice versa. The Freedom Convoy, in my view, was simply using their constitutional right to freely express their views on government action. However, Chief Justice Wagner did not see it that way.

"In the world around us, we see situations that undermine democracy and judicial independence," Wagner observed. "The worst mistake we can make is to say: 'We are exempt from that. It didn't happen with us.' It is a mistake. You have to be on the lookout." He continued,

> We must denounce any circumstance that could undermine our principles such as judicial independence, the rule of law, institutions. I like to say that Canada is not a military power, it is not an economic power. But I think it is a power at the level of judicial and legal values. And that is our strength in Canada because we have succeeded, over the years, in maintaining respect for institutions, in maintaining the rule of law. But it does not live on its own.

Thirteen lawyers took exception with the chief justice's published comments and filed a complaint with the Canadian Judicial Council. They argued that there were four court cases ongoing in the Federal Court addressing the Trucker Convoy, and that one or more might end up at the Supreme Court of Canada. They argued that Justice Wagner's comments raise "a reasonable apprehension of bias and an appearance of partiality."[262]

---

[262] Lee Harding, "Canada's Top Judge Spoke Bias Against Trucker Convoy, Lawyers Say," *The Epoch Times*, May 29, 2022, https://www.theepochtimes.

The complaint also stated that his "remarks will undermine Canadians' confidence in the independence of the Supreme Court of Canada ... and in the judiciary, generally." They went further that the confidence in the judicial system's impartiality and fairness will be undermined.

In the legal community, this is a huge development. To single out the chief justice of the Supreme Court of Canada is not something you do lightly.

The chief justice publicly stated that he approved the use of force against the truckers. His comments were not made in a courtroom after hearing all of the evidence, or after hearing the truckers' side of the story. On what was he basing his stated conclusions? We do not know. And that, respectfully, is the problem. A very serious problem.

It is imperative that all branches of government maintain their respective places in the order of governing. The Freedom Convoy was engaged in a constitutionally protected activity. Unless a case was before it, the judiciary had no prerogative to interfere in commenting on the matter. Recently, in 2019, the Supreme Court of Canada made an approving reference to a 250-year-old statement of, William Pitt (the elder), speaking in the British House of Commons, who described how "'[t]he poorest man may in his cottage bid defiance to all the forces of the crown. It may be frail — its roof may shake — the wind may blow through it — the storm may enter — the rain may enter — but the King of England cannot enter! — all his force dares not cross the threshold of the ruined tenement'."[263] That is equally analogous here. The branches of government must ensure that the rights of Canadians, like right to speak against the king in their house, is not to be violated without out due process of the law.

---

com/canadas-top-judge-spoke-bias-against-trucker-convoy-lawyers-say_4498149.html; Lee Harding, "Lawyers complain about Canada's top judge's comments on truckers' Freedom Convoy," *Western Standard*, May 28, 2022, https://www.westernstandard.news/news/lawyers-complain-about-canada-s-top-judges-comments-on-truckers-freedom-convoy/article_e39feca2-deac-11ec-8f95-57db8e7c78ad.html.

263 R. v. Le, 2019 SCC 34 (CanLII), [2019] 2 SCR 692, <https://canlii.ca/t/j0nvf>, retrieved on 2023-09-05 quoting House of Commons, Speech on the Excise Bill (March 1763), quoted in Lord Brougham, *Historical Sketches of Statesmen Who Flourished in the Time of George III* (1855), vol. I, at p. 42.

In my view, the lawyers were correct to file the complaint against the chief justice. We must have confidence in the rule of law. The chief justice was apparently appalled by the truckers occupying Wellington Street in Ottawa, but (more than that) he seemed to think that they were trying to overturn the institutions of government. They were not. As noted elsewhere, there were some "loose cannons" among the group, but they didn't represent the entire group. There was no armed insurrection; there was no violence. Violence only occurred when the police brutally brought the peaceful protest to an end.

It was the state—not the people—that was violent. The state refused to sit down and have a conversation. To those who would say, "Barry, if you talk to law breakers, you are legitimizing law breaking!" Really? Think about the federal government's willingness to negotiate with those stopping the rail traffic for weeks on end.[264] Stopping the free flow of goods on rail is also illegal, yet the government had no problem parleying with them.

Dr. Brian Lee Crowley, managing director of the Macdonald-Laurier Institute, poignantly stated in a striking op-ed:

> When the law is used to promote or shield specific causes and interests, people only obey the law when it is convenient to do so. And they are sorely tempted to take the law into their own hands when the state cannot be trusted to protect everyone's legal rights impartially. Vigilantism is a sign that public authorities have lost the trust of the people.[265]

In other words, it wasn't the truckers leading the way to anarchy! It was the government because it engaged in an unpardonable sin—treating some differently than others. It used the law as a bludgeon on its political

---

264 John Paul Tasker, "Trudeau asks for patience as rail blockades continue, bars Scheer from leaders' meeting," CBC News, February 18, 2020, accessed May 11,2023,https://www.cbc.ca/news/politics/trudeau-pipeline-protests-house-1.5466878.

265 Brian Lee Crowley, "We undermine the neutrality of the law at our peril," *The Line,* February 9, 2022, accessed May 11, 2023, https://theline.substack.com/p/brian-lee-crowley-we-undermine-the?.

enemies but allowed its "friends," those with whom it ideologically agreed, to ignore the law without consequence. That is a recipe for disaster.

The comments of the chief justice would lead a reasonable person to believe that the truckers had no right to protest. Yes, they were breaking the municipal laws in the street and should duly be fined accordingly, but that is not criminal—it's a parking ticket. Now the Ontario government has passed legislation to make such protests even more consequential. Further, as I've stated elsewhere, all court orders given to the truckers were obeyed. So, it was not "anarchy." Not by a long shot. What was the chief justice's source of news? Did he walk among the people on Wellington before coming to his conclusion?

For there to be public confidence in the judiciary, mutual respect is required. The people must respect the courts, and the courts must respect the people. That means judges are not to pass judgement on the people until they hear the people in a court of law. And the citizenry must allow the courts to speak and offer their reasons for their decisions. Unfortunately, Chief Justice Wagner was not making his comments in the context of a case but simply opining on the news reports and perhaps listening to the rather noisy ruckus coming from outside his office. We have no idea if he walked the streets and talked to the people. And given the very biased reporting on the truckers by the mainstream media, we can safely assume the chief justice was not getting the most accurate accounts if he was limiting his source of information on the truckers to the CBC. He certainly wasn't getting an accurate account from the prime minister, who has shown himself to be rather shy about the truth for some time.

It should be noted that the Ethical Principles for Judges, published by the Canadian Judicial Council (CJC), requires judges to "ensure that their conduct at all times maintains and enhances confidence in their impartiality and that of the judiciary," and "avoid conduct which could reasonably cause others to question their impartiality."[266]

A complaint was made to the CJC, and some weeks later the decision was that there is "nothing to see here," meaning the CJC felt the complaint

---

266 https://cjc-ccm.ca/sites/default/files/documents/2021/CJC_20-301_Ethical-Principles_Bilingual_Final.pdf.

was completely without merit. Here is the operative paragraph sent to those who filed the complaint:

> Considering that your complaint is unsupported, is largely based on a hypothetical scenario, is manifestly without substance, and does not concern judicial conduct, it does not warrant further consideration by the Council.

I, along with Professor Dr. Iain T. Benson of the Faculty of Law at the University of Notre Dame Australia (Sydney), wrote a piece challenging the decision of the CJC. Point by point we highlighted why the CJC had not handled this matter correctly, in our view.

Created in 1971 by Parliament, the CJC is "to maintain and improve the quality of judicial services in Canada's superior courts." Its governance body is chaired by the chief justice. Thus, it is readily seen that there is a conflict when the subject of a complaint is the chief justice, who himself or herself is the chair of the committee! There must be an open and transparent process to ensure there is no conflict. Right now, that doesn't exist if the complaint is about the chair. That needs to be corrected. There needs to be structural change to the CJC, and only Parliament can make such changes.

The "delicate balance" of democracy isn't served when our own chief justice engages in extrajudicial interviews in the popular press. Judges have traditionally refused to be drawn into revealing their private opinions on public matters that may come before the courts.

One can see this in play in the mistreatment of Tamara Lich by the political system intent on punishing her for her political opinions. On Lich's July 8, 2022, hearing, Justice Wagner's comments were referenced by the Crown prosecutor, Moiz Karimjee, as a basis that the trucker protest was an "occupation."[267] The gravitas of Justice Wagner's views was already being used in a court! Such is the consequence of ill-timed remarks.

---

267 Bruce Pardy, "By Freeing Tamara Lich, the Superior Court Restores Confidence in the Rule of Law," *The Epoch Times*, accessed May 11, 2023, https://www.theepochtimes.com/by-freeing-tamara-lich-the-superior-court-restores-confidence-in-the-rule-of-law_4632866.html.

Professor Benson and I sent our critique of the CJC's decision to one of the largest legal publishers in Canada. We felt it was a natural fit. For almost two weeks the publisher's legal department mulled over whether to publish it. Finally, we got their response: "It is a complex and controversial piece in which our editorial group wanted to take a careful look. After much discussion, we have decided that the piece is not for us and we're going to take a pass. We wish you well in getting it placed in another publication."

Within hours it was published by *The Epoch Times*.[268]

Such has been the dramatic effect the truckers had on a judicial system that wasn't prepared for a grassroots uprising against the federal government's overreach. Laid bare for all Canadians to see was the inappropriateness of its own chief justice in making extrajudicial comments against the truckers. The consequences of such comments are yet to be seen.

It also raises the spectre of the politicization of the judiciary. Since the advent of the Charter of Rights, judges have taken upon themselves immense political clout, unheard of before the Charter became law. As author John Robson points out, the "horrendous flaw in our Charter of Rights ... is section one that says you have these rights only until a court says you shouldn't. That sort of thing is dangerous." Robson went on and told me, "You cannot go on and give tyrants that much space because they will take it."[269]

Brian Peckford differs on Robson's view, noting that section one's condition that a government must "demonstrably justify" their limits as understood in "a free and democratic society" is sufficient to protect our rights. However, the judiciary found ways to get around it. "If someone is intent on doing wrong no wording is going to stop them."[270]

Certainly, since Prime Minister Trudeau has taken office, the courts have been in his favour. Consider only a recent decision of the Supreme

---

[268] Iain T. Benson, Barry W. Bussey, "Time to Reassess the Canadian Judicial Council?" *The Epoch Times*, July 24, 2022, accessed May 11, 2023, https://www.theepochtimes.com/benson-and-bussey-time-to-reassess-the-canadian-judicial-council_4618780.html?utm_source=ai&utm_medium=search.

[269] "Magna Carta Must Not Be Forgotten—Interview with John Robson," First Freedoms Foundation, accessed May 11, 2023, https://firstfreedoms.ca/magna-carta-must-not-be-forgotten/.

[270] Personal email with Hon. Brian Peckford, January 27, 2023.

Court of Canada (SCC), written by the chief justice, who proclaimed, "Climate change is real"[271] and allowed the Trudeau government to impose its carbon tax despite its infringement of the rights of the provinces. Although that was not a Charter case, it reflects the tendency of the SCC to support the policies of the current federal government.

It will be fascinating to see what happens in the future if a Charter challenge to the federal government's vaccine mandates make it to the SCC. First, will the chief justice recuse himself because of his statements on the Trucker Freedom Convoy 2022? Second, will the SCC make a scientific pronouncement, like it did on climate change, that the COVID-19 vaccine is safe and effective? Third, will it simply ignore the whole thing by saying that the issue of the vaccines and mandates are now moot? If I were a betting person, which I'm not, I would say the more likely result is that the court will say it is moot and won't hear the case,[272] thus effectively deciding in favour of the government and increasing the power of the executive while avoiding any suggestion that the chief justice recuse himself.

## Tamara Lich

During any moment of national crisis, we depend upon our judicial system being beyond reproach, because the judiciary is tasked with keeping government accountable. The entire country watched what happened to Tamara Lich, during the most significant overreach of the Canadian government in modern times. Indeed, the world watched. Tamara was one of several organizers of the Trucker Convoy. Would the judicial system be seen as the government's check and balance?

On February 17, 2022, the day after Tamara called upon the protestors to forgive the police because "they know not what they do" and to pray for Prime Minister Trudeau, she was arrested during a snowy evening

---

271 "References re: Greenhouse Gas Pollution Pricing Act, 2021 SCC 11, at para. 2, (CanLII)," CanLII, accessed May 11, 2023 https://canlii.ca/t/jdwnw.

272 Much in the same way the SCC refused to hear two recent appeals from BC and Ontario involving churches in the respective provinces who challenged provincial COVID lockdowns, see: https://decisions.scc-csc.ca/scc-csc/scc-l-csc-a/en/item/20021/index.do and https://decisions.scc-csc.ca/scc-csc/scc-l-csc-a/en/item/20025/index.do

in Canada's capital. It was three days after Mr. Trudeau had declared a national emergency.

Tamara was charged with interfering with the lawful use and enjoyment of property ("mischief"), counselling to commit mischief, and obstructing police.[273] In the grand scheme of things, these are very minor, non-violent offenses, but if convicted she will have a criminal record, which is consequential, nonetheless.

While I did practice criminal law, it was limited to my early years. One doesn't have to be a practising criminal lawyer to know that what was done to Tamara Lich in denying her bail for such a long time was simply wrong. I talked with colleagues who shared with me that they'd never had a client experience anything close to what Tamara faced.

To appreciate the extent of Tamara's exceptional mistreatment, we must understand the normal course of events when a person is arrested in Canada. The first thing to remember is that everyone has a constitutional right to reasonable bail (that is, to leave custody of the state on a promise to abide by reasonable conditions and to appear in court for a trial on the charges they face) and a timely bail hearing.

The purpose of bail is to ensure that the public is protected while the person charged awaits trial, since they're waiting in the public realm at large. In most cases, the charged is given "a release order" on the day of arrest. Depending on the alleged offence, the police may release the person without surety but with a promise to appear.

In more serious matters, the person must appear before a justice of the peace (JP) with a surety. A surety is the person who will ensure that the person keeps the bail conditions. If they do not, the surety will have to pay the court the bail money.

Few are aware that a justice of the peace doesn't need legal training. It's a political appointment, yet it's an office that is held in some esteem,

---

[273] Later she was charged with more offenses so that her charges included "one count of counselling intimidation, not committed by one or more persons, a count of counselling the resistance or willful obstruction of a peace officer, not committed by one or more persons, a count of resisting or willfully obstructing a peace officer, one count of intimidation, a count of mischief, and a count of fail to comply with a release order."

especially when you consider the remuneration they receive. In Ontario, for example, the JP salary is $172,010 per year with a pension, a benefits package, and a twenty-two-day yearly vacation allowance.[274] Anyone can be appointed a JP—no special training required. Needless to say these are political appointments.

As Justice Goodman noted, "For the most part, this branch of the Ontario Court of Justice comprising of Justices of the Peace is a lay bench."[275] While they have no legal education, they do go through a significant training process upon their appointment to enable them to carry out their responsibilities. They hold the lowest ranked judicial office that deals with run-of-the-mill matters like bail, search and seizure, and provincial offenses.

Normally the person taken into custody appears before the JP on the day of arrest, or by the next day at the latest. This is particularly the case when it's the person's first-time offense and it's of a minor nature. When Tamara was arrested, the Ontario courts had a special COVID-19 protocol[276] that underscored early release. The protocol "emphasized the need for parties and the Court to work cooperatively and flexibly to maximize the proper and efficient use of court hearing time, particularly in proceedings involving accused persons who are in custody."[277]

## First Court Hearing

Tamara appeared before Justice of the Peace Julie Bourgeois on Saturday, February 20, 2022. That was two days after her arrest—already a day later than most bail hearings. But it wasn't until February 22, 2022, four days

---

[274] "Appointments Process," Ontario Court of Justice, accessed May 11, 2023, https://www.ontariocourts.ca/ocj/jpaac/frequently-asked-questions/#:~:text=What%20are%20the%20salary%20and,two%20(22)%20working%20days.

[275] "R. v. Lich, 2022 ONSC 4390 at para. 33, (CanLII)," CanLII, accessed May 11, 2023, https://canlii.ca/t/jr3cs.

[276] https://web.archive.org/web/20230328210328/https://www.ontariocourts.ca/ocj/COVID-19/COVID-19-protocol-bail-hearings/

[277] See at 1.iii.

from the arrest and two days after the hearing, that Bourgeois released her decision denying bail.

Justice Bourgeois was not impressed with Tamara: "You have had plenty of opportunity to remove yourself and even others from this criminal activity but obstinately chose not to and persistently counselled others not to either."[278] She stated that the offences Tamara faced were "grave" and "a lengthy stay" was possible if convicted. She was not convinced that Tamara wouldn't re-offend, nor did she think Tamara's husband would be an adequate surety.

The offences of which Tamara is accused aren't anywhere near "grave" nor, in my view, will they ever require a lengthy sentence, even if she is convicted. Tamara was surprised that Justice Bourgeois was a Liberal supporter and former Liberal candidate in the 2011 election. "I didn't stand a chance," she said.[279] Her apprehension toward the justice system is understandable.

Her judge, Bourgeois, at the bail hearing and the crown prosecutor, Moiz Karimjee, were both Liberal supporters. However, we have to keep in mind that is how our system works—politicians have a big say on who is appointed. The goal is to have a justice system that it matters not who appoints who but that the judges and prosecutors are professionals and treat everyone alike.

Tamara's treatment was anything but normal.

The week before Tamara's hearing, Ontario Superior Court Justice Hugh McLean had ruled, in a civil court action brought by Ottawa residents and intended to stop honking horns in downtown Ottawa, that Ms. Lich and other defendants were "at liberty to engage in a peaceful, lawful and safe protest."[280] Tamara made it her mission to ensure that the protest

---

[278] Melanie Risdon, "Freedom Convoy organizer Lich denied bail," *Western Standard*, February 22, 2022, accessed May 11, 2023, https://www.westernstandard.news/news/freedom-Convoy-organizer-lich-denied-bail/article_5befa5f7-36f7-531b-8c66-78e18e570a91.html.

[279] Tamara Lich, *Hold The Line: My story from the heart of the Freedom Convoy* (Toronto: Rebel News Network, 2023), 174.

[280] Order of Justice Mclean, February 7, 2022, Zexi Li v, Chris Barber et al, at para. 7, accessed May 11, 2023, https://www.jccf.ca/wp-content/uploads/2022/05/Li-Interim-Order-CV-22-00088514-00CP.pdf.

was indeed peaceful. To the credit of her, her fellow organizers, and the truckers, it was.

Yes, the truckers were violating municipal bylaws by protesting on Ottawa streets. Tamara had no truck in Ottawa. She peacefully protested along with the others over the imposition of vaccine mandates. Consider that she was criminally charged while exercising her Charter freedoms of expression, association, and assembly. But I digress.

One can only imagine the disappointment Tamara faced as she went back to prison. For the longest time she was not permitted a Bible. After a few days she decided to clean up her cell with a toothbrush and soap. The graffiti on the walls disgusted her. She came across these words, "The first 14 days of quarantine are the hardest. Brighter days are coming." Listen to her tell what happened next:

> I started to choke up. And then I started crying. I thought about all the people that were thrown in jail during the pandemic. I'd never considered how hard they must have had it. They would be thrown in these cells for two weeks of isolation—at least two weeks, maybe more. There must have been so many of them. I left that bit of graffiti right where it was.[281]

Justice Bourgeois' decision was reviewed by a higher court.

## Second Court Hearing

On March 7, 2022, Justice Johnston of the Ontario Superior Court of Justice ruled that Justice Bourgeois made a legal error in her analysis of the severity of the offence and her view of a potential lengthy period of imprisonment. He released Tamara on $20,000 bail to a new surety, her sister Dannette, and with very strict bail conditions:

> Do not contact or communicate in any way either directly or indirectly, by any physical, electronic or other means, with the following: [a list of ten prominent leaders of

---

281 Tamara Lich, 175.

the Freedom Convoy including Tom Marazzo] ... except through counsel or in the presence of counsel ... You are not to log on to social media or post any messages on social media ... You are not to allow anyone else to post messages on social media on your behalf or indicate your approval for any future protests so long as this release order is in place ... You are not to engage in organization or promotion of anti-COVID 19 mandate activities and Freedom Convoy activities ... You are not to verbally, or in writing, financially, or by any other means, support anything related to the Freedom Convoy.[282]

That decision came eighteen days after her arrest! Remember, normally the accused is released the day of the arrest, and by the second day at the latest! Was she that much of a threat to the people in Ottawa? I do not think so.

Justice Johnston's bail conditions were, in my view, unduly strict for the circumstance. Tamara wasn't engaged in any violence whatsoever, and there have been no outrageous comments by Tamara on social media that I have seen to date.[283] If the fear was of her organizing another protest, then that could have been stipulated, but to ban her from the city of Ottawa and the province of Ontario seems extreme.

As Tamara drove through Ontario she was filled with anxiety, wanting to make sure she got out of the province in time. She did not want to breach the bail conditions knowing that Mr. Karimjee was keen on putting her back behind bars. She crossed the Manitoba border with one hour to spare in accordance with release conditions.[284]

Tamara's lawyers appealed the bail conditions, but they were struggling to get a court date to hear the appeal. It wasn't until she was offered

---

[282] Superior Court of Justice Release Form, accessed May 11, 2023, https://www.jccf.ca/wp-content/uploads/2022/03/Tamara-Lich-Release-Order_Redacted.pdf.

[283] Barry W. Bussey, "The Cruel Suppression of Tamara Lich's Freedom of Speech," October 14, 2022, https://www.theepochtimes.com/the-cruel-suppression-of-tamara-lichs-freedom-of-speech_4794667.html, accessed June 22, 2023.

[284] Tamara Lich, 181.

the 2022 George Jonas Freedom Award that they found themselves back in court.

The Justice Centre for Constitutional Freedoms (JCCF) awarded her the 2022 George Jonas Freedom Award in recognition of her significant contribution to defending Canada as a free society. The mere acceptance of the award led Assistant Crown Attorney Moiz Karimjee to obtain a court date to incarcerate Tamara again because he reasoned she had violated the bail conditions not to be engaged in activity in Ontario. The gala dinner was to be held in Toronto on June 16.

### Third Court Hearing

On May 19 and 20, Tamara's lawyers argued against the positions of Mr. Karimjee over the bail conditions before Justice Phillips of the Ontario Superior Court. Tamara appeared in court via video link from her home in Alberta.[285] Tamara wanted the bail conditions relaxed because they violated her freedom of expression, especially as the Freedom Convoy was no longer in Ottawa and the threat of it starting again no longer existed.[286] There was therefore no connection between the risk to public safety and the bail terms.

However, Karimjee said Tamara ought to be put back in prison because she breached her bail conditions by accepting the Jonas Freedom Award. Karimjee aggressively argued his position and even asked Justice Phillips to recuse himself from the hearing because Phillips had made critical comments about Karimjee's demeanour in the hearing.[287]

---

285 Aedan Helmer, "'Recuse yourself': Crown prosecutor challenges judge at Tamara Lich bail review," *Windsor Star*, May 19, 2022, accessed May 11, 2023, https://windsorstar.com/news/i-dont-think-its-a-breach-tamara-lich-testifies-during-heated-bail-review-hearing/wcm/b3112704-8cec-484b-bbfc-67aaf6e1f2f0/amp/.
286 "Her Majesty the Queen and Tamara Lee Lich," Ontario Superior Court of Justice, accessed May 11, 2023, https://www.jccf.ca/wp-content/uploads/2022/03/LICH-Notice-of-Application-to-Vary-Bail-Conditions-24-March-22_Redacted.pdf.
287 Helmer, 2022.

In his May 25 decision, Justice Phillips let it be known that "no court would ever seek to control the possession or manifestation of political views. The courts are not a thought police. We seek only to control conduct to the extent that certain behavior will violate or likely lead to violation of the law."[288] Phillips accepted that attending the awards gala was nowhere near the same as organizing another protest, which is what the bail conditions were meant to protect against. "The route between attendance at that function as it has been advertised and problematic 'support' for a demonstration that will by then have been long over is so indirect as to be barely perceptible."[289]

It was "practically impossible to mount a comparable Freedom Convoy in Ottawa again," Phillips wrote. Tamara had not breached her conditions and therefore "she can be trusted to follow release conditions."[290] He recognized that she was off social media, but he made an interesting comment that is worth repeating, if only to show the sentiment against the Freedom Convoy: "It is hard to escape the thought that depriving Ms. Lich of the echo chamber that is social media these days has likely had salutary effect on her and her susceptibility to getting caught up in the sort of toxic group-think that animated the crowd back in February."[291]

Phillips was mindful of the changes to the government's approach toward the mandates—the mask mandates were gone, as were other restrictions. "[T]he temperature in respect of opposition to the official approach has lowered," he observed. "Indeed, as a member of the legal community, I am aware that there are now several court challenges being brought in respect of some of the remaining vaccination mandates. While I am indifferent about the outcome of those endeavours, I see them as good things. Such litigation will serve to ventilate and channel the emotions felt by many about the pandemic and its consequences."[292]

---

288 "R. v. Lich, 2022 ONSC 3093, at para. 6, (CanLII)," CanLII, accessed May 11, 2023, https://canlii.ca/t/jpd6w.
289 Ibid.
290 Ibid., at para. 8.
291 Ibid.
292 Ibid.

Justice Phillips acknowledged a very important principle that we would do well to take note of. Society is best served when the angst in the streets is brought before a reasoned analysis in a court of law. We cannot survive as a society if we're unable to peacefully settle our political differences. The courts play a crucial role in properly dealing with the fallout of the government's mishandling of the vaccine mandate issue that brought the Freedom Convoy to Ottawa in the first place. This is a fundamental principle that is thousands of years old and found to be true, which is why courts must eschew political commentary.

Phillips opined that Justice Bourgeois's decision would have been different with the change in circumstances. She felt that there was a risk of the protest's resurgence, he observed, and that Tamara had no respect for the law; further, there was now "the high quality of the surety."[293]

Likewise, he felt that Justice Johnston was also close to the time of the protest, as "the city was still reeling from the effects of the protest" with the state of emergency, and Tamara having "no history of compliance with court orders and who gave only indication of having little, if any, respect for the law."[294] Therefore, he complimented Justice Johnston's decision.

While he supported his judicial colleagues, he also varied the bail conditions—ever so slightly—but enough to give Tamara better justice. Justice Phillips recognized that there was no evidence that Tamara breached her conditions. But he was concerned that she "is not exactly behaving like someone chastened by the charges." He warned her that "a trial is no sure thing for either side and one of the possible outcomes here is a conviction." Upon conviction, the Crown may argue for a harsher sentence because she has not behaved properly before trial. "The Crown may well rebut the presumption of innocence and Ms. Lich might learn the hard way from Her Majesty the Queen that she who laughs last laughs longest."[295] His point was that Tamara better continue to take these bail conditions seriously or she could be subject to a harsher sentence if convicted.

Justice Phillips reviewed the social media ban and decided that it must continue. Notice how he framed the matter: "[S]ocial media can be

---

293 Ibid., at para. 10.
294 Ibid.
295 Ibid., at para. 13.

a problematic feedback loop where people get egged on and caught up in group activity they would never perform on their own. In a very real way, social media undoubtedly contributed to and even drove the now impugned conduct and Ms. Lich staying away from it is necessary to lower the risk of re-offence to an acceptable level."[296]

Phillips agreed that Tamara could return to Ottawa in the fall to assist her daughter in settling in for university if she didn't go to the downtown core. And he removed the condition that she couldn't be in the province of Ontario. In other words, she was allowed to attend the June 16 JCCF freedom award gala. And, as Tamara noted, "Karimjee had lost again. I think it only made him madder."[297]

## *June 16, 2022, JCCF Gala*

The citation for why Tamara was given the George Jonas Award said it was for inspiring "Canadians to exercise their Charter rights and freedoms by participating actively in the democratic process and took the initiative to help organize a peaceful protest and serve as one of its leaders. The resulting peaceful protest in Ottawa awakened many Canadians to the injustice of Charter-violating lockdowns and mandatory vaccination policies."[298] Indeed, it was a privilege for me to attend the historic event in person.

My friend Samuel Bachand, a JCCF lawyer in Montreal, was kind enough to give me a ticket to the gala. Given the situation and the ever-growing opposition to the Freedom Convoy, the notice I received from JCCF stated, "We advise you to please use discretion and keep the venue location confidential, except to provide to ticket holders and your guests, for security and privacy reasons. Thank you for your understanding." It truly is a sad commentary on Canada that we must be so circumspect in coming together to celebrate freedom.

Security and privacy are increasingly difficult to maintain with social media. The events of that evening were soon to be national news. The

---

296 Ibid., at para. 16.
297 Tamara Lich, 188.
298 "George Jonas Freedom Award," Justice Centre for Constitutional Freedoms, accessed May 11, 2023, https://www.jccf.ca/george-jonas-freedom-award/.

brief interaction Tamara had with fellow convoy organizer Tom Marazzo was posted on social media.

The evening was a great who's who in the world of freedom-loving activists and lawyers. As my first post-COVID event with so many people, it was exhilarating to meet up with legal colleagues I hadn't seen in a couple of years. When lawyers get together, we talk shop, and I had the opportunity to share my new non-profit—First Freedoms Foundation (www.firstfreedoms.ca). They in turn shared their continued work on the cases that mean so much for Canadians.

The JCCF, more than any other organization in the country,[299] has been the vanguard for freedom during the COVID-19 pandemic, but also for defence of the truckers. They have single-handedly raised the funds to finance court action after court action in the defence of freedom in Canada, including paying for legal representation to advise and represent the truckers in Ottawa in January-February 2022, and numerous court actions arising from that time and situation, like paying for the criminal defence of wrongfully accused persons like Chris Barber and Tamara Lich. John Carpay and his JCCF team have done Canada a great service.

Yet it must be said that the JCCF is not without controversy, and its zealous approach got ahead of them. In July of 2021, Carpay admitted to hiring a private investigator to observe government officials in Manitoba in regard to whether they themselves were following the COVID restrictions they had imposed on the entire population. Carpay had surveillance conducted on the premier, the chief medical officer, and Manitoba Chief Justice Glen Joyal. Carpay has publicly apologized for including Joyal in this surveillance. Eighteen months after the events in question, Carpay was surprised to face criminal charges in late December 2022. He spent

---

[299] Of course, there are others who have been assisting in protecting the rights of Canadians. For example, The Democracy Fund, https://www.thedemocracyfund.ca/ and its Fight the Fines campaign has done admirable work in assisting Canadians during this time frame. Also, of note is the work of the late Carol Crosson of the Rights & Freedoms Advocates, https://www.freedomsadvocate.ca/.

twenty-three hours in jail. He is pleading not guilty to accusations of intimidating a justice system participant and obstruction of justice.[300]

Many people have lost sight of the fact that lawyers routinely hire private investigators to conduct surveillance, for example to uncover insurance fraud or in spousal disputes in family law contexts. Hiring a private investigator is neither illegal nor immoral nor unethical—it is a means of determining the truth of matters. However, the optics of a lawyer requesting surveillance on a judge are problematic. As explained by Bruce Pardy, who sat on the JCCF board at the time, in an op-ed: "Surveilling a sitting judge is wrong. Justice must be done and must manifestly appear to be done. Any hint that a party or lawyer might be attempting to influence a judge outside of the courtroom, even if that is not the motivation, is an affront to the integrity of the judicial process."[301]

In due course, we can expect to find out more from Carpay as to what led to such a lack of judgement. It's admirable that he has taken ownership of the mistake and is courageously weathering the storm. Although we're in a "cancel culture" where every mistake is magnified to destroy anyone who has stepped offside of acceptable behaviour, we mustn't lose sight of the admirable work that has been done by JCCF, tainted as it may be by this incident. It's a serious matter and there are serious consequences if he's found guilty.[302]

---

[300] Dan Vadeboncoeur, "Alberta lawyer charged for having Manitoba judge followed during COVID-19 restriction case involving churches," CTV News, January 2, 2023, accessed May 11, 2023, https://winnipeg.ctvnews.ca/alberta-lawyer-charged-for-having-a-manitoba-judge-followed-during-the-pandemic-1.6215217.

[301] Bruce Pardy, "Even in a COVID snitch society, surveilling your judge is wrong," National Post, July 20, 2021, accessed May 11, 2023, https://nationalpost.com/opinion/bruce-pardy-surveilling-a-judge-was-wrong-but-we-must-keep-a-close-eye-on-government-officials.

[302] He has already suffered a negative decision from the Manitoba Law Society, which barred him for life from practicing law in Manitoba and fined him $5,000.00. See "Justice Centre statement on the conclusion of Manitoba Law Society proceedings," August 21, 2023, https://www.jccf.ca/statement-on-the-conclusion-of-manitoba-law-society-proceedings/, accessed August 30, 2023.

Despite this, I am a believer that we are to give credit where credit is due. I thanked John personally for his work. While he appreciated the words of support, he let me know that it wasn't him alone but the efforts of a great team.

One cannot but think of Keith Wilson[303] and Eva Chipiuk, lawyers who worked with JCCF, who were on the frontlines during the convoy in Ottawa, working day and night as they negotiated with the police and politicians. Such dedication for the cause of freedom is to be applauded.

The awards program went without a hitch. Tamara gave a stirring speech on her experience in solitary confinement, having to sleep on a cement floor without a pillow or a blanket while her clothes were wet from the snow. She held no resentment. But she spoke powerfully on the importance of freedom.

"We know that democracy, that system of government that Churchill said was the worst form of government except for all the others which have been tried," Tamara said toward the end of her speech. "We know it has its origins in Athens, but a very important question is often missing and that is, "What gave rise to Athens? What gave rise to all the philosophy, the math, the fundamental ideas, some 3000 years ago that started Western civilization?"

The answer she said came when a Persian general answered the queen of Persia's questions, "Who governs these Greeks? Who commands their army?" The general responded, "No one. People say they are no man's slaves or servants."

> That was the spirit of freedom that propelled the Greeks. That is the spirit that started Athenian democracy and the fundamental basis of our civilization ... it is about human flourishing and humanity's survival. Anyone who diminishes this by calling it exaggeration or hyperbole will lead you to a path of extinction. The true path is hard but is the only way forward. You must fight for your ancestors,

---

303 See my interview of Keith Wilson, "Fighting Mandates: Livestream with Keith Wilson, QC," First Freedoms Foundation, accessed May 11, 2023, https://firstfreedoms.ca/fighting-mandates-livestream-with-keith-wilson-qc/.

fight for your children and fight for yourselves. The future is ours. The people are awakening to a force that cannot be suppressed. Glory be to freedom. Glory be to Canada, and glory be to all of you! Thank you.[304]

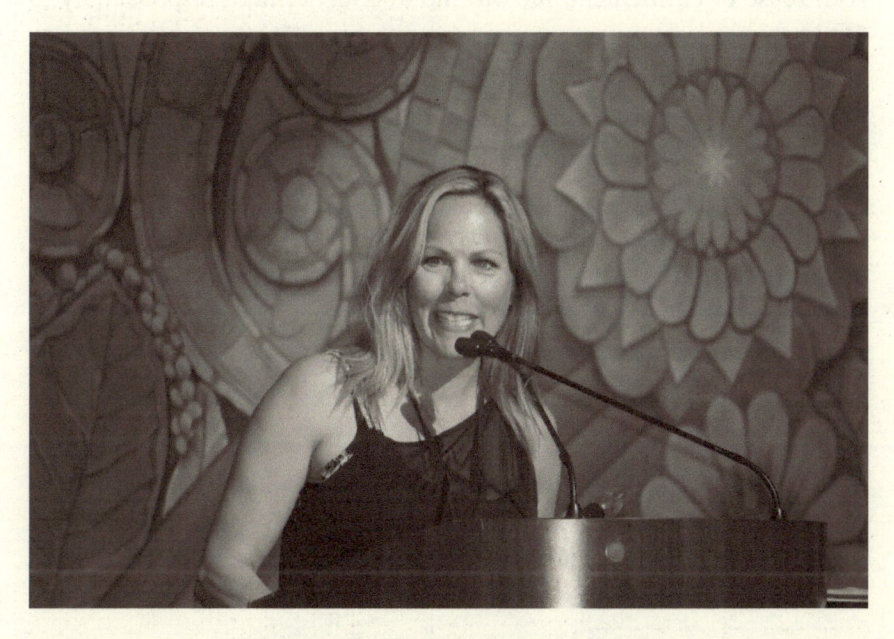

*Tamara Lich Giving Her Powerful Speech*

After her speech, Tamara was given a resounding standing ovation. She was celebrated as the Canadian hero she is—not Justin Trudeau's type of hero or the hero of the Cathedral but one for the average Canadians who stood up against the imposition of medical procedures against their will. This one lady stands as their symbol of opposition. Peaceful opposition. Opposition that is very fitting for the country that once had an international reputation as a no-nonsense peacekeeping nation.

Somehow over the last seven years, we've become a nation that has lost its nerve, no longer confident in its own history. The current focus on the past is on all that the modern view finds embarrassing. We are now a country of identity politics and remorse over every possible conception

---

304 Thats Facts, "Tamara Lich Delivers a Speech for the Ages," YouTube, June 20, 2022, 5:07, https://www.youtube.com/watch?v=MEbYKaCdQTM.

of offence against such identities. No longer are we Canadian but multi-hyphenated people groups with little to no understanding of our history of freedom and the institutions that allowed us to enjoy unparalleled prosperity. We have become a country that has lost its way, possessing a keen sense of entitlement but with no duty or sense of responsibility to future generations.

Just as this book was in its final stages, an uproar against Lt. Gen. J.O. Michel Maisonneuve made the news over his speech after receiving the Vimy Award at a gala in Ottawa. In many ways he lamented Canada's drift as I have just outlined it. Among his "offensive" commentary was his call for leadership and service where people take responsibility for their own actions and stop fighting over "who gets to wear the coveted victim's cloak."[305]

He got a standing ovation from the military officers in attendance, but not surprisingly, he received derision from some in the Cathedral.[306] This is but the latest example of why the truckers' pushback was so necessary—it provides an opening for more, not less, dialogue.

Tamara, of Metis heritage and raised by adoptive parents in Western Canada, a grandmother, and an activist against the globalist anti-Canadian

---

305 Lt. Gen. Michel Maisonneuve, "'Making Canada better': An excerpt from the anti-woke speech by a general that caused an uproar," *National Post*, November 17, 2022, accessed May 11, 2023, https://nationalpost.com/opinion/the-speech-by-a-general-attacking-cancel-culture-and-green-policies-that-caused-an-uproar.

306 See Thomas Juneau (@thomasjuneau), "This speech by retired LGen Michel Maisonneuve was an embarrassment and a good illustration of the culture of entitlement," Twitter, November 10, 2022, 9:58 AM, https://twitter.com/thomasjuneau/status/1590720582634856448;
David Pugliese, "Canadian Forces officers applaud speech slamming Canada's climate change policies, cancel culture, weak leaders," *Ottawa Citizen*, November 15, 2022, accessed May 11, 2023, https://www.thepost.on.ca/news/national/defence-watch/speech-slamming-canadas-climate-change-policies-cancel-culture-and-weak-leaders-applauded-by-canadian-forces-officers; John Robson had this to say: "I applaud Lt.-Gen. Maisonneuve for ruffling feathers instead of smothering debate." I agree. See John Robson, "The retired general who spoke truth about Canadian wokeness," *National Post*, November 16, 2022, accessed May 11, 2023, https://nationalpost.com/opinion/he-retired-general-who-spoke-truth-about-military-wokeness.

Laurentian imposition on the average working class, became the lightning rod, and she stood firm. She was rightly celebrated. The entire room sought a picture with her. The lineups were extensive.

Immediately after her speech, she was congratulated by PPC Party Leader, Maxime Bernier, and his wife, and as Tamara walked by Tom Marazzo, with whom she'd worked in Ottawa to organize the protest during the three weeks, she bent down, and they chatted for all of three seconds as he thanked her for the speech. A video was taken by someone and posted on social media. That three-second interchange, along with a picture that included Tamara and Tom, caused one of the strangest events in Canadian legal history.

I had the privilege of having Tom on my Freedom Feature program, and he shared how unprecedented the treatment of Tamara was. Remember, one of the bail conditions was that she couldn't be in the presence of fellow convoy organizers. They were specifically listed in the court order. However, she was allowed to meet with them if in the presence of legal counsel.

As Tom told me,[307] "The lawyers were the ones who sponsored the dinner!" There were scores of JCCF lawyers in attendance, including Tamara's criminal lawyer. "We were surrounded by Tamara's lawyers. I was put at the dinner table with her. I had hardly any communication with her because there were too many guests of the dinner that wanted to talk to Tamara, to shake her hand, to take pictures with her. So, she was busy that night."

Beforehand, Tom confirmed with her lawyers whether it was permissible for him to attend. They said that his being there would not violate the bail conditions, as both he and Tamara were "in the presence of counsel." Their meeting at the gala was not to plan another protest but to honour Tamara receiving the award.

At the table, John Carpay, the president of JCCF, sat at Tamara's left, and on her right sat her husband, and then Tom sat next to him.

"I thought it was strange," Tamara recalls, "but I had to assume that meant everything would be fine. I mean, they wouldn't sit me right at the

---

307 You can find my interview with Tom Marazzo at https://firstfreedoms.ca/trudeaus-tiananmen-square/.

same table with Tom Marazzo if they thought it would end up with me being sent back to jail. Right?"[308]

Tom continues the story of what happened: "She gave her speech. It was a brilliant speech. She delivered it very well and when she stepped off the stage, I just congratulated her on such a great speech. That's it. Three seconds. She sat down."

No more to it than that.

Yet when a picture and video of their three-second interaction was put on social media, all kinds of trouble broke out. The Ottawa police and Crown prosecutor went into action yet again on the premise that Tamara "broke" her bail conditions.

"And the Crown tried to make the case that within those three seconds," said Tom dramatically, "Tamara and I plotted a successful strategy to overthrow the entire planet."

After the June 16 dinner, Tamara and her husband drove all the way back home to Medicine Hat, Alberta. Given that the unvaccinated weren't permitted to fly or go by train, the Lichs had no choice but to drive to Toronto and back.

After she arrived home, the Ottawa police made plans to transport Tamara back to Ottawa to appear before a court on the claim that she had broken her bail condition of not communicating with Tom Marazzo. It was done with great dramatic effect. It seems that the drama expertise in the PMO has filtered through the bureaucratic ranks, much like one would expect from a Hollywood blockbuster, as the police detectives and lawyers plotted to capture the criminal and bring her to justice.

Monday, June 27, as Tamara was making her way home, after checking in with her sister Dannette to comply with her bail conditions, she saw flashing police lights behind her.

"'Oh crap, he must have clocked me speeding.'"[309]

Not so.

"'Ma'am when I run your plates, it's coming back that there's a warrant for your arrest.'"[310]

---

308 Tamara Lich, 190.
309 Tamara Lich, 193.
310 Tamara Lich, 194.

She had to go with the officer and left her truck on the side of the road for her husband to pick up. By Wednesday she was at the Calgary airport, put in a wheelchair in shackles, and put on a plane to Ottawa.

A national warrant for Tamara's arrest was issued, and two Ottawa homicide detectives were dispatched and accompanied her on the flight to the city from which she had earlier been banned. There she was incarcerated yet again.

We must stop and think about this for a moment. Compare her treatment to that of forty-two-year-old David Alexander Zegarac, who with his Jeep struck four people among the Freedom Convoy protesters at the Manitoba legislative buildings back in February. The Manitoba protesters were not connected with those in Ottawa but were acting in sympathy with what was happening. It was late in the evening of February 5, 2022, when Zegarac plowed into the protesters. He was caught a half-hour later, arrested, and put in jail overnight. He was released the next day on a $10,000 bail, had to leave Winnipeg, not sit in a driver's seat of a vehicle, not own or possess any weapon, and not contact the victims, according to the media report.[311] A bit of a difference from how Tamara was treated, don't you think?

### Fourth Court Hearing

Tamara's case was brought before another justice of the peace, Justice Paul Harris, on July 4. Tamara wasn't allowed to appear personally because she wouldn't submit to a COVID test. At this hearing, Crown prosecutor Karimjee presented the court with a video clip from the dinner, showing Tamara in a three-second congratulatory interaction with Tom.

Tamara's defence counsel, Lawrence Greenspon, asked the Crown's only witness, Ottawa homicide detective Chris Benson, if he was aware that some lawyers from the JCCF and her defence lawyer were present at

---

311 Danton Unger, "Man accused in hit-and-run at Manitoba Freedom Convoy protest granted bail, barred from entering Winnipeg," CTV News Winnipeg, February 7, 2022, accessed May 11, 2023, https://winnipeg.ctvnews.ca/man-accused-in-hit-and-run-at-manitoba-freedom-convoy-protest-granted-bail-barred-from-entering-winnipeg-1.5771619.

the June 16 dinner. The detective didn't even know who her lawyers were and couldn't identify them, nor could he identify JCCF's president and lawyer John Carpay, who sat next to Tamara at the head table.[312] "It seemed to me," Tamara recalls, "he wasn't really into helping Karimjee put me back in jail."[313]

The detective's evidence was also remarkable in that he testified that it was the first time in his experience that a country-wide warrant was issued to arrest a person for breaching a bail condition. Such was the importance to the government of keeping Tamara in jail. At this point, we can't but conclude that this has all the hallmarks of a political enterprise.

Several days later, Justice Harris decided not to allow Tamara bail. Harris said, "It is absolutely ridiculous to think the intention of the court-ordered condition not to communicate could be superseded simply by a lawyer's presence."[314] The conditions did not envision, in Harris's view, for her to be sitting at the same table with Marazzo and posing for a photo. "To add even more fuel to fire, Ms. Lich choose to pose arm-in-arm with Mr. Marazzo. One would find this puzzling." "Such actions most certainly erode public confidence in the administration of justice."[315]

"I was completely shaken," says Tamara. "I was going back to prison, apparently until my criminal trial, whenever that was going to be. I was having trouble keeping up hope after hearing Harris tear into me like that." [316]

In fact, the failure of Harris to release Tamara has done more to bring the administration of justice in disrepute than anything we have seen in a long time.

---

312 As reviewed by Justice A. J. Goodman, "R. v. Lich, 2022 ONSC 4390 at para. 18, (CanLII)," CanLII, accessed May 11, 2023, https://canlii.ca/t/jr3cs.
313 Tamara Lich, 197.
314 Erika Ibrahim, "'Freedom Convoy' organizer Tamara Lich denied bail, ordered detained until trial," *Toronto Star*, Friday, July 8, 2022, accessed May 11, 2023, https://www.thestar.com/politics/2022/07/08/freedom-convoy-organizer-tamara-lich-to-learn-whether-shell-remain-in-jail.html.
315 Glen McGregor, "'Freedom Convoy' organizer Tamara Lich to stay in jail until trial," CTV News, July 8, 2022, accessed May 11, 2023, https://www.ctvnews.ca/canada/freedom-convoy-organizer-tamara-lich-to-stay-in-jail-until-trial-1.5979392.
316 Tamara Lich, 197.

Justice Harris' lack of legal education is evident in his handling of the case. As noted, the purpose of bail is to protect the public while recognizing that the charged is presumed to be innocent until proven otherwise. The greatest erosion of public confidence was to consider as a breach of bail for a three-second congratulatory moment (and in the presence of counsel) after another court had allowed Tamara to go to Ontario to receive the award and make a speech, not to mention the immense expense for the government of sending two detectives out to fetch her and fly her back to Ottawa. It's simply incredible that a court would hold Tamara deserving of this kind of treatment.

Karen Selick, now a retired lawyer, noted that Harris's "decision effectually imposed a prison term on someone who hasn't yet been tried for the offences she is accused of and is legally entitled to be presumed innocent until her guilt is proven. Yes, there is a reverse onus for breach of a bail condition, but the penalty JP Harris imposed is vastly disproportionate to the breach alleged—namely, a three-second interaction with Tom Marazzo in the presence of other people, possibly including her counsel. The probability they plotted a further convoy in that time period is zero."[317]

The one saving moment for Tamara came when "Robert," a court officer, waited with her at her cell for the vehicle to take her to the detention centre. He told her he was from Poland and that his congregation was praying for her. She was in their view a political prisoner. "'I just want to thank you for everything you've done.'" [318]

"Those few words from Robert changed everything for me that day," Tamara recalls. "They gave me new strength ... he told me it broke his heart to put handcuffs on me. He looked at me and said, 'Don't give up.' I promised I wouldn't." [319]

For the next month Tamara languished in prison, moved from one cell to another due to the outbursts of mentally unstable inmates. She had

---

[317] Karen Selick, "Tamara Lich decision undermines confidence in justice system," *Western Standard*, July 12, 2022, accessed May 11, 2023, https://www.westernstandard.news/opinion/selick-tamara-lich-decision-undermines-confidence-in-justice-system/article_a77fa30a-01f9-11ed-abe9-07e928c09191.html.
[318] Tamara Lich, 198.
[319] Tamara Lich, 198.

writing supplies and a Bible. She wrote out Bible passages, poems and quotes for inspiration and comfort and kept a diary. She called family and friends as often as she was allowed.

July 9 her writing included, "Morning spent reading the Bible. Trying to be strong but am a little emotional when thinking about my daughters."[320]

July 11, she noted she did not have a great sleep. "I need a different mat. At this point I think the hard steel frame would be better. Spent my morning reading the Bible (Ezra and Job. I am really liking Job so far). Wrote my grandma …."[321]

On it went day after day.

Her imprisonment, so unjustified, defies credulity.

### Fifth Court Hearing

Two more days of hearing were held in Ottawa on July 25 and 26.

During the hearings Karimjee emphasized that her charges could bring a ten-year sentence. "He was always bringing up firearms," Tamara observed. "I think as a way to try and paint me as violent and dangerous."[322] Justice Goodman called him out on that asking whether Karimjee knew of a case of a ten-year sentence for a mischief conviction. There was none.

"Karimjee's strategy had backfired," says Tamara, "He had made a big deal of the ten-year sentence and when the judge called him on his crap, he had nothing to back it up."[323]

Then on July 28, Justice Goodman of the Ontario Superior Court issued his decision releasing Tamara, again.

Justice Goodman noted that the justice of the peace must provide "some cogent and reasoned analysis of the evidence … to support the findings."[324] The court is called upon "to make a prediction about the accused person's

---

320 Tamara Lich, 200.
321 Tamara Lich, 201.
322 Tamara Lich, 210.
323 Tamara Lich, 210.
324 "R. v. Lich, 2022 ONSC 4390 at para. 35, (CanLII)," CanLII, accessed May 11, 2023, https://canlii.ca/t/jr3cs.

future conduct, as well as the impact of a decision to release on public confidence in the justice system."[325]

Goodman held that JP Harris erred in requiring Tamara's lawyers to provide direct evidence that there were lawyers at the gala on June 16: "[T]here was an air of reality that legal counsel may have been in close proximity" when Lich and Marazzo were chatting. As Tom said, the gala was organized by lawyers!

Goodman also took the JP's "it is absolutely ridiculous" statement to task, noting that the wording of the bail condition was broad so that as long as legal counsel was present, then Lich and Marazzo were allowed to communicate.[326] Goodman was not impressed: "Thus, properly considered, the claim that counsel were present was not "absolutely ridiculous" or a "misguided excuse" as characterized by the Justice of the Peace."[327] Further, he noted that the JP "may have proceeded to demean the arguments advanced by defence counsel."

Demeaning good faith arguments is not the role of a JP!

Goodman concluded that "the plain language" of the bail condition permitted Tamara and Tom to communicate if "it took place in the presence of counsel. Period. The police and Crown were aware that Ms. Lich would be attending the gala event sponsored by the [JCCF]. With respect, in my view, the Justice of the Peace overemphasized its scope and effect."[328]

Justice Goodman held that the JP also didn't recognize the change in circumstances since Tamara's first arrest, as did Justice Phillips in the previous decision. In other words, the bail was originally premised on the idea that there was a fear that Tamara might re-ignite the protest in Ottawa again. But that was no longer the case. Time had moved on. The truckers had moved on.[329]

---

325 "R. v. Lich, 2022 ONSC 4390 (CanLII)," CanLII, accessed May 11, 2023, https://canlii.ca/t/jr3cs, quoting from *The Law of Bail in Canada*, 3rd ed. (Toronto: Carswell, 2010) at §5:20.
326 Ibid., at paras. 49–51.
327 Ibid., at para. 52.
328 Ibid., at para. 55.
329 Ibid., at paras. 56–60.

Goodman rejected outright the JP's claim that Tamara wasn't prepared to follow court orders. Tamara was faithfully following the bail conditions. She had done nothing that should lead to denying her bail.

JP Harris wrongly stated that Tamara faced up to ten years in jail if convicted. Goodman put a quick slap to that idea, as he noted the previous judges Johnson and Phillips held the view that it is "very doubtful" that Tamara would face any jail time.[330]

Reading Justice Goodman's decision, I came away with the idea that JP Harris had vastly overstated the case against Tamara and had too readily taken the exaggerations of the Crown, Mr. Karimjee, to comprise the truth of the matter. There was no legitimate reason to fear for the "vulnerable victims" of the Ottawa protest because of Tamara and Tom's three-second communication. As Goodman pointed out, it "remains a very live question as to whether there has been a breach of the release order at all" by the three-second communication![331]

Goodman looked at Tamara and warned, "'You're under a microscope ... [a]nd you need to be very careful.'" Then he ordered the bailiff, "Take those shackles off." [332]

With that, Tamara was released on bail yet again. She and her counsel are fully aware that the eagle eyes of the state are scanning the terrain for any twitch to justify another pounce on getting her before the court.

"Karimjee seemed to only win when he was dealing with justices of the peace, who didn't really know the law," Tamara rightly says, "Whenever he came up against real judges, he couldn't convince them of his case." [333]

Tom Marazzo notes that the thing he finds "beautiful" and "hilarious" is that the government "thought that by going after Tamara that maybe they were going to somehow break her, break her spirit, or use her as an example of 'look we could crush you.'"

"It's like, could you have picked the worst person?" asks Tom. "Because Tamara is as hard as nails and she wasn't ever going to be defeated by ... the

---

330 Ibid., at para. 78.
331 Ibid., at para. 99.
332 Tamara Lich, 215.
333 Tamara Lich, 211.

likes of this prosecutor, or Justin Trudeau, or anyone else. There's no way they were going to break Tamara. That's not possible. She's unbreakable."[334]

## The Trial

As this book goes to print the trial of Tamara Lich and Chris Barber is ongoing. Day one was September 5, 2023, and it appears that a decision in the matter may go well into January 2024. Such is the fate of high-profile trials that have huge significance. On trial is not simply Tamara and Chris. Rather, it is the full extent of what is and is not acceptable in Canada for protesting government violation of constitutional rights. The Cathedral is also waiting to see if their low esteem of the Truckers is legitimized.

From my early observations it is highly unlikely that Tamara will be found guilty of criminal mischief and the other charges.[335] Already the Crown decided to "stay" the charges on her breaching her bail conditions.[336] While the Crown said it was due the fact that they want to centre on the other charges, in my view, it simply meant that the Crown recognized it did not have a chance on convicting her.

Further, from my following of the press reports it does appear that Justice Heather Perkins-McVey is doing our justice system great service by her questioning of the Crown and her investigation into Crown documents that were redacted when in her view they should not have been.[337] That is but one example of her professional and admirable approach to ensure that justice is carried out. No doubt she is more than aware of the fact that tens of thousands of Canadians are watching her every move.

---

334 See my interview with Tom Marazzo at https://firstfreedoms.ca/trudeaus-tiananmen-square/https://firstfreedoms.ca/trudeaus-tiananmen-square/.
335 She is charged with, mischief, obstructing police, counselling others to commit mischief, and intimidation.
336 Laura Osman, "Crown drops bail violation charge against 'Freedom Convoy' organizer Tamara Lich," The Canadian Press, October 16, 2023, https://edmonton.citynews.ca/2023/10/23/cp-newsalert-crown-drops-bail-violation-charge-against-convoy-organizer-tamara-lich/
337 David Fraser, "Judge orders Crown to disclose internal police documents in convoy trial," CBC News, October 31, 2023, https://www.cbc.ca/news/canada/ottawa/judge-orders-crown-to-disclose-internal-police-documents-in-convoy-trial-1.7014149

Now consider the complete waste of taxpayers' money that was expended in tracking Tamara down across the country for such utterly fooling charges of her breaching her bail conditions. Never have we seen such disregard of the basic right of the inviolability of the person in Canada.

Even if she were convicted on any of the other charges, I cannot see how she will spend anymore time behind bars. She has paid and has been put through enough.

## Conclusion

I cannot but conclude that Tamara's treatment by the Crown possesses the air of political interference. For forty-nine days she suffered incarceration while trying to obtain a lasting release on bail. That must be a new Canadian record. It was all so unnecessary.

I'm not privy to any direct political interference by the prime minister in this case, comparable to what happened in the Jody Wilson-Raybould case. However, it's suspicious how the Crown prosecutor took such an unusual interest in aggressively pursuing Tamara. Or, as Justice Goodman so politely puts it, "Mr. Karimjee is passionate about the case and forcefully represents the Crown's interests on behalf of the community."[338] What would motivate such a "passionate" response by the Crown? One is left to speculate.

It was imperative to get Tamara freed on bail rather than allow her to be locked up until trial,[339] in terms of the best interests of the community. The mistreatment of Tamara smacks of a government more concerned than anything else about sending the message to any non-government-supported activist that they best not act against any government narrative.

I would hate to say that our judicial system has been politicised in the process, but it has come awfully close at the justice of the peace level. I think we would agree that the Superior Courts handled the matter in a very judicious manner—worthy of great respect. The actions of the Crown in this case, however, are unacceptable. The Crown slanted toward politicization in a way unheard of in Canada's modern times.

---

338 "R. v. Lich, 2022 ONSC 4390 (CanLII)," at para. 93.
339 Which finally got underway on September 6, 2023.

Consider Tom Marazzo's view, which I'm sure reflects many in Canada. He reminded me of the cost the taxpayers had to pay for the entire re-arresting of Tamara at her home, all because of "this Crown, or should I say 'clown' prosecutor, [who] is a Liberal card-carrying member, and a donor to the federal Liberal Party of Canada. You can't tell me that this is not politically motivated. It absolutely is politically motivated."

Again, perception is crucial when it comes to justice. Justice is to be done and *seen to be done*. "I mean, come on!" said Tom. "There were no reasonable grounds that they were going to get a conviction based off of a photograph. How did this serve the public's interest to even take these actions against Tamara in the first place? It's absolutely the intimidation of the public."

The Trucker Freedom Convoy has laid bare the good, the bad, and the ugly of our justice system. Seeing what has happened to Tamara may well lead to changes in how we do bail in this country. Surely, we can see that the system is broken. The expense that the Crown incurred to chastise, harass, and literally imprison Tamara because of its hypersensitive interpretation of the bail conditions is way over the top. It is unjust.

We've seen two instances of justices of the peace taking very questionable approaches toward Tamara. They both refused to let her out on bail despite there being no reasonable concern of her breaching bail conditions or of her being a harm to the public interest.

What is evident, however, is that judges, like all of us, live in the community, and we must expect them to come to their own conclusions about the politics of the time in which they live. They will have their own inherent bias. The tenor of the times as exhibited by the prime minister, his ministers, the mainstream media, academia, and the Cathedral is that the Trucker Freedom Convoy was a dangerous event. All support of the convoy must be crushed, in their view.

Chances are the JPs didn't speak to the various truckers and protesters who lost everything from the government's mandates. They were snug in their homes with no fear of losing a paycheque and didn't experience the pain that the protesters felt. Nor did they likely experience the protest itself. Therefore, they can be excused for having not seen the goodwill and cheer of the crowd. They also couldn't see the tens of thousands of people who critically assessed their own experience against the government's constant message of fear and demonization over COVID-19.

The judiciary was not part of the Trudeau-labelled "fringe minority." They weren't the ones labelled "racist, misogynist, and anti-science" by the prime minister. They had no fear of continuing to be a minority in an increasingly hostile environment, where they weren't allowed to travel or leave the country. They suffered no loss of their homes due to decisions made on conscience. They simply couldn't relate. Further, they had no appreciation of the fact that this protest was a non-violent one with a carnival-like atmosphere, not the typical smash-and-dash burning of police cars or the like.

The judiciary is reclusive by nature. This exclusivity insulates the judges from the street. That's a good thing although perhaps this makes them more susceptible to being influenced by the "echo chamber" that is the news on Canadian TV and major news websites these days, and therefore unaware of "the other side" of the story. We don't want political judges. Nor do we want judges who opine every time they're presented with an opportunity to speak on controversial matters that may well come before them in court down the line. That insulation can only go so far. Ultimately, the judiciary is in the world but not of the world, in the sense of not being partial. Impartiality is a must.

We saw the judiciary in Tamara's case reflect on the intricacies of the lower court decisions. They weighed those decisions in the balance of justice and found them wanting. That's how it should be. That's how it must be if we're to live in a free country.

The Great Canadian Trucker Protest woke us up to the reality of the judiciary's role in ensuring that justice is not only *done* but also *seen to be done*. We now await the ongoing trial verdicts.

# 8. Exposed the Failure of the Academics

AS I WALKED through the crowds in Ottawa, I was struck by one conversation I had with a truck mechanic from Windsor, Ontario. He was very proud of the fact that he and his wife had sacrificed to ensure that both of their children were able to go to university without debt: "This is a big deal for us. We are not educated people. We are the lower middleclass, but we wanted what we thought was best for our children. But now our children are suffering the craziness of the university bureaucrats. My children cannot attend classes because they are not vaccinated!"

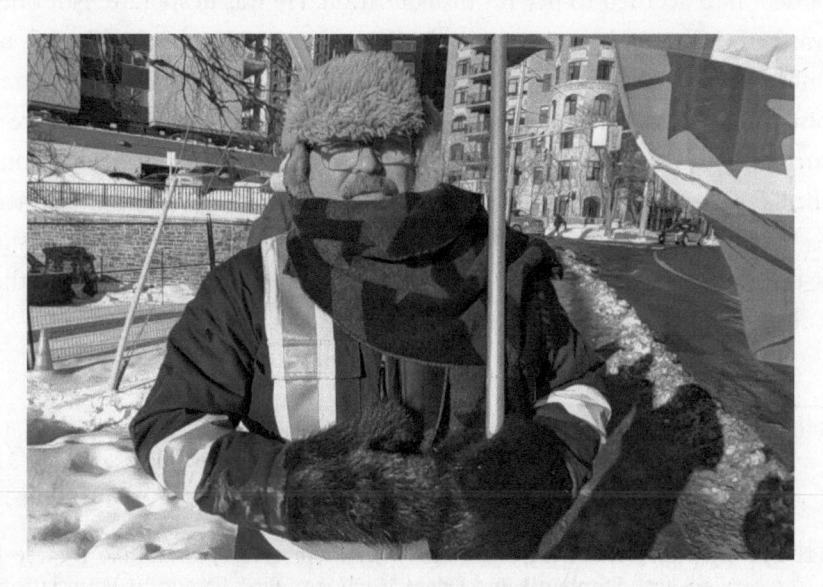

*My Children Cannot Attend Classes*

I could see his disgust and outright frustration over what he and his family were facing because of the university's policy. Incidentally, as I write this, an eruption has occurred at one of my alma maters, Western University in London, Ontario, which decided that all students must have their vaccines up to date and must wear masks for the 2022–2023 school year. Only a few kilometres across the city, Fanshawe College requires neither.[340] One must conclude that the science at Western is different than the science at Fanshawe. "Science" has become, like most things in our society, whatever those in authority say it is—which, of course, doesn't give us much confidence. We must do our own due diligence.

The Trucker Freedom Convoy emboldened students to speak out. A student named David contacted me just as the truckers were beginning to agitate against the imposed vaccine trucker mandate.[341] David was in turmoil. He had one course left to complete his four-year astrophysics degree at Ryerson University in Toronto, but unless he agreed to be vaccinated, he was going to be booted out of the program.

Imagine the upheaval he was going through. He faced an uncertain future without the university diploma that means much for employment in the aerospace industry—not to mention the tens of thousands of dollars of debt he'd accrued to pay for his education. He was desperate. Not only was he facing expulsion from university, but so was Stephanie, his wife of only a few weeks when I met them. She dreamt of being a physical therapist, but with only one semester left to complete her bio-medical degree, she refused "the jab." She had investigated the claims being made about the COVID-19 "vaccines" and determined they were not what they claimed to be. She was troubled by the idea that as a healthy young person, she had little to fear from the COVID-19 virus, yet the government and the university insisted that she take the jab or be expelled.

---

340 Ashley Hyshka, "Western revokes COVID-19 vaccine policy, mask mandate remains in effect," CTV News, November 29, 2022, accessed May 11, 2023, https://london.ctvnews.ca/western-revokes-covid-19-vaccine-policy-mask-mandate-remains-in-effect-1.6173756.

341 See my interview of David and his wife Stephanie, "No Jab, No Degree—Interview with Stephanie and David Machuca," First Freedoms Foundation, accessed May 11, 2023, https://firstfreedoms.ca/no-jab-no-degree/.

David wanted to talk to someone to find some middle ground: an arrangement to study online. No one would answer his questions. Ryerson bureaucracy hid behind the "policy of the university." That wasn't good enough for David. He wanted to know why last year, at the beginning of the COVID crisis, the students a year ahead of him were able to complete their final course online, but this year he was not. The only difference was the availability of a vaccine.

Yet the danger of COVID to young people his age remains negligible. According to data, David has a huge probability of recovering from the virus, should he be infected.[342] If the intention is to protect others who may be at higher risk, forcing David to get the shot does not help them either, since the vaccine doesn't prevent transmission of the disease.

David and Stephanie are also conscientious objectors. Not only are they unconvinced by the claims of the government's "science," but they're also opposed to the vaccine based on their deeply held religious beliefs. To them, religion is not about rules; it is a profoundly personal relationship. They spoke to me about their view that their bodies are the temple of God, and they don't want to put anything in their bodies that would dishonour God's temple.

David and Stephanie, along with four other university students, drove over two hours to come to my house to share their experiences. They described their fruitless appeals to bureaucrats who sent them emails saying there was nothing they could do because of university policy. To these students, such a policy has the effect of a law threatening to end their educational careers and ruin their chances to earn a living.

As I listened to six of Canada's bright, courageous, and intelligent young people, I shook my head at the tyranny of the faceless bureaucracy that now dominates Canada. High and mighty deciders of policy think it somehow righteous to destroy the lives of conscientious young people who dare question the rationality of taking a vaccine that is proving to be

---

342 Angelo Maria Pezzullo, Cathrine Axfors, Despina G. Contopoulos-Ioannidis, Alexandre Apostolatos, John P.A. Ioannidis, "Age-stratified infection fatality rate of COVID-19 in the non-elderly population," Environmental Research, Volume 216, Part 3, 2023, 114655, ISSN 0013-9351, https://doi.org/10.1016/j.envres.2022.114655.

much less effective than claimed for a disease that would likely have no impact on their health.

I assisted them in preparing their religious exemption letters based on my years working on human rights cases. Unfortunately, all but two of those I helped were denied the exemptions. One student at Seneca College got his religious exemption. The other was David, studying astrophysics at Ryerson. David wasn't granted religious exemption per se, but through the efforts of his professors, he was able to do the course online and finish his degree. His wife was not so blessed—although because of the eventual change in policy at Ryerson, she was able to sign up again in September for the following school year. A totally unnecessary inconvenience.

I found it rather disconcerting to see that the correspondence rejecting the exemption applications from colleges and universities were strikingly similar. The documentation of the federal government lawyers as developed in Transport Canada for air carriers look eerily familiar.[343] They are biased toward rejecting religious exemption applications. I'm left wondering if there wasn't some government legal help given to the educational institutions as well. Although some may accuse me of being conspiratorial with this question, it certainly seems logical, given other revelations that have come to light in past months.

There are so many moments over the three years of the COVID-19 pandemic I found myself saying, "No, it can't be. Surely that's not the case. I don't want to promote 'conspiracy theories.'" But then I find out that my suspicions were, indeed, reality. For example, I questioned whether the "science" that the prime minister talked about really did say that the unvaccinated couldn't travel. Now we know it did not. It's thoroughly shameful that in a stated health crisis we must second guess what we hear from our elected and once trusted institutional leaders.

The academic world claims to be our society's "critical thinkers." I have spent a considerable amount of my life studying in universities; I understand the importance of critical thinking. The academic pursuit is one that I thoroughly believe in. I want to know and understand things myself. And though I have a lot of formal education, I recognize that I am but a boy on

---

[343] See the affidavit of Jennifer Little as noted above at:

the beach throwing a stone into the sea of knowledge that is out there yet to discover.[344]

My PhD dissertation delved into Thomas S. Kuhn's work *The Structure of Scientific Revolutions*,[345] wherein he describes the "paradigm shifts" that occur in science. It's not all about what is found in a test tube. Science involves a huge amount of the "human factor"—those "aha!" moments of discovery. The scientific data are there for all to see. What the data mean is that there is a divergence of views. It's not surprising to have different scientists with different interpretations, and different consequences flow from those different interpretations.

We had many "aha!" moments during the COVID-19 crisis. A very few brave, courageous academics who followed the science and not the politics spoke out against what they perceived as the mischaracterizations, and in some cases outright lies, told by politicians and their public health advisors—who should've known better. The brave few soon felt the ire of their colleagues and administrators for speaking out.[346]

The academic institutions showed themselves to be uncritical—except when it came to nonconformists![347] Instead of pursuing their own

---

344 A take from Sir Isaac Newton who said, "I don't know what I may seem to the world; but as to myself, I seem to have been only like a boy playing on the sea-shore and diverting myself in now and then finding a smoother pebble or a prettier shell than ordinary, whilst the great ocean of truth lay all undiscovered before me." As noted in Joseph Spence, *Observations, Anecdotes, and Characters, of Books and Men*, (London: John Murray, 1820), 158–159.
345 Thomas S. Kuhn, *The Structure of Scientific Revolutions*, 2nd Ed., Enlarged, (Chicago: The University of Chicago Press, 1970).
346 For example, Daniel Caudle, "Controversial U of G prof criticizes school's vaccine mandate: A letter penned by Byram Bridle says he has been banned from the campus for a year," *Guelph Today*, September 27, 2021, accessed May 11, 2023, https://www.guelphtoday.com/local-news/controversial-u-of-g-prof-criticizes-schools-vaccine-mandate-4456348, and Graeme McNaughton, "Guelph Immunologists raise concerns on U of Guelph prof's views on COVID-19 vaccine safety," *Guelph Mercury Tribune*, June 21, 2021, accessed May 11, 2023, https://www.thestar.com/local-guelph/news/2021/06/21/immunologists-raise-concerns-on-u-of-guelph-prof-s-views-on-covid-19-vaccine-safety.html
347 For an interesting discussion, see "Death by a 1000 Cuts—Interview with Jennifer Kabbany," First Freedoms Foundation, accessed May 11,

inquiry, they decided to go with the interpretation of the science that the government proclaimed. The practical reason is rather obvious, since much of the educational budgets come from government sources. As we've seen with the federal government's practice in the Canada Summer Jobs file, institutions will only get the money when they agree with the government's ideology. Plus, we can't discount the fact that all the pharmaceutical corporations that hand out grants to universities have a keen interest in ensuring that the universities are in tune with the "science" they advocate. Of course, we must accept, by faith, that there is no conflict of interest. We must "trust the experts."

Or maybe it is a case of "belief perseverance," the concept that despite evidence to the contrary, we will continue to hold to our beliefs. Religion often has a "belief perseverance" component to it, and I can't but wonder if we're not witnessing the same phenomena in those advocating the government narrative on COVID—even in the so-called "critical thinking" universities.

Jeffrey A. Tucker strikes at the heart of academia's willingness to go along with the COVID narrative, saying the issue comes down to the "fungibility" of an academic career. An academic's career isn't easily exchangeable. It's very difficult for an academic to go from one institution to another. Their marketplace is small, and it requires a huge amount of time and resources to be qualified to teach at the university level, but there are few opportunities. Therefore, "career paths absolutely require compliance with prevailing narratives. Any deviation could lead to potential doom for them. The spirit of going along is the driving force of everything they do."[348] Tucker points out that the academic career requires advancement based on "who you know and how much they like you." The academic "must play the game or else face career death." They cannot risk offending their colleagues or their administration. Stepping out of line ruins their careers.

---

2023,https://firstfreedoms.ca/death-by-a-1000-cuts-interview-with-jennifer-kappany/.

348 Jeffrey A. Tucker, "Why Did So Many Intellectuals Refuse to Speak Out?" Brownstone Institute, October 6, 2022, accessed May 11, 2023, https://brownstone.org/articles/why-did-so-many-intellectuals-refuse-to-speak-out/.

This means that those who speak the truth are typically those who can afford to do so without any fear of loss. They are retired, or otherwise financially independent, and have no career aspirations to worry about. Their family's livelihood is not on the line if they speak the truth. Ultimately, very few people are able or willing to sacrifice their personal comfort for speaking the truth. It's rare in any context, but perhaps even rarer in the academic community.

But truth, like water, has a way of leaking out.

The Trucker Freedom Convoy opened the hearts of young people in the universities to recognize that they weren't the only ones to question the COVID-19 rules of the academic world. The truckers might be blue-collar workers without fancy degrees, but they knew something was off. By comparison, only a few academics were willing to put their careers on the line and critically analyze what was occurring on their doorstep.[349]

The challenge to the academic community is profound. Right now, academics think that their institutions are too big and important to fail. But if it turns out that a significantly sized group of Canadians begin to question the utility of higher education, and if the universities are more interested in "progressive" woke politics than in meaningful critical study, then higher educational institutions shouldn't expect the blue-collar workers, whom the trucker protest represented, to keep paying university bills for their children or through their taxes. A once sleeping bear has been disturbed by academic intransigence.

Professor Jonathan Haidt, a keen observer of the right/left differences of support toward universities in the USA, concludes that the left-leaning bias of higher education has created an existential threat for the university establishment: "We are losing the support of half the country," he told Jordan Peterson. "This is unsustainable."[350] Unsustainable because

---

[349] Canadian Academics for Covid Ethics, accessed May 11, 2023, https://www.academics4covidethics.ca/, see also, "Open letter to the president of the University of Guelph from Dr. Byram Bridle," Justice Centre for Constitutional Freedoms, accessed May 11, 2023, https://www.jccf.ca/open-letter-to-the-president-of-the-university-of-guelph-from-dr-byram-bridle/.

[350] Jordan B Peterson, "The Perilous State of the University: Jonathan Haidt & Jordan B Peterson," YouTube, November 16, 2017, 45:00– https://www.

fifty per cent of the population who pay the taxes for the universities are questioning their value.

If we in Canada think that a political movement to curb the left-wing bias in universities[351] couldn't happen here, we only need to consider the example of the Canadian truckers.

Change is in the air. The Trucker Freedom Convoy is but the first major pushback against the Cathedral that the university establishment supports. There's no reason to think that the taxpaying public won't soon turn its sights on the huge amount of public funding that's funnelled every year to a higher education regime that attacks the very common sense, civic, and moral traditions that created those institutions in the first place.

For now, the university establishment may have won a battle. But the Trucker Freedom Convoy horns are loud. The cry for freedom from academic tyranny will only get louder.

---

youtube.com/watch?v=4lBegL_V6AA,
351  For an engaging discussion of concern even on the left of the left-wing bias in Canadian universities, see my interview with Paige Thombs, self-declared as "very left-leaning and openly gay" in "No Space For Conservative Thought— Interview With Paige Thombs," First Freedoms Foundation, accessed May 11, 2023, https://firstfreedoms.ca/no-space-for-conservative-thought/.

# 9. Exposed the Utter Complicity of Mainstream Media

IT'S FAIR TO say that the mainstream media, by and large, carried the government narrative on COVID-19. For two years prior to the Trucker Freedom Convoy, the media parroted Prime Minister Trudeau's daily update from what Rex Murphy so aptly described as "the Liberal Government at the Bottom of the Cottage Doorsteps."[352]

During the early stages of the pandemic, this kneejerk reaction can be understood as a means of protecting the public from an unknown, potentially catastrophic disease. After a couple of months, however, it had become clear that the disease was not as apocalyptic as first feared. Yet any view that questioned the government narrative was suspect. Indeed, it was portrayed as conspiratorial by the media.

The country had witnessed several political scandals before the COVID pandemic. One example was the prime minister's handling of the Jody Wilson-Raybould affair, which shook our confidence in his honesty (this is described in detail in a previous chapter). Yet the mainstream media focused on his every word without questioning the veracity of his daily claims about the pandemic and the necessity of his various measures to "keep Canadians safe." There was no cost/benefit analysis of the government's COVID measures. Any concern for the economy, the public's mental health, or the loss of freedom was seen as insensitive.

---

352 Rex Murphy, "COVID-19 and our new Government at the Bottom of the Cottage Doorsteps," *National Post*, May 6, 2020, accessed May 11, 2023, https://nationalpost.com/opinion/rex-murphy-covid-19-and-our-new-government-at-the-bottom-of-the-cottage-doorsteps.

Before the convoy, the mainstream media actively censored and suppressed any opposing view. For example, it was racist to say that the virus came from the Wuhan lab. CBC ran a story claiming that that *The Epoch Times* was racist because it dared to suggest that the virus came from the Wuhan lab.[353] That story did not age well, as CBC's original headline stated that *The Epoch Times* said that China made the virus as a bioweapon. "*The Epoch Times*, a newspaper that has polarized people over its content, is coming under fire for advancing a conspiracy theory about the origin of the coronavirus—and having it delivered straight into people's mailboxes unsolicited."[354]

The "conspiracy theory," as labelled by CBC, is currently viewed by US authorities as the "more likely" scenario.[355] Rather than allow for open debate about such matters, the media developed its own group-think and shot down any opposing view as "racist." The failure to permit free speech will be a dark spot for our legacy media for years to come. It's not conspiratorial to say that opposing voices were literally silenced. The Orwellian nature of our media must not be forgotten.

When the Trucker Freedom Convoy got rolling, the mainstream media came out with their typeset blazing at the alleged violence, intimidation, and harassment by the truckers toward the people of Ottawa. It seemed to be a joke among the journalists to make fun of the "backward," uneducated truckers who were seen as science deniers. Overall, the press was all

---

353 Andrea Bellemare, Jason Ho, and Katie Nicholson, "Some Canadians who received unsolicited copy of *Epoch Times* upset by claim that China was behind virus," CBC News, April 29, 2020, accessed May 11, 2023, https://www.cbc.ca/news/canada/epoch-times-coronavirus-bioweapon-1.5548217.
354 Ibid., Editor's Note.
355 Michael R. Gordon and Warren P. Strobel, "Lab Leak Most Likely Origin of Covid-19 Pandemic, Energy Department Now Says," *Wall Street Journal*, February 26, 2023, accessed May 11, 2023, https://www.wsj.com/articles/covid-origin-china-lab-leak-807b7b0a; John Robson, "Lifting the Taboo on Discussing COVID's Possible Lab-Leak Origin Signals a Return to Sanity and Civility," *The Epoch Times*, February 27, 2023, accessed May 11, 2023, https://www.theepochtimes.com/john-robson-lifting-the-taboo-on-discussing-covids-possible-lab-leak-origin-signals-a-return-to-sanity-and-civility_5084356.html.

too willing to parrot the "fringe minority with unacceptable views" spirit of the prime minister.[356]

A simple review of the media coverage reveals the journalists' bias against the truckers in the way they framed their reporting. Here are a few examples. An article by Christopher Reynolds[357] was entitled, "Truckers should have done more to prepare for vaccine mandate, experts say." Notice the reference to "experts." The COVID era is the era of the ubiquitous "expert" magnified in the press. Reynolds referenced "experts" who faulted the truckers for not accepting a vaccine mandate that, according to the article, was supported by most of the public.

Like Reynolds, Jason Warick of the CBC referred in his piece to the "experts." His title: "Illogical for truck convoy to claim freedoms threatened by vaccine mandate, say experts."[358] According to this piece, the "experts" claimed the truckers' position made "no sense." Among the experts quoted were Associate Professor Alexander Crizzle, at the University of Saskatchewan, who said the truckers should accept the vaccination "as just one more thing." In other words, it's the cost of doing business. Another expert, Professor Ahmed Shalaby of the University of Manitoba said that the rules are meant to protect everyone, including the truckers; Shalaby was also concerned that the truckers were being distracted on the roads by the crowds waving flags. Also cited in the article is trucker Sean Tiessen, who is quoted as saying the mandates were "draconian, fascist." He insisted, "If I don't want to get a shot, that's my right and it's none of your

---

356 Brian Lilley, "Media's handling of trucker convoy one-sided, inflammatory, shameful
Can we really be shocked that public trust in the media continues to fall?" *Toronto Sun*, January 28, 2022, accessed May 11, 2023, https://torontosun.com/opinion/columnists/lilley-medias-handling-of-trucker-convoy-one-sided-inflammatory-shameful.

357 Christopher Reynolds, "Truckers should have done more to prepare for vaccine mandate, experts say," CTV News, January 21, 2022, accessed May 11, 2023, https://www.ctvnews.ca/politics/truckers-should-have-done-more-to-prepare-for-vaccine-mandate-experts-say-1.5749984.

358 Jason Warick, "Illogical for truck convoy to claim freedoms threatened by vaccine mandate, say experts," CBC News, January 28, 2022, accessed May 11, 2023, https://www.cbc.ca/news/canada/saskatoon/truck-convoy-vaccination-freedoms-1.6330176.

f--king business." So, put side by side, the university "experts" are logical, according to Warick, but the truckers are "salty" and, well, just illogical.

Another CBC journalist, Nil Köksal, suggested falsely that the truckers were supported by Russia.[359] Joy Henderson's opinion piece in the *Toronto Star* said that the truckers were white supremacists who got a free pass in Canada compared to Indigenous and Black protesters.[360] Nothing like upping the ante against those evil trucker types!

Saleema Nawaz of the *Montreal Gazette* said:

> With its brazen display of swastikas and confederate flags in the nation's capital, the hostile harassment of residents and local businesses and riotous occupation of downtown streets by what seemed to be a mix of hooligans and would-be militia members, the trucker convoy has vividly brought home the dangerous reach of misinformation.[361]

Nawaz observed, "Listening to the protesters, one thing became evident: we are not all working with the same set of facts. Too many people have been misled by online conspiracy theories and far-right narratives."

One thing is true: there can be no doubt that we are "not all working with the same set of facts." While Nawaz bemoaned, as did the prime minister, that there were multiple "swastikas and confederate flags," there was only evidence of one of each. When the crowd saw the Confederate

---

359 Cosmin Dzsurdzsa, "CBC anchor invents conspiracy about Russia orchestrating freedom convoy," *True North*, January 29, 2022, accessed May 11, 2023, https://tnc.news/2022/01/29/cbc-anchor-invents-conspiracy-about-russia-orchestrating-freedom-convoy/.
360 Joy Henderson, "While Canada cracks down on Indigenous and Black protesters, White supremacists get a free pass in Canada. Just look at the convoy," *Toronto Star*, January 29, 2022, accessed May 11, 2023, https://www.thestar.com/opinion/contributors/2022/01/29/while-indigenous-and-black-people-are-killed-for-speaking-up-white-supremacists-get-a-free-pass-in-canada-just-look-at-the-convoy.html.
361 Saleema Nawaz, "Trucker convoy spotlights urgent need for media literacy," *Montreal Gazette*, March 1, 2022, accessed May 11, 2023, https://montrealgazette.com/opinion/columnists/nawaz-trucker-convoy-spotlights-urgent-need-for-media-literacy.

flag, they told the person to leave[362] because that was not what the protest or protesters were about. The Nazi flag bearer was never seen beforehand or afterwards. Was this a "hit-and-run" photo-op designed to smear the convoy? Who knows. There seems to be a lack of interest among the mainstream media to find out. Meanwhile, independent media want to know.[363]

Even though the protest ended over a year ago, the Trucker Freedom Convoy continues to be a target for journalist insults and insinuations: a sort of shorthand to dismiss or discredit anyone who was involved or even sympathetic toward the protestors. Consider the September 2022 piece written by John Ivison of the *National Post*, who called out Pierre Poilievre for supporting the convoy. Although Ivison was critical of the government's use of the *Emergencies Act*, he was also critical of the convoy, condemning Poilievre for dabbling in conspiratorial waters."[364]

Ivison's account drips with sarcasm.

Look out, "convoy supporters"! You're under suspicion for dipping your toes into "conspiratorial waters."

---

362 "Watch: Canadian trucker convoy protesters confront masked man with Confederate flag, tell him to leave," *Post Millennial*, January 30, 2022, accessed May 11, 2023, https://thepostmillennial.com/canadian-trucker-convoy-confront-masked-man-confederate-flag.

363 Candice Malcolm, "Everything we know so far about the Nazi Flag guy," *True North*, January 30, 2022, accessed May 11, 2023, https://tnc.news/2022/01/30/everything-we-know-so-far-about-the-nazi-flag-guy2/.

364 John Ivison, "Poilievre should know better than to tear down Canadian institutions," *National Post*, September 7, 2022, accessed May 11, 2023, https://nationalpost.com/opinion/john-ivison-poilievre-should-know-better-than-to-tear-down-canadian-institutions.

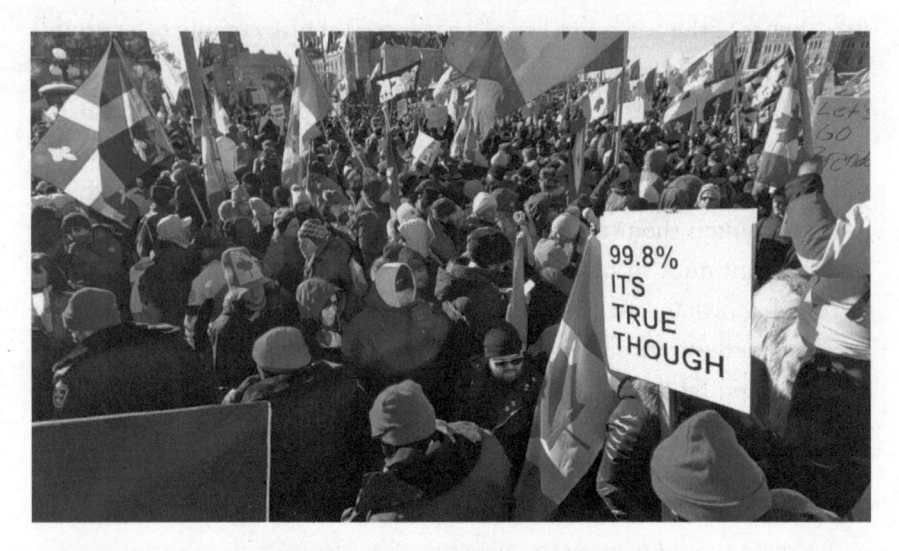

*Truth A Rare Commodity In Today's Age*

The Trucker Freedom Convoy has become a dividing line, in the same way the vaccinated versus unvaccinated demarcation occurred. Yet the convoy organizers I've read and listened to made it clear that the protest was non-violent with no interest in conspiratorial theories. It was simply a call to end the government overreach as illustrated by the mandates and restore people's basic freedoms of speech, conscience, and mobility.[365]

What is it about this protest that drives the media to take such a negative view of it? Was it that truckers were perceived as "denying science"? If so, what about the scientists like Dr. Byram Bridle, who engaged in the protest? The usual comeback is, "He's not legitimate." Why? "Well, because he doesn't support the vaccine. Only those who support the vaccine are correct." As Bruce Pardy points out, if you don't support the progressive narrative, you are wrong—full stop. It's a vicious cycle of condemnation for having the wrong opinion.

That's the problem. The ideological commitments of the press have blinded their ability to critically assess the broader picture. Peter Menzies

---

[365] "What is Going On in Ottawa? Freedom Feature Interview with Davina Peters, Nadine Ness, and Don Hutchinson," First Freedoms Foundation, accessed May 11, 2023, https://firstfreedoms.ca/what_is_going_on_in_ottawa_freedom_feature/.

observes that this one-sided approach leads to a loss of public trust. He explains, "traditional news media are under siege largely because the public has lost faith in their ability to be good at the objective practice of their craft and see them as putting their own wants, needs, beliefs and crusades ahead of the public interest."[366]

Still a mystery to me is the mainstream media's lack of sympathy when the government imposed the Emergencies Act and then later sent in the riot squad dressed for war against unarmed protesters. One can only imagine the media reaction if these powers had been assumed by the Stephen Harper government. Then again, as Bruce Pardy points out, "repressive tolerance" justifies violence if it's used to implement the policies of the so called "progressive" group.

Consider the events of the final days of the protest:

> February 14, 2022: According to the Prime Minister of Canada, public order was under threat. A national emergency had to be declared because protestors with unacceptable views had "occupied" the city of Ottawa. So menacing were the truckers, with their bouncy castles and hot tubs, that none of the nation's existing laws could combat such a dire crisis. Obviously, dialogue was out of the question. The only way to free Ottawa was to take away all the rights that Canadians once cherished.
>
> February 18–20, 2022: Police from around the country were deployed *en masse* for the takedown of those unarmed truckers and their fellow protesters. Batons, "chemical irritants," mounted police, and commandeered tow trucks were all part of the arsenal called forth to bring peace, order, and good government.

---

366 Peter Menzies, "Objectivity: What Journalists Hate but the Public Still Craves," *C2C Journal*, August 31, 2022, accessed May 11, 2023, https://c2cjournal.ca/2022/08/objectivity-what-journalists-hate-but-the-public-still-craves/.

February 21, 2022: When the House of Commons voted on the continued use of the Emergencies Act, the Prime Minister implied that the outcome would be a matter of confidence, meaning he would dissolve parliament and call another election if his government lost the vote.[367] The Liberals dutifully supported the motion, as did the NDP led by Mr. Singh. The government won 185–151.

February 23, 2022: Just before the Senate was to hold their vote on the Emergencies Act, the Prime Minister—perhaps realizing that the Senate was likely to vote against the Act—decided that he had enough "tools" to deal with the situation and no longer needed an additional three weeks of emergency powers.[368]

From one dizzying extreme to the other—first dismissing the protestors as an insignificant "fringe," then proclaiming them to be one of the greatest threats ever faced in Canadian history—the press rallied behind the prime minister with each twist and turn.

Andrew Coyne, a well known and distinguished journalist, reacted to lifting of emergency powers by mocking those of us who called out the abuse of power. Coyne tweeted, "So ... not martial law then. Not the beginning of an endless night of repression. Not Tiananmen, or Hitler's Germany, or any of the other unbelievably silly things grown adults worked themselves into saying. Ottawa is ending the use of the Emergencies Act."[369]

Consider Mr. Coyne's derision toward the "unbelievably silly things grown adults worked themselves into saying."

---

367 Mia Rabson & Marie Woolf, "*Emergencies Act* motion passes after heated House of Commons debate," *Canada's National Observer*, February 22, 2022, accessed May 11, 2023, https://www.nationalobserver.com/2022/02/22/news/emergencies-act-motion-passes-house-commons-debate.

368 Nick Boisvert, "Trudeau ends use of Emergencies Act, says 'situation is no longer an emergency', CBC News, February 23, 2022, https://www.cbc.ca/news/politics/trudeau-event-feb23-1.6361847.

369 Andrew Coyne (@acoyne), "So ... not martial law then. Not the beginning of an endless night of repression. Not Tiananmen, or Hitler's Germany," February 23, 2022, 4:49 PM, https://twitter.com/acoyne/status/1496603089578692609?lang=en.

Was it "silly" to be alarmed when the prime minister refused to engage in any kind of negotiation or de-escalation before invoking the most powerful and punitive authority possible in our democracy so that he could put down a peaceful protest? (Regarding the government's insistence that the protests amounted to a violent siege, it's worth reiterating that, yes, the protests were disruptive. Yet there was no torching of vehicles or smashing of shop windows, no tearing down of statues or burning of churches, no axe-wielding assaults on police officers.)

The prime minister deemed a gathering of truckers and sympathizers so "dangerous" it warranted the complete and chilling suspension of our rights and freedoms. The Emergencies Act opened a panoply of powers for state forces to engage in surveillance, imprisonment, detention, and freezing of bank accounts, all because citizens didn't accept the ideological commitments of the prime minister. And opposition to such egregious behaviour is somehow "silly?"

In truth, it's becoming increasingly difficult to engage in public dialogue when the mainstream media has become the propaganda arm of the government. Given the huge subsidies the government is giving to the media companies, perhaps that's to be expected.

The Trucker Freedom Convoy smoked out the media in more ways than I have room to expand upon. I look forward to those brave scholars who will take it upon themselves to conduct a thorough empirical investigation of the data to show exactly how askew the reporting of mainstream media was on the convoy. Perhaps the "woke" nature of Canadian mainstream media has played a major role.[370]

The problem with any "misinformation" in media is that people who trust the media will be convinced of the perspective being portrayed. In other words, if people aren't questioning the validity of their newspapers, they're more apt to be deceived if their trusted media source goes rogue. There's already a sense that in polite company you don't disclose that you

---

370 David Rozado and Aaron Wudrick, "Northern awokening: How social justice and woke language have infiltrated Canadian news media," MLI, March 8, 2023, accessed May 11, 2023, https://macdonaldlaurier.ca/northern-awokening-how-social-justice-and-woke-language-have-infiltrated-canadian-news-media/.

supported the Trucker Freedom Convoy. Given the way things are going, it just might be the end of your career and your friendships, as we are seeing in the police forces.

Even after the protest, the media have continued their role as propagandists for the government. In July 2022, the prime minister went to Calgary for the Stampede, where he was, allegedly, surrounded by adoring masses. That's what we were told. Pictures flooded the government-subsidized press of the prime minister in his cowboy garb with crowds of admirers supposedly at the Stampede. The Canadian Press's report was picked up by other paid press with headlines like, "'Happy Stampede': Prime minister mobbed by admirers at Stampede events" (*National Post*),[371] and "Prime Minister mobbed by admirers at Stampede pancake breakfast," (*Calgary City News*).[372]

The truth was that Trudeau went to a pancake breakfast put on by his own Liberal MP, George Chahal, held kilometres away from the actual Stampede grounds.[373] It was a staged event, which is fine, of course, but to say or imply that he was at the Calgary Stampede was rather rich. Even less plausible was the "mob" of enthusiastic fans in a region of the country known for its animosity toward the Trudeau family name.[374] Trudeau's spin is characteristic of his government. Remember what Catherine McKenna said about repeating your talking points: "people will totally believe it!"[375]

---

[371] Colette Derworiz and Bill Graveland, "'Happy Stampede': Prime minister mobbed by admirers at Stampede events," *National Post*, July 10, 2022, accessed May 11, 2023, https://nationalpost.com/pmn/news-pmn/canada-news-pmn/happy-stampede-prime-minister-mobbed-by-admirers-at-stampede-pancake-breakfast.

[372] Bill Graveland, "Prime Minister mobbed by admirers at Stampede pancake breakfast," CityNews, July 10, 2022, accessed May 11, 2023, https://calgary.citynews.ca/2022/07/10/trudeau-mobbed-stampede-pancake-breakfast/.

[373] Arthur C. Green, "'Trudeau you're a traitor' Calgary Stampede crowd heckles PM," *Western Standard,* July 11, 2022, accessed May 11, 2023, https://www.westernstandard.news/news/trudeau-you-re-a-traitor-calgary-stampede-crowd-heckles-pm/article_42cfdb10-00f4-11ed-ab83-7b010e68c0c9.html.

[374] Consider the story of Pierre E. Trudeau in "Prime Minister Trudeau faced demonstrators heaving tomatoes and …," UPI, August 9, 1982, accessed May 11, 2023, https://www.upi.com/Archives/1982/08/09/Prime-Minister-Pierre-Trudeau-faced-demonstrators-heaving-tomatoes-and/2710397713600/.

[375] Lorrie Goldstein, "Screeched-in McKenna commits a classic political gaffe," *Toronto Sun*, May 27, 2019, accessed May 11, 2023, https://torontosun.com/

Since the invention of the printing press, the powerful have recognized the power of propaganda. The people must "get the right message." Of course, controlling the people is easier when they are fed lies, or better yet, half-truths, like the prime minister being mobbed by crowds at the Calgary Stampede.

We are living in a time when the office of the Canadian prime minister is a bully pulpit with access to a huge presence in the mainstream media that is heavily subsidized by government funding.[376] The press dislike being reminded of their dependence on the government. They argue that they are professionals and would not report based on who gave them money.

I understand the sensitivity to this issue, but I say if the shoe fits, wear it. From my own observations on the ground in Ottawa compared to the reporting I saw in the press; the differences were irreconcilable. Like it or not, I say the paid-for press is drawing the government's water. I wish it were not so. But in my view, it is.

The government money to the media, says reporter Paul Wells, is "enough to shatter our credibility with some of our readership and some of our audiences ... when someone says you're in the tank of the government, after all they're paying part of your paycheck, I had no rebuttal."[377] He disagreed with that characterization, of course, but he had no credible response.

Tom Marazzo's view, a view that's becoming the position of a growing number of Canadians, is that "by and large the only reason Justin Trudeau can get away with what he has done and what he continues to do is because he funds the mainstream media. They just lap it up and regurgitate what

---

opinion/columnists/goldstein-screeched-in-mckenna-commits-a-classic-political-gaffe.

376 Tom Parry, "Journalists question Liberal government's $600M media bailout plan," CBC News, May 23, 2019, accessed May 11, 2023, https://www.cbc.ca/news/politics/journalists-question-media-bailout-1.5147761.

377 Candice Malcolm, "Canada's top political journalist goes independent (ft. Paul Wells," *True North*, April 20, 2022, accessed May 11, 2023, https://tnc.news/2022/04/20/canadas-top-political-journalist-goes-independent-ft-paul-wells/.

he says. He controls the narrative through the media ... mass formation psychosis can only be made possible through the media, and it works."[378]

Even many conservative journalists and commentators[379] were only too quick to label the truckers as extreme. I don't know if they walked the Ottawa streets or not—it was very cold to do so—but I fear many were conducting laptop journalism and not walking the streets and talking with the people.

This may not be entirely fair to all journalists, given the truckers' explicit instructions not to talk with mainstream media. I hold the view that the truckers were justified in fearing that the CBC and others would twist their words and misrepresent them, but they also left the media with nothing but speculation. Treating the press as enemies ensured they would be antagonists. Therefore, it's reasonable to suggest that those among the mainstream media that did attempt to reach out would have been rebuffed.

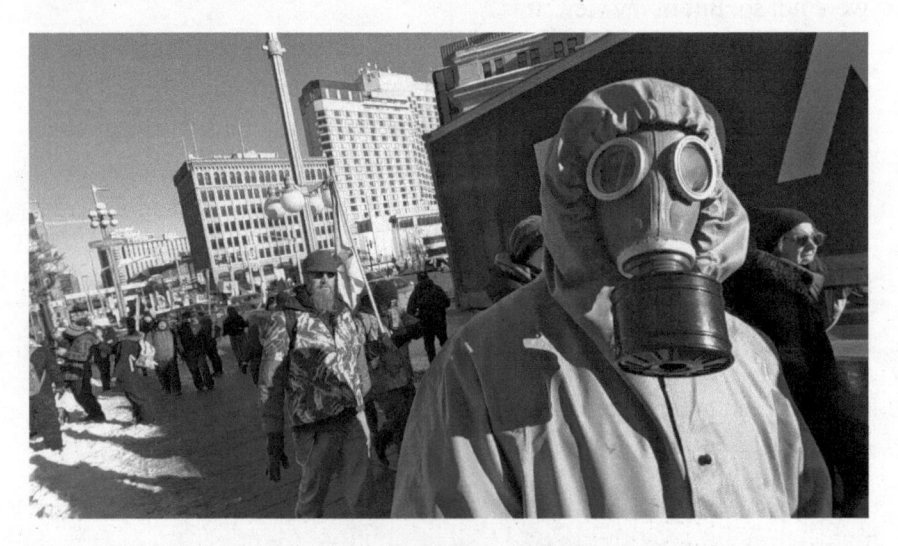

*The Only Way To Be Safe Is Having The Right Equipment!*

---

378 See Barry W. Bussey, "Trudeau's Tiananmen Square—Interview with Tom Marazzo," First Freedoms Foundation, accessed May 31, 2023, https://firstfreedoms.ca/trudeaus-tiananmen-square.

379 Tasha Kheiriddin, "The more Tories support the convoy protest, the less appeal they will hold for voters," *National Post*, February 4, 2022, accessed May 11, 2023, https://nationalpost.com/opinion/tasha-kheiriddin-the-more-tories-support-the-convoy-protest-the-less-appeal-they-will-hold-for-voters.

Consider another very scary situation—the freezing of bank accounts. How can we ever forget the "hand in glove" approach between the prime minister and minister of Finance as they announced the freezing of bank accounts of those who gave money to the truckers? Then somehow there was a "leak" of the donor list from the "GiveSendGo" online giving platform. The pro-government press took it upon themselves to publicly humiliate (and potentially threaten) anyone who gave money to the truckers for fuel and food. Even US Democratic Congresswoman Ilhan Omar tweeted at the time: "I fail to see why any journalist felt the need to report on a shop owner making such a [sic] insignificant donation rather than to get them harassed. It's unconscionable and journalists need to do better."[380] And what a blowback she received for that comment, despite its truth. Again, the message seems quite clear that violence (or behaviour that opens the doors for it to occur) seems all right if it's done "on the right side."

CBC released the names and businesses of donors without regard for their privacy, careers, or even personal safety. Thanks to these efforts, individuals lost their jobs[381] or were threatened with physical violence. For example, a café owner in Ottawa[382] was forced to close her café for a while because people, encouraged by the press and the inflammatory language of the prime minister, threatened to "throw bricks" or "come and get" her employees. She gave a mere $250 to the convoy. Her real transgression was holding the wrong opinion.

In the same way that the unvaccinated were attacked by a tribal mentality, so too were those who gave money to the trucker protest. It was

---

380 Ilhan Omar (@IlhanMN), "I fail to see why any journalist felt the need to report on a shop owner," Twitter, February 16, 2022, 5:57 PM, https://twitter.com/IlhanMN/status/1494083595689943045.

381 Robert Benzie, "Tory staffer suddenly departs Queen's Park after donating $100 to convoy protests," *Toronto Star*, February 15, 2022, accessed June 20, 2023, https://www.thestar.com/politics/provincial/2022/02/15/tory-staffer-suddenly-departs-queens-park-after-donating-100-to-convoy-protests.html

382 Blair Crawford, "Threats close Stella Luna Gelato Café after owner's name appears in GiveSendGo data leak," *Ottawa Citizen*, February 15, 2022, accessed May 11, 2023, https://ottawacitizen.com/news/local-news/threats-close-stella-luna-gelato-cafe-after-owners-name-appears-in-givesendgo-data-leak.

a gross abuse, mob rule by the mainstream media, the so-called "fourth branch." The media have long claimed that they fulfill an important role in keeping the three branches of government (executive, legislative, and judicial) honest and true to democratic principles. That may no longer be the case. More and more they are an arm of the executive, pushing the government's narrative, repeating the government's media releases and press conference talking points.

We are moving into very dangerous waters, especially given the government's ever-advancing regulation over the internet such as the now passed Bill C-11,[383] which is but the beginning of a multiyear project to control information and ultimately to control our speech. The internet was the one place we could all go to find different opinions and discussions. Now, the government is claiming the right to control the internet. CRTC will, as Peter Menzies pointed out, will be spending the next year or so to develop regulations of what we can see and not see on the internet.[384]

Soon any expression deemed "hateful" by an all-knowing government will send shivers down the spine of those who are so labelled.

What refuge or justice will remain for those who disagree with government? Will the present vindictive spirit be turned against those who doxxed small business owners or froze the bank accounts of peaceful protestors? Or will we have the courage, integrity, and wisdom to restore the strength and stability of this great country by returning to the rule of law and the defence of freedom?

The mainstream media's detestation of the Truckers' Convoy revealed once and for all that they are not for the little guy but for the "big guy" who pays their bills. That realization now must play an important part in saving Canada's right to a free press. Given this government's recent passage of the Online Streaming Act,[385] the Online News Act,[386] and the

---

[383] Online Streaming Act, Bill C-11, (Royal Assent), April 27, 2023 https://www.parl.ca/DocumentViewer/en/44-1/bill/C-11/royal-assent, accessed June 22, 2023.

[384] Freedom Feature interview Peter Menzies, with https://firstfreedoms.ca/now-that-bill-c-11-is-law-whats-next-interview-with-peter-menzies/, accessed June 22, 2023.

[385] https://www.parl.ca/DocumentViewer/en/44-1/bill/C-11/royal-assent

[386] https://www.parl.ca/DocumentViewer/en/44-1/bill/C-18/royal-assent

soon to be the "online harms act" will put the government in control of the internet. The internet, which won the free speech public square, is now under threat. The trucker protest reminds us that our freedom demands eternal vigilance.

# 10. Exposed the Complicity of the Banks

THE GENEROSITY OF Canadians was on full display as the Trucker Freedom Convoy made its way across the country. In Winnipeg, thousands of people lined the roads to cheer the convoy and provide sandwiches and other food despite the bitter cold.[387] This came in handy, as the unvaccinated in the convoy weren't permitted to eat in restaurants. The convoy lifted Canadians' spirits, and as one story noted, "Trudeau's problem is not the Truckers; it's the Canadians making sandwiches for the Truckers."[388] The warm selflessness generated by the convoy came as a stark contrast to the bitterly cold greed and control of the government.

---

387 "Trucker convoy opposed to COVID-19 vaccine mandates reaches Winnipeg," Chek News, January 25, 2022, accessed May 11, 2023, https://www.cheknews.ca/trucker-convoy-opposed-to-covid-19-vaccine-mandates-reaches-winnipeg-944047/. "Some waved signs while others handed out sandwiches, snacks and water as the truckers slowly rolled by. Some brought family members and cheered as the thermometer stayed below -20 C."

388 Rita Smith, "Trudeau's problem is not the Truckers; it's the Canadians making sandwiches for the Truckers," January 30, 2022, https://roadwarriornews.com/trudeaus-problem-is-the-canadians-making-sandwiches-for-the-truckers/

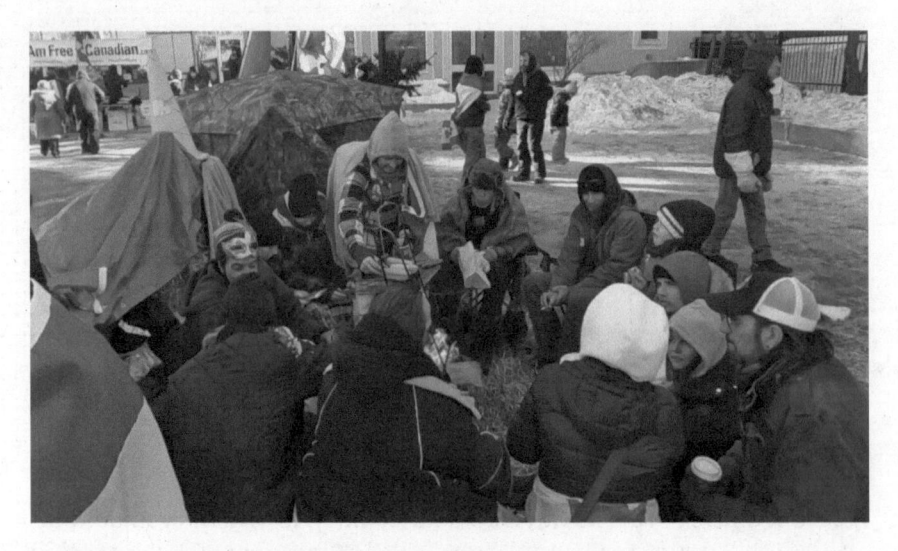

*Strangers Brought Together Despite The Cold*

When the federal government froze bank accounts of those who donated money to assist the Trucker Freedom Convoy, a bitterly cold chill came over me and most of my friends and acquaintances. How was it possible that a "free and democratic" country could stoop so low as to financially punish its own citizens just because they held different views from the government? For that is what happened.

The government tried to spin the protest as an insurrection. It was not an insurrection. An insurrection doesn't involve the deployment of people handing out donuts and hot chocolate at the foot of Parliament Hill. One would expect much more lethal tools for a real insurrection, such as tanks and troop carriers, with some form of fighting force to remove a government—not tractor trailers and protestors, and ball hockey on Wellington.

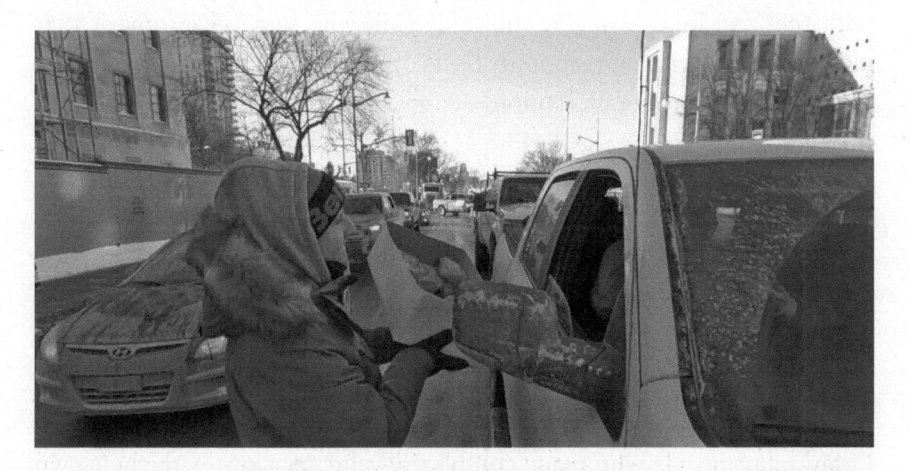

*Canadian Weapons Of Mass Donuts!*

This protest was not an insurrection against the government. There was no chance that the government was going to fall. The prime minister wasn't going to be taken prisoner and held for ransom—although his decision to leave the capital for an "undisclosed location" at Meech Lake gives some indication of the fear he seemed to have about the arrival of the "fringe minority" with "unacceptable views." Therein lies the issue: the protest was a peaceful insurrection against government over-reach.

The government sought to force its own view of the world on its citizens. COVID-19, said the government, was an existential threat that must be put down at all costs, including the cost of truckers losing their incomes if they refused to accept the vaccine mandate. The truckers rejected the government's COVID-19 narrative. For that, the truckers and their supporters were given the comeuppance cabinet thought they deserved—freezing their bank accounts and property.

"[P]rivate property," Richard M. Weaver observed, "... is ... the last metaphysical right remaining to us."[389] The relationship to what we own has never been so explicitly attacked by such a vindictive Canadian government as when bank accounts were frozen during the convoy. Nothing can erase the scene of average Canadians stepping in to supply the convoy

---

389 Richard M. Weaver, *Ideas Have Consequences* (Chicago: University of Chicago Press, 1984), 131.

with fuel and food, while at the same time, the same government that wrought havoc with our economy by its disastrous lockdowns accused the convoy of disrupting our economy. A government so unable to see itself maliciously destroying the livelihood of truckers by removing their vehicle insurance and other government approvals.

The government's outrageous freezing of bank accounts instilled fear in the average Canadian to such a degree that some were afraid to use their debit and credit cards for fear of being traced. This had a huge impact on charitable giving, as people are fearful and hesitant to donate to legitimate causes that may be politically controversial. Consider that donations made to the convoy were one hundred percent legal as the convoy travelled to Ottawa, but people who made completely valid decisions with their own money were then treated as criminals with the release of personal information unlawfully obtained and imposition of the Emergencies Act.

It rammed us head-on with the realization that our financial security hangs on a thread. For the first time, thoughtful Canadians became acutely aware that there is serious liability to their own property if they hold "unacceptable views." Until that moment, as citizens of a free country, we understood that our property was secure, regardless of our opinions. Aside from lawfully imposed taxes, the government could never take our property just because of our political, or even moral, views. Whether we obtained that property by inheritance or by hard work, the result was the same: it was ours. No government could breach that right of ownership.

That understanding of the basic right to private property, that trust in a democratic government's respect for private property, is now irretrievably broken in Canada.

"You don't have an absolute right to own private property in Canada," David Lametti said when asked about the legality of taking Russian assets in Canada.[390] The Trucker Convoy supporters now know what it is to be treated as enemies of the state.

---

390 Cristin Schmitz, "Constitution doesn't bar seizing, selling Russian assets in Canada for Ukraine rebuilding: Lametti," *Law360*, June 9, 2022, accessed September 6, 2023, https://www.law360.ca/articles/37167/constitution-doesn-t-bar-seizing-selling-russian-assets-in-canada-for-ukraine-rebuilding-lametti

You probably know some people who began taking money out of their bank accounts for fear that their beliefs might provoke the party in power to seize their assets. Friends of mine shared how they can no longer trust the banks; they began a steady withdrawal of funds. Other friends have left the country altogether. Faith in their own government has been broken.

There's a rumour going around that Trudeau ended his invocation of the Emergencies Act due to the pressure he received from the big banks. As the story goes, the bankers saw an immediate run on the banks locally and internationally by investors. I have yet to see evidence that supports this rumour. Even if it were true, I call out the banks and the entire establishment for not openly pushing back to defend private ownership in a free society. At a minimum, the banks should have gone before the federal courts and obtained a ruling, even during the emergency declaration, to protect Canadians' basic right to property. That they did not do.

Instead, what we have seen from the evidence of the POEC hearings is that the big banks had a primary role in calling for the Public Order Emergency to begin with! That's perhaps one of the more shocking revelations from the hearings. Chrystia Freeland, minister of Finance, stated that by the second weekend of the "occupation" in Ottawa, she was hearing from "business leaders" about the trucker protests.[391]

The Ambassador Bridge blockade caused her department to look at "what was in the finance toolbox" to address the protests. One was FINTRAC, which monitors all financial transactions for money laundering and terrorist activity. The other was the *Bank Act*. However, she felt everything that could be done was being done.[392] The problem, in her mind, was that FINTRAC wasn't an enforcement agency—it simply monitored financial transactions. It deals with twentieth-century financing but not with twenty-first-century development, such as crowdfunding.[393] The *Bank Act*, according to Freeland, would require a long time to get an amendment

---

391 Chrystia Freeland, POEC, Volume 30, 12. Of note was that Ms. Freeland began her testimony with a litany of descriptions of her roles in government that had absolutely no relevance to the POEC hearings. It was remarkable.
392 POEC, Volume 30, 15–16.
393 Ibid., 16.

through Parliament to freeze bank accounts in response to the destructive impact on the economy.

Freeland spoke with Brian Deese, an advisor to President Biden, who was "very, very, very worried" about the Ambassador Bridge blockage due to the car plant supplies.[394] Of interest here is that Alan Kestenbaum, from Stelco and thereby also concerned about international trade, suggested that Freeland back away from the vaccine mandate for the sake of the industry as US companies will want to move car parts manufacturing back to the USA. He feared the government's strong-arm approach would only create a public backlash especially when the vaccine was of limited value. He said, "Does it really pay to carry on the policy in support of a mandate for a vaccine that doesn't prevent the spread of omicron, and which seems to be vanishing naturally anyway?[395] This was a common-sense suggestion, but Freeland would have none of it—it wasn't "relevant" she said![396]

Over the weekend of February 12, the CEOs of the Bank of Montreal and the Toronto Dominion Bank reached out to Freeland to express their concern about the damage being done to the Canadian economy. Then on February 13, Freeland chatted with a number of Canadian Bank CEOs prior to the Incident Response Group meeting, when the final decision to invoke the Emergencies Act was made.

According to Freeland's testimony, it's evident that the bankers were scratching their heads as to how they could assist the government in shutting down the convoy protest. As Freeland put it, "no one has any line of sight" to deal with the crowdfunding platforms, including crypto.[397] She expressed concern that if banks were perceived as having "agency" to freeze people's bank accounts, they would be accused of taking a political position against the protest.[398] The decision should, therefore, be shouldered by the government. The implication appears to be that the banks wanted something done but did not want to freeze the accounts on their own but hide behind a government mandate.

---

394 Ibid., 20.
395 Ibid., 28.
396 Ibid., 30.
397 Ibid., 34.
398 Ibid.

Freeland's notes of the call also included the suggestion that the Canadian public needs to be educated on how the protest was "an attack on democracy."[399] Imagine that—exercising one's freedom of expression and freedom of speech is a threat to democracy according to our bankers![400] Such is the thinking of the government and the big banks when it comes to groups with which the prime minister is not ideologically aligned.

Further, it appeared the bankers were also suggesting that the military be brought to the border, even after the borders were cleared, to send a message that this would not happen again.[401] Evidently when it comes to making money, the banks had no problem with using military might to ensure that the economy continued unhindered. Never mind Charter rights.

Freeland's notes also stated that she was "very resolute in ending this occupation of our democracy" and that she "will never" negotiate "with those who [held] our democracy hostage."[402]

Note that the intra-departmental discussion she described took place during the border blockages. The bank CEO discussions happened after the borders were opened and just before the IRG meeting on February 13, when the decision to invoke the Emergencies Act was irrevocably made. At that point, only the Ottawa protest remained. How could that be said to hold our Canadian government hostage? Parliament was still meeting. Cabinet was meeting. The borders were opened, so the economic issue was resolved. The Ottawa businesses that closed in the inner core could have been opened but were not. The government bureaucracy was largely working from home as a result of the COVID-19 pandemic, so there was presumably no disruption to their productivity. So then, why the need for such dramatic language and drastic measures?

One trucker explained to me that if the way to a delivery is blocked "'I don't throw up my arms and think, 'This is never going to get there.' If

---

399 Ibid.
400 For a powerful lecture on freedom of speech, see Professor Ryan Alford's 2022 Diefenbaker Lecture, First Freedoms Foundation, accessed May 11, 2023, https://firstfreedoms.ca/2022-diefenbaker-lecture/.
401 POEC, Volume 30, 35–36.
402 Ibid., 42.

that was the case, I'd be out of business ... Canada and the U.S. have the longest border in the world and we would simply choose another route. [The government was] worried that if they open one impeded route the protest would move to a different border crossing. So what! The truckers would use the previously closed route to move freight. This is part of the economics of transport."

Freeland testified that "operating in the fog of war," the government operated with "open-source information." The analogy Freeland made to "war" is telling. Obviously senior members of the government saw themselves in a battle with their protesting citizens. What was this "war"? Was it not a battle of ideas? Was it not over government overreach? I take "open-source" to mean newspaper articles that claimed foreign extremists were funding the convoy.[403]

Freeland wanted to ensure the convoy ended peacefully without any "blood on the face of a child,"[404] and she felt the freezing of bank accounts was the economic incentive necessary to get everyone to leave the "illegal protest," since the country was "in jeopardy." She claims to "regret" having to freeze people's accounts, all the while giggling at the prospect, but when weighed in the balance, only around fifty-seven people were disadvantaged compared to protecting "hundreds of thousands of Canadian jobs and families."[405] Therefore, for her, it was worth it.

Like so many other institutions during this COVID-19 pandemic, the banks have utterly failed to stand up for the property rights of the Canadian public. Although the banks are prepared to fly the flags of one protest group after another, they didn't stand up for the marginalized who suffered under Mr. Trudeau's assault on their property.

The banks have shown that they do not side with the most hurting. Perhaps we shouldn't be surprised, as the banks will always win—whether the people are prosperous or poor. Bankers simply follow the money.

We must be prepared now more than ever to be resourceful to survive ideological and political assaults from our own government. Resourcefulness includes developing personal skills to provide the necessities of life and

---

403 POEC, Volume 30, 48.
404 Ibid., 53.
405 Ibid., 54.

having the means to exchange goods for currency that others, in turn, will accept. The protestors became a community of resources. Neighbours were helping neighbours. And given the moves toward digital currency, we need to act on the age-old wisdom of our parents and grandparents: don't keep all your eggs in one basket. History is replete with examples of people doing just that and despite the odds stacked against them they survived.

The Trucker Freedom Convoy made it abundantly clear that we can't rely on the banks to protect our financial interests in times of crisis. We must be independently capable of making our own way.

# 11. Exposed the Complicity of the Healthcare System

HEALTHCARE PROVIDERS MAKE sacrifices every day on our behalf. Of that there can be no doubt. Those working in the designated COVID-19 care hospitals struggled with the waves of patients during the pandemic. The vaccine mandates hit the healthcare system at a weak point. The system, already burdened prior to the pandemic, at the time was teetering on the brink of another capacity crisis.[406]

Many healthcare workers refused to take the vaccine for the same reasons that motivated others, including conscience, logic, and personal health factors. Their refusal was met with an unrelenting administrative decision to dismiss them.[407] In British Columbia alone, some 2,500 healthcare workers lost their jobs.[408] Tensions are rising within the system[409] as

---

406 Robyn Doolittle and Tome Cardoso, "Canada's hospital capacity crisis will remain long after the pandemic is over," *The Globe and Mail*, April 2, 2022, https://www.theglobeandmail.com/canada/article-canada-hospitalizations-covid-19-pandemic/

407 See, "No Jab No Job—A Nurse's Perspective on Mandates—Interview with Nurse Judy Bacalso," First Freedoms Foundation, accessed May 11, 2023, https://firstfreedoms.ca/a-nurses-perspective-on-mandates-freedom-feature/.

408 Susan Lazaruk, "COVID-19: About 2,500 B.C. health-care workers lost jobs over refusal to vaccinate," *Vancouver Sun*, March 22, 2022, accessed May 11, 2023, https://vancouversun.com/news/local-news/about-2500-health-care-workers-lost-jobs-over-refusal-to-vaccinate.

409 Sharon Kirkey, "'I can't do this anymore': How to fix Canada's nursing crisis: Without enough nurses, the entire health system would collapse. But they're fleeing the profession in droves," *National Post*, October 11, 2022,

the overburdened workers take early retirement or find work elsewhere, like some I know who have left for the United States. The firing of healthcare workers because of the vaccine issue has not benefited the system.

A close friend of mine retired early as a physician due to the profession's vaccine emphasis. "Barry," he commented, "all you have to do is consider the coercive approach on the vaccine to know that something is amiss. I have never seen anything like it."

The Trucker Convoy challenged the public's unquestioning acceptance of the pronouncements of the public health experts. The POEC commission evidence revealed that health authorities did not advise the federal government to implement the travel vaccine mandates. At first glance, if there is any profession that would not need a vaccine, it would be the truckers.

Why?

Because virtually their entire day is spent in the cab of a truck. On most days, they interact personally with as many people as Tom Hanks' character did in the movie *Castaway*. Further, when the COVID pandemic began, the truckers were put in the same category as healthcare workers. They were seen as on the frontline, diligently working for the benefit of everyone in the country who still needed to have their groceries delivered. Indeed, the person who became their harshest critic, Prime Minister Justin Trudeau, tweeted on March 31, 2020,

> While many of us are working from home, there are others who aren't able to do that—like the truck drivers who are working day and night to make sure our shelves are stocked. So when you can, please #ThankATrucker for everything they're doing and help them however you can.[410]

---

accessed May 11, 2023, https://nationalpost.com/health/canadas-nursing-crisis.

410 Justin Trudeau (@JustinTrudeau), "While many of us are working from home, there are others who aren't able to do that," Twitter, March 31, 2020, 8:01 PM, https://twitter.com/justintrudeau/status/1245139169934016517?lang=en.

Yet just before the 2021 election, the Trudeau government let it be known that the truckers would have to be vaccinated. Truckers wondered where the healthcare executives and medical associations were getting their evidence to support this. The healthcare system adopted the government narrative and absolutely refused to allow any medical doctor to offer an opposing opinion.

"[Doctors] have basically been told," noted law professor Pardy, "that they are not allowed—Not allowed!—to express medical opinions about certain public policies that run against the official narrative. That is an extraordinary thing to contemplate in the here and now." The principle had been, until COVID-19, "that only the doctor who has examined the patient is in a position to make a diagnosis."[411]

How was this mindset seen as acceptable for a profession that prided itself in "following the science?" Science required, at a minimum, that there be critical assessments of those scientists and practitioners whose opinions were contrary to the accepted view.

When government mandated the vaccines, they claimed that there would be medical and religious exemptions. The reality was, such exemptions were extremely rare, and nearly non-existent if application was made for religious reasons.

Anecdotally, a friend with severe medical conditions told me that in meeting with their cardiologist, they were informed that, "Yes, under normal circumstances I would give you a medical exemption, but I fear for my medical license if I were to give you the exemption."[412]

Unbelievable! The medical profession, rather than allowing its members to "practise" medicine, was intent on ensuring that none of the sort would happen. The whole idea of "practise" is that the medical practitioner has the professional responsibility to determine for herself, based on her own knowledge and experience with treating disease, her own response to the case presented to her.

---

[411] Interview with Prof. Bruce Pardy on Freedom Feature, "The Experts Don't Own Us," https://firstfreedoms.ca/the-experts-dont-own-us-interview-with-bruce-pardy/
[412] A nurse, who remains anonymous, told me this was her experience.

Over the course of the pandemic, Canadians have become so conditioned by repeated warnings from our public health officials that, unless we look back, it can be difficult to recall what life was like before COVID-19. This loss of corporate memory gives the advantage to a government that keeps the populace in a constant state of fear as it implements its agenda without any checks or balances. Destabilization of the populace was due in no small part to healthcare professionals who chose silence rather than speaking up, often shamed or intimidated into compliance by the heavy hand of their professional regulators.

As a result of the constant media bombardment with the government narrative, many Canadians were convinced that if they deviated from public health orders, they would be seen as responsible for the collapse of our healthcare system. We've heard the same dire warnings over[413] and over.[414]

States of emergency were extended repeatedly to prevent our hospitals from becoming overwhelmed. Looking back on this government-propagated fear, we cannot but shake our heads that we were so hoodwinked into thinking that using our own common sense—like getting out and exercising in fresh air and taking vitamins C and D, along with Zinc, instead of being cooped up in our apartments—was somehow making us responsible for the already-existing failures of the healthcare system!

Patty Hajdu, a graphic designer, was elected as a member of Parliament in 2015, and Trudeau felt she would make an ideal federal minister of Health for Canada. Many were taken aback when she opined that the use of vitamin D as a therapeutic for COVID was "fake news."[415] Such a conclusion, based no doubt on her "expertise," struck most critical-thinking

---

413 Licia Corbella, "Canada's health care system overrun by administrators and lacks doctors," *Calgary Herald*, January 22, 2022, accessed May 11, 2023,https://calgaryherald.com/opinion/columnists/corbella-canadas-health-care-system-overrun-by-administrators-and-lacks-doctors.

414 Alanna Smith, "'Boiling point': Alberta doctors warn of health system collapse as COVID cases climb," CBC News, September 9, 2021, accessed May11,2023,https://www.cbc.ca/news/canada/calgary/alberta-doctors-health-care-collapse-covid-1.6169269.

415 True North Wire, "Hajdu says Vitamin-D COVID-19 protection is 'fake news,'" *True North*, April 22, 2021, accessed May 11, 2023, https://tnc.news/2021/04/22/hajdu-says-vitamin-d-covid-19-protection-is-fake-news/.

people in the country as non-ensical. And indeed, "the facts are that Hajdu's statement was the fake one."[416]

We can certainly sympathize with our hard-working health professionals during this COVID crisis. Think of the stress that those working in the hospitals designated as COVID-care centres experienced. They saw more than their share of suffering from the disease. It was no joke.

However, we must also acknowledge the experiences of other health professionals who did not have a heavy COVID patient load. Dr. Charles Hoffe, for example, noted that at the hospital in Lytton, British Columbia, there were hardly any major disruptions. He felt undeserving of all the accolades the public poured out for him and his colleagues for being on the "front lines."[417]

We can admit that for many, there was a heavy burden. They are, unquestionably, exhausted (as are, incidentally, most people in most vocations, from teaching to trucking). But to blame a collapse of the healthcare system solely on coronavirus is misleading at best.

First, the notion that obeying regulations will "protect the healthcare system" assumes that following the ever-changing government policy is effective. Yet when we looked around, we saw wave after wave of infection, even among those who followed all the guidelines to a T.

Second, Canadians forget that our healthcare system was stretched to the limit before COVID-19. In a March 11, 2020, CBC article[418] it was

---

416 Editorial, "Staying healthy during COVID-19," *Toronto Sun*, Dec 19, 2021, accessed May 11, 2023, https://torontosun.com/opinion/editorials/editorial-staying-healthy-during-covid-19; see also, Nathan Jeffay, "1 in 4 COVID patients hospitalized while vitamin D deficient die—Israeli study," *Times of Israel*, June 17, 2021, accessed May 11, 2023, https://www.timesofisrael.com/1-in-4-hospitalized-covid-patients-who-lack-vitamin-d-die-israeli-study/.

417 "Don't Give in to Fear—Interview with Dr. Charles Hoffe," First Freedoms Foundation, accessed May 11, 2023, https://firstfreedoms.ca/dont-give-in-to-fear-interview-with-dr-charles-hoffe/.

418 Kelly Crowe, "Canadians being urged to help 'flatten the curve' of COVID-19," CBC News, March 11, 2020, accessed May 11, 2023, https://www.cbc.ca/news/health/canada-covid-19-coronavirus-spread-hospital-surge-capacity-ventilators-1.5493178.

admitted that "Most of the country's hospitals are *already operating at 100 per cent* capacity, a *largely normal* situation in Canada's health-care system" (emphasis added). The same CBC piece quoted a Toronto physician saying, "We're at capacity most of the time." So, any extra change was going to cause stress—consider all the new COVID protocols that came into effect just with the PPE!

Ontario's minister of Health promised[419] in January 2020 that "current overcrowding in hospitals won't be an issue." It remains an issue.[420]

In other words, we had a pre-existing crisis that was used to push Canadians into perpetual panic over a disease that has proven to be far less lethal than initially feared. (Early news reports cited an alarming fourteen per cent fatality rate; the reality is about one per cent but it's primarily a concern for the very old.)[421] Yet our government, for reasons that only they know, has chosen to blame Canadians for "overwhelming" a system that was already at the breaking point.[422]

It's not hard to see why the Truckers' Convoy opposition to a vaccine mandate would cause a total upset to the narrative. This entire situation is a bit like a government announcing that instead of using tax dollars to fix potholes or deal with congested thoroughfares, it's going to ban all vehicle

---

419 Liam Casey, "Quarantining a Canadian city over coronavirus would be illegal: experts," *Global News*, January 25, 2020, accessed May 11, 2023, https://globalnews.ca/news/6453641/coronavirus-quarantine-illegal-canada/.
420 "Ontario's health care system in need of major surgery: It's time to stop providing Band-Aid solutions to what is a long-term systemic crisis," *Ancaster News*, August 8, 2022, accessed May 11, 2023, https://www.thespec.com/local-ancaster/opinion/2022/08/08/ontario-s-health-care-system-in-need-of-major-surgery.html.
421 Maria Pezzullo, Cathrine Axfors, Despina G. Contopoulos-Ioannidis, Alexandre Apostolatos, John P.A. Ioannidis, "Age-stratified infection fatality rate of COVID-19 in the non-elderly population," *Environmental Research*, Volume 216, Part 3, 1 January 2023, 114655, accessed May 11, 2023, https://doi.org/10.1016/j.envres.2022.114655. It was not a concern for the younger generation: "At a global level, pre-vaccination IFR may have been as low as 0.03% and 0.07% for 0–59 and 0–69 year-old people, respectively."
422 Robyn Urback, "When do we admit Canada's health care system just isn't working?" *The Globe and Mail*, January 5, 2022, accessed May 11, 2023, https://www.theglobeandmail.com/opinion/article-when-do-we-admit-canadas-health-care-system-just-isnt-working/.

traffic on the roads until they're safe to drive on—a goal that will never be achieved without the necessary repairs. It's a solution that places all the blame on drivers while conveniently allowing the government to escape any responsibility.

Government escaping responsibility is a common theme throughout the Trudeau regime. And when you think of all the scandals—whether it's the Aga Khan conflict of interest, or the SNC-Lavalin scandal, or the WE Charity, or pushing the RCMP to favour its political gun control interests, or invocation of the Emergencies Act—each time the government has said it did nothing wrong. The truckers went to Ottawa to tell a different story.

It should be obvious that the right response to our overstrained healthcare system was not to punish people for needing health care. Instead, government should have taken the initiative to build resilience and increase capacity. (And by that I don't mean giving tens of millions of dollars to SNC-Lavalin for "mobile health units" that have never been deployed!)[423]

The truckers, those "salt of the earth" types, came to Ottawa fully aware of how they were being blamed for causing problems with health care because they were unvaccinated, or supported those who were not. They challenged health care's willingness to be co-opted for political purposes and parrot the government narrative.

Perhaps one of the most effective solutions to our health care problem is referenced by Licia Corbella[424] that Canada's "bloated, bureaucratic" healthcare system is overburdened by an excessive number of administrators: "The problem with administrators is they never look inward.

---

[423] Robert Fife, Steven Chase, "Mobile hospitals that cost Ottawa $300-million sit in storage while Omicron strains Canada's health system," *The Globe and Mail*, January 14, 2022, https://www.theglobeandmail.com/politics/article-federal-mobile-hospital-units-sitting-in-warehouses-as-omicron-surges/

[424] Licia Corbella, "Frustrated doctors say they are 'hindered,' not helped by too many managers," *Calgary Herald*, January 26, 2022, accessed May 11, 2023, https://calgaryherald.com/opinion/columnists/corbella-frustrated-doctors-say-they-are-hindered-not-helped-by-too-many-managers; See also Susan D. Martinuk at https://www.amazon.ca/Patients-Risk-Exposing-Canadas-Health-care/dp/1777657741.

Administrators never recommend that administration be cut."[425] Now there's a thought to consider.

The truckers came to Ottawa with a message: Canadians are going to start holding our public officials to account. And that requires transparency and honesty—not hiding behind professional doublespeak that limits rather than enhances freedom. Scapegoating the unvaccinated, the "fringe minorities," for systemic problems that already existed in our healthcare system is not how we will be a free and healthy society. If the last two years are any indication, it's unlikely that change will come unless Canadians begin to rethink the conversation.

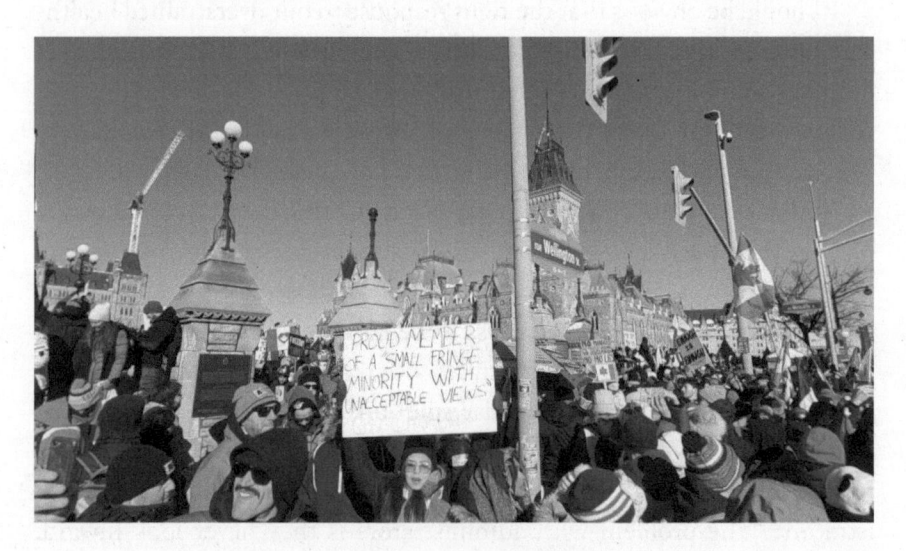

*Another Proud Member Of The Small Fringe Minority*

Things may be open now, but if we want to escape the current cycle of lockdowns for good, then it's up to us to hold our public officials and politicians to account. A shift in attitude and approaches starts with a willingness to acknowledge and address the issues honestly and openly. It's past time to stop scapegoating[426] "fringe minorities" and start working together

---

425 Ibid.
426 Jared McBrady, "Othering Unvaccinated Persons," Brownstone Institute, January 10, 2022, accessed May 11, 2023, https://brownstone.org/articles/othering-unvaccinated-persons/.

on productive and helpful solutions that will allow us to move forward as a free and healthy society.

The Trucker Freedom Convoy brought attention to the public health authorities and government for their failure to own the struggles they were unnecessarily causing Canadians. That willingness to challenge the accepted narrative proved to be one of many ways the truckers helped save Canada from a terrible fate wrought by unchecked power and its beaming headlights will protect us going forward by making us aware of our responsibility not to always accept what the "experts" say but think for ourselves in analyzing the complete context.

# 12. Exposed the Complicity of the Police

FEBRUARY 13, 2022, I stood among the protestors in front of the flatbed trailer at the intersection of Metcalfe and Wellington Streets. The Peace Tower rose in the background. Skies were clear and the temperature was biting cold, but the crowd was warm and lively. Little did we know that in the halls of government, the prime minister had met with the Incident Response Group (IRG) and the final decision was made to invoke the Emergencies Act the next day, February 14, 2022—a "Valentine's Gift" from the PMO to the protesters.

There I stood, listening to the rousing speeches, including those of Maxine Bernier[427] and Brian Peckford. Among the group on the stage was Mark Foreman, a former member of the RCMP. He read the oath he took on becoming a Mountie and the code of objectives of the RCMP and commented on the important role of the police:[428] "Maintaining the confidence of Canadians in the Royal Canadian Mounted Police is essential," he said. Then for emphasis, "Essential!"

"This tunic has been stained in the past," he continued. "Officers like myself went to Native reserves and—" He struggled emotionally to continue, but like many in that circumstance, he took a moment to catch his breath and continued—"took children from their parents. I'm a parent. I can't imagine how it must have felt. We cannot let that happen again!

---

427 See "It's Time to Fight For Freedom—Maxime Bernier Interview," First Freedoms Foundation, accessed May 11, 2023, https://firstfreedoms.ca/its-time-to-fight-for-freedom-maxime-bernier-interview/.
428 I recorded him with my camera and quote from that recording.

We're on the top of a very slippery slope. We can't let it go on. I know what's right. I know you know what's right. I had to come here this morning."

This former officer was transparent in his awe of the magnitude of the historical moment. He went on, "Early this morning I was sitting, and something reached inside my chest, and it felt like I was going to pop. And I knew exactly what I had to do. I didn't hear a voice or anything. It just popped in my head. I don't care what you think. You can roll your eyes at me. But I think it was God."

"God." To many today, the mere mention of "God" automatically disqualifies a speaker. However, for the protesters, that was not the case. One of the huge differences between the protesters and the Cathedral is that the protesters are not afraid to mention "God."

Here was a police veteran who identified with the people and with the Judeo-Christian cultural framework that many in the protest understood to be the philosophical underpinning of the country's history, and they were not ashamed of it. It was rather the celebration of the philosophical and religious underpinning of the rights that were being violated for which the protest emerged.

"I had to come here and wear this serge, on this Parliament Hill, because there is nothing more iconic than that flag and this red serge. The entire world recognizes both of those things, and we need to show the world that we are going to lead by example what freedom is."

Then he turned his attention to the "media outlets out there, you will not listen to them"—he pointed to the audience— "listen to me! A retired Mountie. I took an oath. I'll tell the truth ... I have been to protests. I have never seen a protest like this. I saw kids down the street playing and I knelt with them and said 'Hi' to them, and they're not scared. There is no fear here."

Little did he know that two government ministers, David Lametti, minister of Justice, and Marco Mendicino, minister of Public Safety, joked about bringing in army tanks,[429] and that the military were put on notice

---

[429] Ian Bailey, "Politics Briefing: Texts about using military during convoy protests were a 'joke,' Justice Minister Lametti says," *The Globe and Mail*, November 23, 2022, https://www.theglobeandmail.com/politics/

that they might be called upon to use the country's absolute power on the peaceful protest of citizens.[430]

Foreman then turned his attention to his police colleagues. "I just want to say a little more to the police officers out there. Remember we took an oath to the Constitution. We didn't take an oath to a government. I didn't take an oath to a police chief. I will follow my police chief's orders ... if they are lawful. So, Officers, if you truly feel in your heart that your orders are not lawful, then you shouldn't follow them. I have your back, and all of these people have your back."

While Foreman may have the officers' "back," the reality is he's not signing their paycheque. The trucker sympathizers in the police forces had much to lose if seen as disloyal to their police chief. It takes a very rare police member to stand up to the institution and put conscientious conviction, even if the rule of law is at stake, ahead of the security of their career. This is especially true when the police member is young with a whole life ahead of him or her. It's not easy to stand out and suffer the loss of income, pension, and other benefits. Even more so if the member has a family dependent upon his or her income.

As it turned out, there were police officers who did voice their support for the truckers, and they paid dearly for it. Constable Erin Howard of the Durham Regional Police Services posted support of the Trucker Freedom Convoy on Twitter on January 24, 2022. She was charged with two counts of misconduct, insubordination, and breach of trust for that post and her support to the truckers at a Nathan Phillips Square rally earlier. She pled guilty to one count of discreditable conduct, and the other charges were dropped. She was demoted for three months.[431] Some say it wasn't enough; others say it was too much. Therein is the dilemma police face.

---

article-politics-briefing-texts-about-using-military-during-convoy-protests/, accessed June 22, 2023.

430 Lee Berthiaume, "Military was told to prepare to intervene in 'Freedom Convoy' protests: official," The Canadian Press, December 1, 2022 https://www.ctvnews.ca/politics/military-was-told-to-prepare-to-intervene-in-freedom-convoy-protests-official-1.6177166, accessed June 22, 2023

431 Michelle Mandel, "Durham cop demoted three months for outspoken 'Freedom Convoy' support," *Ottawa Sun*, December 6, 2022, accessed May 11, 2023, https://ottawasun.com/news/local-news/

"The greatest tool a policeman has is critical thinking and thinking for themselves," Clay Farnsworth of Police on Guard[432] told me.[433] "Police work is not black and white, cut and dried. You have to be able to think on your feet." One would surmise that part of that thinking is to ensure that when they are following orders, such orders are in accordance with the law.

In Tamara Lich's gripping book, she notes that there were many in the police force, court officers, and prison guards who expressed sympathy toward her.[434] She noted that as she was handcuffed and shackled to be sent to Calgary for the flight to Ottawa, "one officer came over to me and thanked me, saying that we had helped to give a future to his kids. 'There's a lot of us behind you,' he said. 'Stay strong.'"[435]

Following orders is what police must do. But what if those orders are themselves illegal? We mustn't be surprised that in our form of government politicians are required to keep their distance from the police. While politicians make law through the legislature, and the judiciary interprets that law and makes law through their judicial decisions (which we call the "common law"), the police are independent enforcers of the law. Police are never to be politicized. Politicians must not interfere with the work of the police. That is key to maintaining a peaceful and uncorrupted society. Everyone is to be treated equally before and under the law.

Prime Minister Trudeau has favourite protesters. He told us so. The Trucker Freedom Convoy was his least favourite. He told us so. They were the "fringe minority ... with unacceptable views." Unacceptable, of course, because they didn't jive with his ideological positions. Yet he had no authority to coerce the police into carrying out his desire against the truckers.

---

mandel-durham-cop-demoted-three-months-for-outspoken-freedom-convoy-support/wcm/8b20e00c-3350-48d9-af19-4e9b989b14dc.
432 Police on Guard for Thee, accessed May 11, 2023, https://policeonguard.ca/.
433 "Police On Guard for Thee: Freedom Feature with Clay Farnsworth, Freedom Feature," First Freedoms Foundation, accessed May 11, 2023, https://firstfreedoms.ca/police-on-guard-for-thee-freedom-feature-with-clay-farnsworth/.
434 Tamara Lich, 177.
435 Tamara Lich, 195.

It was evident from the POEC hearings that Mr. Trudeau wanted the police to act far more quickly in getting rid of the trucker protest. As he stated from the very beginning, he thought of the Emergencies Act as a means to get rid of the protest. For him, the police were always coming up with a plan, but the plans weren't being carried out—at least not as he thought they should be. He wanted the Ottawa streets cleared, whereas it appeared to him the police were willing to allow the protest to continue. From my reading of the testimony of the police at the POEC, they were being respectful of the protesters' Charter rights. Not so the government. Mr. Trudeau wanted the protest gone.

Our Charter rights are only as good as the respect given them by the executive branch of the government. In Canada, the executive is known as the "King's Privy Council of Canada,"[436] which is the federal cabinet chaired by the prime minister. The prime minister is, for all practical purposes, where "the buck stops." It's no exaggeration to say that the character and personality of the government takes on the character and personality of the prime minister.

Therefore, if the prime minister is dismissive of the Charter rights of those he doesn't appreciate, such a stance will be reflected in how the government behaves. That is not how it should be. We intuitively expect the government to respect the Charter for the benefit of both its political allies and enemies. Unfortunately, under the current government, there is a serious blurring of the line of Charter rights for Prime Minister Trudeau's political enemies.

Every Canadian prime minister and his or her subordinates must strategically analyze how close to the constitutional (of which the Charter is but a part) boundaries they're willing to go in taking away Charter protections to enhance a political goal. Much of our ability to exercise our freedoms is dependent upon the good faith of our government. We may exercise our rights if the government respects them. What we saw in the Trucker Freedom Convoy was a government that was more than willing to limit those rights without any sense of obligation to protect them—a matter still to be sorted out in the courts. Prime Minister Trudeau wanted

---

[436] Of course, at the time of this protest, it was the "Queen's Privy Council of Canada."

the protesters out of Ottawa, and all his subordinates were expected to make it happen.

It is of utmost importance for the Canadian public to put in the prime minister's office one who deeply cherishes the first freedoms of all Canadians, regardless of ideology. Be mindful, as I reference Solzhenitsyn earlier, that the line between good and evil runs through every human heart.[437] The human heart that governs us must be true to duty and truth as any legitimate scale of weights. The tendency of human beings to rationalize must be acknowledged. As Professor Jonathan Haidt points out in his psychological research,[438] we make decisions by our emotions and then use our intellect to justify those decisions. Indeed, Mr. Trudeau's emotional decisions since taking office are on full display, including his expectation that his closest advisors ensure that his directives are carried out and rationalizations are established justifying those decisions after they are made.

As an aside, the same mentality was evident throughout the COVID-19 pandemic. Those in power made decisions, ostensibly based on "science." However, I suggest that many decisions were political in nature—such as Mr. Trudeau's travel mandates. Nevertheless, we all witnessed numerous government entities willing to curb freedoms of assembly and mobility by issuing lockdowns and huge fines to violators. There was scant attention given to basic rights.

Yet in many cases these fines were dropped by the authorities as the court dates loomed. However, the public objective was met. A huge segment of the population self-censored and followed government orders. The fines worked in controlling people. Even the mere threat of fines had that restraining power upon people to do as they were told and not exercise their rights. Police showing up at the doors of returning travellers let it be known that "big brother" was watching. Everyone got the message. With many tickets for non-compliance being dropped at the last minute, the government can claim an effective compliance of the population with their regulations.

---

437 Solzhenitsyn, *The Gulag Archipelago Two.* Supra Note
438 Jonathan Haidt, *The Righteous Mind: Why Good People Are Divided by Politics and Religion*, (New York: Pantheon Books, 2012).

During the Trucker Freedom Convoy, one cannot help but be sympathetic with the police services as they struggled with the competing demands from the PMO and Ottawa City Hall on the one hand, demanding removal of the protesters, and the Charter imperative that the state respect the rights of all citizens.

As already canvassed, I believe that the Emergencies Act was wrongly invoked. Nevertheless, the invocation meant that the police forces—the RCMP, the Ottawa Police Services (OPS), and the Ontario Provincial Police (OPP), along with police from other provinces and cities—were given extraordinary powers to end the protest.

The POEC hearings revealed that many in the police forces recognized that the government improperly invoked the Act and that they didn't need any extra powers to clear Ottawa of the protest. We learned that on February 6, 2022, the Deputy Minister of Public Safety, on a call with the OPP Commissioner, OPS Chief, and others, demanded that they diffuse the protest "to satisfy the political objectives of the government."[439]

As Donald Best, former Toronto Police investigator, told me, "It was all political." There was no need for the Emergencies Act. "When I consider the tremendous overreach of freezing people's assets, destroying their businesses, destroying their lives, with no due process, no appeal, no court order, just the government targeting political opposition. What country is this again?"[440]

It has been recognized[441] for some time in Canada that when it comes to public protests, there is considerable grey area as to how police are to act. That means police must make up their own rules of engagement as they go

---

439 "Summary of Call with City of Ottawa, Federal Government and Provincial Government," February 6, 2022, (11:00am EST), accessed May 12, 2023, https://commissionsurletatdurgence.ca/files/exhibits/ONT00000311.pdf?t=1668245255.
440 Political Policing—Interview with Donald Best, https://firstfreedoms.ca/political-policing-interview-with-donald-best/
441 See Robert Diab and Wesley Pue, "The Gap in Canadian Police Powers: Canada Needs 'Public Order Policing' Legislation," SSRN, August 6, 2009, accessed May 12, 2023, https://ssrn.com/abstract=1388602 or http://dx.doi.org/10.2139/ssrn.1388602

through a protest. This leaves citizens in a no man's land, not knowing the limits of their rights.

As a result of the Trucker Freedom Convoy, legislation has been passed limiting the use of trucks in public protest. For example, in Ontario, the Progressive Conservative government passed legislation that prohibits protesters from impeding the flow of goods on the province's transportation infrastructure if it disrupts "ordinary economic activity or interfer[es] with the safety, health or well-being of members of the public."[442]

During the Trucker Freedom Convoy, sympathetic members of the police were giving internal information to the lawyers representing the truckers. Donald Best pointed out that such behaviour is totally unacceptable. "I'd have the handcuffs on him right away," Best said. If an officer can't carry out his orders, then he should simply inform his superiors that he's not to show up, according to Best. That's how Best and his colleagues did it when they couldn't take part in the Morgentaler abortion clinic protests many years ago. "But we didn't give information to the other side," said Best. That would be betraying the oath they took on becoming an officer.

Best, like Foreman, remains very troubled by the heavy-handedness of some police officers during the pandemic and during the Trucker Freedom Convoy: "We will never forget the scenes of 220-pound police officers armed to the teeth, handcuffing visibly pregnant mothers in front of their screaming children—for the 'criminal' offense of failing to be vaxxed or failing to wear a mask at a hockey game, or pushing their kid on a swing in a closed park," says Best.

"I'll never forget that," he continues, "that kind of overreach and the terrible abuses that we saw during the convoy, those are forever there." Best noted that even "as a retired police officer," to think that "the police just forgot about Rule of Law, forgot about Peel's Principles of Policing, and the law itself, and they just did whatever the elected officials told them to. And that is a prescription for totalitarianism. It's terrible, and we saw that."

Each "police officer has the authority to independently launch any investigation they want ... we do that (as a society), so that the power

---

[442] "Keeping Ontario Open for Business Act, 2022," Legislative Assembly of Ontario, accessed May 12, 2023, https://www.ola.org/en/legislative-business/bills/parliament-42/session-2/bill-100.

that be cannot, without consequences, and without good reason, stop an investigation ... [T]hat foundation of how we run our police forces is why [they]... are not as thoroughly corrupt as some other countries."

As Best notes, politicians are not to direct the police forces on how to police. Of course, politicians try to influence the police all the time in accordance with their political objectives, as was revealed in the POEC hearings. For example, we know that during the Trucker Freedom Convoy in Ottawa, there were no safety concerns to force an early end to the protest. In fact, the city's crime rate went down.

However, that didn't stop the politicians from wanting the convoy protest to end. It was a problem politically for the prime minister and for Ottawa's mayor. Within the OPS leadership there was some serious feuding going on. Donald Best notes that long before the convey showed up, the OPS was struggling with the arrival of Police Chief Sloly. Sloly didn't rise through the OPS ranks but was parachuted into the position to deal with complaints that the OPS was racist. In one op-ed, Sloly noted, "We've significantly increased our capacity to drive the principles of equity, diversity and inclusion in every aspect of our organization."[443] As to the specifics of what was going on within the OPS, the intrigue may take an entire book to unravel. However, the convoy appears to have exacerbated an already dysfunctional police force leadership.

The convoy created another layer of complexity to an already struggling Ottawa police force. Now the members had to struggle with a prime minister who had so divided the country that a huge protest was on their doorstep, and Trudeau criticized their policing. Clearly some members sympathized with the truckers, and while trying to deal with the protest, had to deal with a dysfunctional office and demanding federal government.

After invocation of the Emergencies Act, Peter Sloly resigned[444] and Steve Bell, a long-time member of the OPS, was named the interim police

---

443 Peter Sloly, "Ottawa police are committed to resolving bias and systemic racism," *Ottawa Citizen*, September 4, 2020, accessed May 12, 2023, https://ottawacitizen.com/opinion/sloly-ottawa-police-are-committed-to-resolving-bias-and-systemic-racism.

444 Matthew Lapierre, "Ottawa police Chief Peter Sloly resigns amid criticism over handling of convoy protests," *Ottawa Citizen*, February 16, 2022, accessed May 12, 2023, https://ottawacitizen.com/news/local-news/

chief. Bell immediately took a very hard stance against the convoy and was instrumental in ending the protest within days, as police shipped in from across the country violently ended the protest.

"The sheer level of violence that was put on to Canadian unarmed citizens" shocked Tom Marazzo. [445]

Chris Deering served Canada in Afghanistan and suffered injuries from an IED explosion that killed two of his fellow soldiers. During the last day of the convoy, he was among a number of veterans protecting the National War Memorial when the police took him to the ground and beat him.

During the POEC hearings, Chris described what happened to him:

> I gave myself to the police. And as the police took me down, again, he knew, he kneed me in my side, kicked me in my back. I was laying down. I was in the fetal position on my back. He kicked me in my ankle and my foot. As I was laying down, I had my hands completely up. I'm saying, "I'm very peaceful. I'm peaceful. I'm not resisting." I was then punched four or five times in my head. I had a knee on my back to keep myself down. I was on the ground for one-and-a-half to two minutes. My hands were zip tied. The officers slowly picked me up and then we slowly proceeded to the processing line.[446]
>
> We get to the processing line. The day was minus 20. I had no gloves on ... the duration of the processing line was one-and-a-half to two hours ... I asked the policeman who was on both sides of me, I said, "Do you mind, you know my conditions, is it okay if I sit or kneel because I'm in chronic pain?" It was obvious. My face was flushed, and I had cried multiple times, and I don't cry ever ... [I]t was the worst pain I had felt since I'd been blown up. The fact

---

ottawa-police-chief-peter-sloly-resigns-amid-criticism-over-handling-of-convoy-protests

445 Interview with Tom Marazzo on Freedom Feature, https://firstfreedoms.ca/trudeaus-tiananmen-square/

446 POEC Hearings, transcript, Friday November 4, 2022, 96.

that I couldn't sit, or stand was, to me, cruel and unusual punishment. We would go 15, 20 minutes without even moving. I also asked if I could have my medication ... I was denied my medication to comfort my duress ... They then placed me in the back of the squad car.[447]

They read me what I was being charged with, which was public obstruction and mischief. So, I said I understood. The police officer then—the police officer then left the vehicle for five minutes. He came back and he said, "Well, today's your lucky day. You're not being charged."

I said, "That's great." I said, "Can I know what's—why that changed?" He said, "No, you don't need to know that." So at that time, I felt that it was my understanding that I'm free to go because I'm not being charged with anything. Then the next five, 10 minutes they put me in a paddy wagon with no direction. They didn't say, "Go in here." So, again, I mean, I had no choice. I go in the paddy wagon. I'm there for 25 minutes. I don't know where I'm going, don't know how long I'm there.

Eventually, the paddy wagon does fill up over the next couple of hours. Then they drive us around for approximately half an hour to 40 minutes. It was very hard to tell because there's no windows, of course, in the paddy wagon; you know, there's no concept of time. They then drove us to a Public Works building that was 10.2 kilometres away from Parliament Hill. When they let us out of the paddy wagons, they gave us our possessions back. They gave us no paperwork. The police officer came out and he gave us a stern warning and said, "You don't come back to Ottawa, or you'll be charged." They gave us all our possessions back and—sorry; most of us, due to the cold, our cell phones had died. No one had any money; no one

---

447 Ibid., 96–97.

had any masks. We couldn't go into the building to make a phone call. So, we were stranded. So, we were forced to walk to a Wendy's that was—and I forget the approximate distance; we had to walk from that Public Works building in the snow, in the freezing cold to a Wendy's.

I never thought that I would get dumped out of the seat like trash by ... the police.[448]

"Nobody," says Marazzo, "expected that the law enforcement in this country would have such a disgusting disregard for Canadian citizens. You can see all of the video of them kneeing and butt-stroking people. Just brutal beatings of Canadian citizens."

Not every police officer approved of such treatment. As Marazzo points out, "There was also a lot of Ottawa Police officers, and OPP and other police in other jurisdictions that told their bosses, 'I'm not going to Ottawa. If you try to send me to Ottawa to turn on citizens like that I'm going to go on sick leave. Or I'm taking the day off. I'm going on vacation. But do not send me to Ottawa because I won't participate in that.'"

Clay Farnsworth, of Police on Guard, and Donald Best both shared with me that it's not uncommon for police to refuse to participate in actions they deem unacceptable and a violation of their basic decency. Yet in Ottawa in mid-February 2022, hundreds of police officers had no qualms about executing the will of a prime minister who demanded that the streets be cleared of the Trucker Freedom Convoy. Some revelled in their participation. They made fun of the protesters and couldn't wait to take part.

To our collective shame, texts of RCMP members delighting in the brutality were made public.[449] "Time for the protesters to hear our jackboots on the ground," RCMP officer Andrew Nixon wrote. Fellow officer Robin

---

448 Ibid., 126–127.
449 Doug Mainwaring, "Two of the RCMP officers, and the image of mounted police trampling a demonstrator at the Freedom Convoy." LifeSiteNews, February 21, 2022, accessed May 12, 2023, https://www.lifesitenews.com/news/leaked-messages-show-canadian-police-delighting-in-crushing-freedom-convoy-report/.

Thibault jokingly warned Nixon, "this is a kinder, gentler RCMP." Nixon responded, "Okay, we can give out free hugs and unicorn stickers."

When video of the mounted police trampling the protesters was posted on Facebook, Scott Peever wrote, "That's awesome."

"We only think we're living the dream," Chris Russell said.

"That's what we need to do!" Nixon wrote.

"Just watched that horse video—that is awesome!!!" Marca wrote. "We should practice that manoevre [sic]."

At the time the RCMP stated that "this material is not representative" of its members and they were looking into the matter. To this day, I don't know what, if anything, has been done about it. However, it again reveals Solzhenitsyn's wisdom—the dividing line of good and evil runs through every human heart.

## Constable Kristina Neilson

Constable Kristina Neilson of the OPS donated to the Trucker Freedom Convoy. That turned out to be a poor decision for her career, since someone hacked the crowdfunding donor list and gave it to mainstream media, who were more than willing to dox the donors. Constable Neilson was made an example, in line with the harsh words of the OPS interim chief Steve Bell: "If somebody was helping to support the unlawful demonstrators in our streets that had such traumatic and terrible consequences on our population and was deemed to be illegal, I'll seriously question their ability to deliver community safety and wellbeing in this city moving ahead."[450]

Neilson's earlier career was with the Canadian Armed Forces, serving three tours with the navy. She gave a $55 donation to the convoy, first to the GoFundMe platform, but when that was stopped, she resubmitted the same amount to the GiveSendGo platform. Once discovered by the

---

450 Matthew Lapierre, "Interim Ottawa police chief considering action against officers who allegedly supported 'Freedom Convoy'," *Ottawa Citizen*, March 7, 2022, accessed May 12, 2023, https://ottawacitizen.com/news/local-news/interim-ottawa-police-chief-considering-action-against-officers-who-supported-freedom-convoy.

OPS, she was charged with discreditable conduct. She appeared before the internal police tribunal and admitted to the donation.

On November 4, 2022, the trials officer released his decision[451] that she would lose forty hours of pay. She also had to participate in a program of "restorative justice," which essentially means she will meet with community members who were "harmed" by her donation to the convoy. "I think in China, they used to call this a 'Struggle Session,'" Donald Best quipped.

For the trials officer, retired Superintendent Chris Renwick, this was a very serious matter that required a sentence that deterred any other officer from doing anything similar. Renwick noted that the OPS and various levels of government deemed the convoy "an unlawful occupation and fundraising prolonged it." He continued, "The public expects police officers to uphold the law and, foremost, to protect the public. If individual officers fall short of this responsibility through misconduct, then the misconduct must attract an appropriate and proportional sanction."[452]

Renwick found "that the seriousness of Cst. Neilson's behaviour is an aggravating factor for consideration."[453] However, he was satisfied that she "learned from her experience and based on her post-charge conduct, is most unlikely to find herself before a tribunal on similar misconduct."[454] He did not stop there.

To let it be known that Cst. Neilson was but an example for, and a warning to, all other police officers, Renwick stated:

> I view General Deterrence as a much more aggravating factor. It requires a clear message aimed at all members of the OPS and other services across Ontario that have or may express sympathies to any controversial causes that serve to undermine public trust and confidence in the impartiality of the police. Any individual police officers deviating from neutral objectivity and the consistent,

---

451 "Renwick Decision in Neilson Case," November 4, 2022, accessed May 12, 2023, https://www.ottawapolice.ca/en/news-and-updates/resources/Documents/Disciplinary-decisions/Decision-Neilson.pdf.
452 Ibid., 4.
453 Ibid., 5.
454 Ibid.

fair, and impartial application of rule of law must clearly understand that it will result in corrective and/or punitive sanctions.[455]

Take Mr. Renwick's reasoning at face value. Neilson must be made an example because police officers must have "neutral objectivity" and the "consistent, fair, and impartial application of rule of law." They cannot express "sympathy" to "any controversial causes" that "undermine public trust and confidence in the impartiality of the police."

This raises the question, "Are all 'controversial causes' equal?" Consider that Prime Minister Trudeau doesn't see all causes equal. He specifically let it be known that Indigenous protests and Black Lives Matter protests are acceptable but that the Trucker Freedom Convoy 2022 was not acceptable.[456] The truckers were the "fringe minority" with "unacceptable views."

We cannot help but wonder what would have happened had the January–February 2022 protest been by Indigenous or Black Lives Matter activists, and Cst. Neilson had donated to those causes. Would Cst. Neilson be charged with "discreditable conduct"? Have there been police officers who gave funding to other protest groups? Were they charged? In other words, are we now at a place where police officers aren't to give any money, make any statement on "controversial causes," for fear of violating the "neutral objective" principle, like what we expect of judges? Or is this principle limited to the causes that the Cathedral disapprove of?

It is my position that the police and the government of Mr. Trudeau underestimated the frustration and resolve of the people to push back against the government's over-reach and ill treatment of the unvaccinated. It wasn't ready for the protest. The OPS was caught up in its own internal matters, and Mr. Trudeau couldn't believe that any person or group would dare question his wisdom and the wisdom of those in the Cathedral that he represented.

---

455 Ibid.
456 See Brian Lee Crowley's criticism of this in, "Law for All—Interview With Brian Lee Crowley," First Freedoms Foundation, accessed May 12, 2023, https://firstfreedoms.ca/law-for-all/.

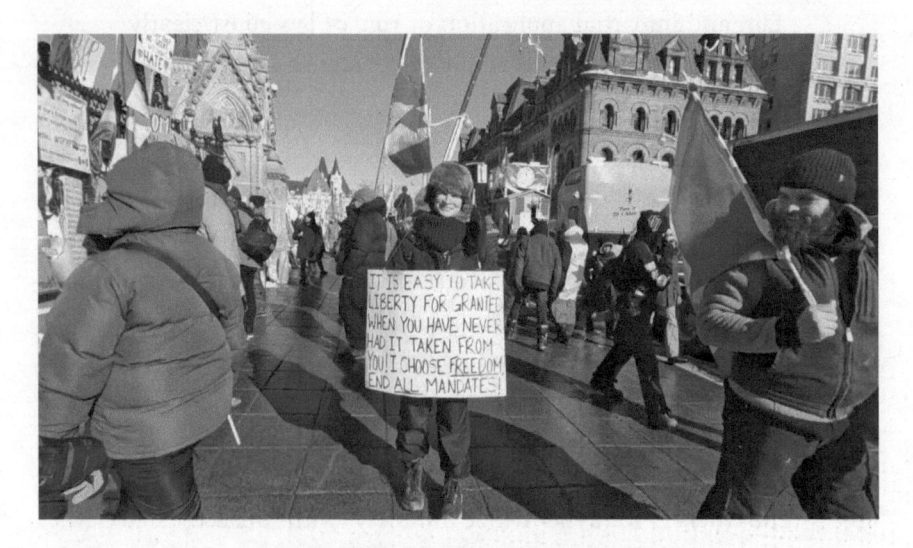

*It Is Easy To Take Liberty For Granted*

Imagine what would have happened had Mr. Trudeau respected the truckers' views instead of showing his petulance. The violence of the Trucker Freedom Convoy 2022 came not from the truckers but from the police officers who scoffed at the plight of their victims and who then harassed their own members who dared show the truckers some respect by pitching in a few bucks for them to buy a meal.

The people now know that the police can be compromised like any other state institution. It's why a group like Police on Guard is so very important. They represent those who understand the importance of having a police force that is not compromised by politics. As Clay Farnsworth noted, "The only consistency coming out of our House of Parliament is the inconsistencies."[457] Such an environment of instability on the political front requires this country to take seriously what we have seen in how the government and its police forces treated protesters differently based on the ideological commitment of the Cathedral.

We remain a divided country. The police in Ottawa, from the many different police departments, were under a lot of political and social strain

---

[457] "Police On Guard for Thee: Freedom Feature with Clay Farnsworth," First Freedoms Foundation, accessed May 12, 2023, https://firstfreedoms.ca/police-on-guard-for-thee-freedom-feature-with-clay-farnsworth/.

coming from different directions. Their mistreatment of the protesters, prodded by Mr. Trudeau and his ministers, the press, and others of the Cathedral, will be long remembered by Canadians who only wanted to peacefully demonstrate against a government that had gone too far.

The truckers showed Canada and the world that the lessons learned from the civil rights protests of years past remain important for us today. Peaceful protests that end in state violence solidify the fact that the state has lost the argument and support of the people. The elites may think they have won, but it's a pyrrhic victory in the long run.

The truckers showed the complicity of the police and woke its members to the political reality.

# 13. Exposed the Complicity of Politicians

POLITICIANS, LIKE BANKS, are risk averse. They give support to a cause only if they know they can win. They're very skittish about leading the charge unless there's a large following behind them. And it's not just any following they want, but usually a following from the Cathedral. Currently, the top figurehead of Canada's Cathedral is Prime Minister Justin Trudeau.

Mr. Trudeau is everything that the left "woke" mandarins want. On every major front, from climate change to the numerous issues of sexuality, he speaks the hippest "woke" jargon. But as with many politicians, he talks the talk but struggles with the walk. Our first self-declared "feminist" prime minister with a tattoo of an Indigenous Haida raven on his shoulder (which also contains a tattoo of the planet), has it all—that is, if you ignore him wearing blackface, or booting out Jody Wilson-Raybould, or travelling by private jet as his carbon footprint grows exponentially. But for the Cathedral, he is their "peoplekind" because he uses their vocabulary, and he showers money on causes they support.[458]

The Trucker Freedom Convoy had enough of the "woke" politician; it had enough of the political class that wanted to control their lives. The convoy leaders wanted to meet with the politicians so that their cause would get a fair hearing. Despite the prime minister's aversion to them, they wanted to speak to him and come to some resolution of their

---

[458] "Canada invests $100M in 'historic' action plan for 2SLGBT communities: Majority of money will help fund community organizations over 5-year term," CBC News, August 29, 2022, accessed May 12, 2023, https://www.cbc.ca/news/politics/federal-action-plan-lgbtq-1.6564977.

concerns. However, the vocabulary made it very difficult. "Freedom" to the truckers was just that—freedom to live their lives without government control. "Freedom" for the Cathedral meant "domestic extremist terrorism." Not even the reality of bouncy castles could change their minds. In their view, such castles were a ruse to catch the naive unawares.

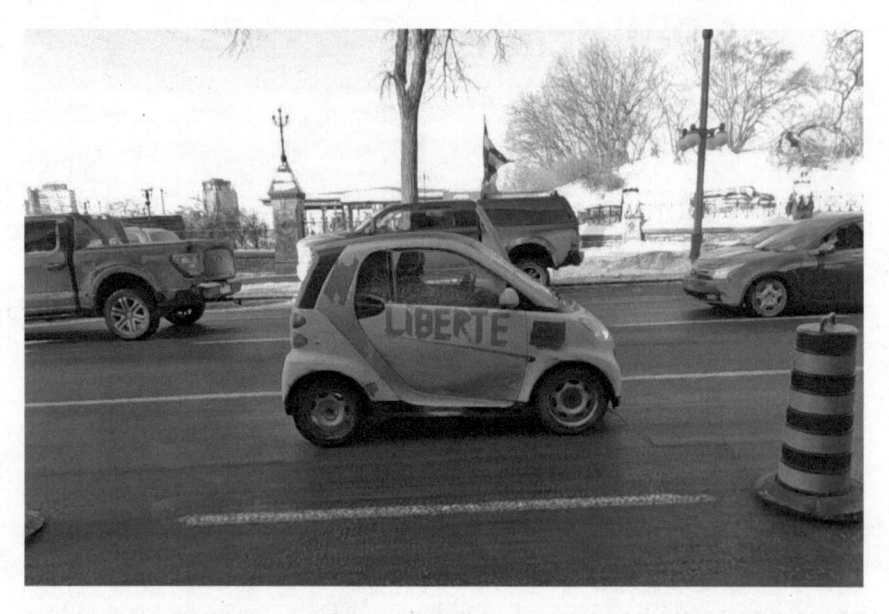

*Liberte*

The prime minister made it very clear that he wasn't going to parley with the convoy leaders. To talk with them would mean facing the scorn of his "woke" followers. The Liberals and the NDP—parties that once advocated for the rights of workers—shivered at the thought of having anything to do with the convoy. The more those political parties identify with the Cathedral, the less they understand, let alone represent, the working class who keep our economy going.

Even Erin O'Toole, the then-leader of the Opposition Conservatives, at the beginning of the convoy, waffled in his attitude toward the truckers. O'Toole's goal was to bring the Conservative Party into closer alignment with the Cathedral, as he hoped to increase his political market share. It didn't work out well for him as he straddled the ever-increasing divide.

With the convoy driving to Ottawa, O'Toole wouldn't commit to supporting them. He said, "It's not for the leader of the opposition or a political party to attend a protest on the hill or a convoy."[459] A far cry from Trudeau's position that he attends only those protests he agrees with. O'Toole continued, "It's up to politicians to advocate for solutions in a cost-of-living crisis, in a supply chain crisis in a way that's responsible and respectful of the public health crisis we're in." He sought to get "as many people vaccinated as possible, including truckers."

As O'Toole wavered, his caucus got restless. Pierre Poilievre tweeted for the end of government COVID-19 measures and to "Reopen our businesses, let our truckers drive and restore freedom for all."[460] Poilievre was not alone. Martin Shields,[461] Andrew Scheer,[462] Leslyn Lewis,[463] and Garnett Genuis[464] were among the growing number of Conservatives stating their support for the truckers.

O'Toole, who had lost the 2021 election by taking the Conservative Party toward the left, didn't have the political capital to weather the

---

[459] Catherine Levesque, "As opposition to trucker vaccine mandate grows, Erin O'Toole dodges questions," *National Post,* January 24, 2022, accessed May 12, 2023, https://nationalpost.com/news/politics/erin-otoole-dodges-questions-on-trucker-vaccine-mandates.

[460] Traceitback#LETREALWOMENSPEAK (@traceitback), "From Pierre Poilievre: COVID has become a never-ending excuse for power-hungry authorities to replace our freedom with their control," Twitter, January 23, 2022, 11:17 PM, https://twitter.com/traceitback/status/1485466689999310850.

[461] Martin Shields, (@MartinBowRiver), "I am in Ottawa awaiting the trucking convoy on its way to the capital," Twitter, January 24, 2022, 2:51 PM, https://twitter.com/MartinBowRiver/status/1485701746332557314.

[462] Warren Steinley (@WarrenSteinley), "Nice to listen to a new trucker who sees the impacts of the Trudeau Liberals failed polices daily," Twitter, January 24, 2022, 8:09 PM, https://twitter.com/WarrenSteinley/status/1485781927382581248.

[463] Dr. Leslyn Lewis (@LeslynLewis), "I'm proud of the Truckers. Peaceful protest is a cornerstone of our democracy," Twitter, January 25, 2023, 10:37 AM, https://twitter.com/LeslynLewis/status/1486000209427681295.

[464] Garnett Genuis (@GarnettGenuis), "I stand with truckers across North America, who want to be able to bring essential goods to people who need them," Twitter, January 22, 2022, 3:16 PM, https://twitter.com/GarnettGenuis/status/1484983342227283971.

Trucker Convoy. His caucus was in revolt. One MP said that the "straw that broke the camel's back" was O'Toole's "ham-fisted response to this trucker convoy."[465] The hammer came down when O'Toole's ally, MP Bob Benzen, called for a review of O'Toole's leadership.[466]

Benjamin Dichter, one of the convoy organizers, chimed in, "If they (the Conservatives) were smart, they would pull Erin now. Right now. Get him out of there. We all think that Pierre resonates with the vast majority of Canadians in his opposition to Justin Trudeau."[467]

The convoy wasn't even a week in Ottawa before it shook Canadian politics to the core. O'Toole was out as leader on the evening of February 2, 2022, and his caucus appointed Candice Bergen the interim leader.[468] She held that post until Pierre Poilievre was elected the next leader on September 10, 2022.

If Poilievre eventually forms the next government, he will owe his position, in part, to the Trucker Convoy. Hopefully he will be different from other politicians, who speak one way during the campaign season, and another once elected. That is yet to be seen. Mr. O'Toole promised to be a "blue" conservative only to be a "red" conservative (or perhaps a red liberal) in practice. Poilievre, being the keen politician he is, will no doubt learn from the O'Toole experience. He has no choice if he's to remain as leader and as prime minister, if the latter should come to pass.

However, when three of his caucus met with European parliamentarian Christine Anderson, who was touring Canada, Poilievre decided to disassociate himself from Anderson because of her views on immigration. Anderson gained popularity among those who supported the truckers

---

465 Stephen Maher, "The Conservative revolt has begun," *Maclean's*, February 1, 2022, accessed May 12, 2023, https://www.macleans.ca/politics/the-conservative-revolt-has-begun/.

466 Bob Benzen (@BobBenzen), "Today, I am calling for a caucus review of Erin O'Toole's leadership of the Conservative Party of Canada," Twitter, January 31, 2022, 7:30 PM, https://twitter.com/BobBenzen/status/1488308784703414272.

467 Maher, February 1, 2022.

468 Marieke Walsh, Robert Fife, and Ian Bailey, "Erin O'Toole ousted as Conservative Party leader after caucus leadership vote," *The Globe and Mail*, February 2, 2022, accessed May 12, 2023, https://www.theglobeandmail.com/politics/article-erin-otoole-loses-conservative-party-leadership-vote/.

because of her outspoken criticism of Prime Minister Trudeau. The conservative MPs were "silent" after Poilievre's statement that Anderson's views were "racist."[469] Such is the nature of politics.

People are watching how the politicians understand the Trucker Freedom Convoy. Those in the Cathedral have already made their judgement: the truckers and all they stand for are to be despised. The Canadian flag on a pickup truck triggers fear in their hearts.

The Trucker Freedom Convoy was not your typical Canadian protest. Consider how the Trudeau government responded with brutal force, how the media propagandized the government talking points and its misshaped narrative against the people and the mission of the protest. That experience has fuelled the angry embers burning in the hearts of many Canadians. It's a political fire against the Canadian establishment like nothing else in modern times. Labelling the protesters as "fringe" only fed that fire.

Those in the Cathedral have much to chatter about right now. Their entire cultural project is being placed on the public scales and being weighed in the balance of the people. The common-sense, no-nonsense types are evaluating the "experts," and they are not happy with the cost of all of the putdowns, the job losses, and the lost family opportunities to gather for special life events over the pandemic years, especially as more revelations appear of political malfeasance being behind much of the "science" for the vaccine mandates and lockdowns. While those in the Cathedral argue that rejections of government health mandates are based on "conspiracy theories," time is revealing that such "theories have actually become true."[470]

The Trucker Freedom Convoy and its supporters aren't the fools the Cathedral think they are. And it behooves Mr. Poilievre and other

---

469 Stephanie Taylor, CTV News, March 1, 2023, accessed May 12, 2023, "Two Conservative MPs silent after Poilievre says they 'regret' meeting German politician," https://www.ctvnews.ca/politics/two-conservative-mps-silent-after-poilievre-says-they-regret-meeting-german-politician-1.6294470.

470 Bruce Pardy, "It's time to drop the hysteria and learn to live with COVID," Probe International, accessed May 12, 2023, https://journal.probeinternational.org/2022/01/10/its-time-to-drop-the-hysteria-and-learn-to-live-with-covid/.

politicians to be careful not to take the truckers' support for granted. It is a movement, as we have seen, that is gracious and non-violent, but they are not sheep.

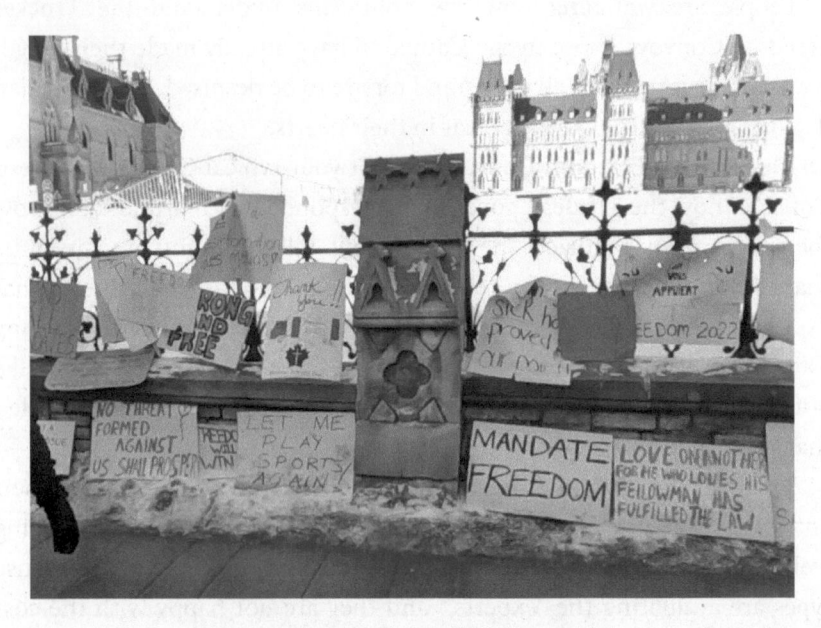

*The People Poured Out Their Hearts' Cry*

Tom Marazzo observed[471] that when Candice Bergen took over as interim leader of the Conservatives, she did a photo-op with the truckers in a café, but then the "next day she went into the Commons and said, 'Ok truckers you proved your point now go home.'"[472] Wow! That really helped nobody. You just abandoned all hope that the Conservatives were actually going to be an effective opposition of any kind now. They were playing politics with us ... It frustrates me that a lot of them are running

---

471 "Trudeau's Tiananmen Square—Interview with Tom Marazzo," First Freedoms Foundation, accessed May 12, 2023, https://firstfreedoms.ca/trudeaus-tiananmen-square/.
472 For her actual statement in the House of Commons see CTV News, "Bergen to convoy protestors: 'Take down the barricades," YouTube, February 10, 2022, :51, https://www.youtube.com/watch?v=g_ft0l61pNI.

around saying that they supported the Convoy. You know what, actions speak louder than words."[473]

Marazzo explains that after invocation of the emergency powers, the convoy organizers and their legal counsel wrote the "Roadmap to Freedom." They recognized that the Liberals and the NDP weren't going to listen, but they hoped that the Conservatives would at least give it some consideration. Marazzo personally emailed it to Pierre Poilievre and requested a closed-door meeting but never received a response. He surmises that the Conservative leadership was preventing any ongoing connections with the convoy because of the declaration of emergency.

It was a crucial moment of truth for the convoy. Would the politicians stand up against the abuse of power by the Liberal government? While the Conservatives voted against the extension of powers, the NDP voted with the government. The Cathedral had won the battle. It remains to be seen if Canadians will allow them to win the war.

The Trucker Freedom Convoy motif has become a powerful political symbol. That symbol is more legitimate because the convoy was non-violent. There's no question that had it turned violent on the part of the truckers or protesters, then it would have been a very different story. The violence of the police is a shame on the country and has tarnished Mr. Trudeau and the Liberal Party brand in the minds of many Canadians and the onlookers the world over.

All symbols can be commandeered for political purposes that may, or often may not, be to the benefit of the original cause. Politicians, like banks or businesses, will jump on any social movement that can benefit, or perceive to benefit, their bottom line. Just because a politician takes on the vocabulary of the Trucker Freedom Convoy doesn't mean they're the real thing. As Marazzo said, "actions speak louder than words." When Justin Trudeau says he is a "feminist," one must hear the opinion of people who worked with him, like Jody Wilson-Raybould to know if he's genuine. The point is this: be mindful of the virtue-signalling politician.

---

[473] "Trudeau's Tiananmen Square—Interview with Tom Marazzo," First Freedoms Foundation, accessed May 12, 2023, https://firstfreedoms.ca/trudeaus-tiananmen-square/ at minute 36.

Marjory LeBreton, the former Tory Senate leader, revealed that she stepped down from the board of directors of the Conservative riding association in Carleton, Pierre Poilievre's local riding, because of Poilievre's support for the trucker convoy.[474] Going forward, politicians will have to be on their toes, ensuring that they are who they say they are, because opposition is coming.

Pierre Poilievre was armed with his "secret weapon," Jenni Byrne,[475] who whispered to him what he must do to win. Her strategic expertise in the "ground war" of politics, much like the no-nonsense of the truckers, fit hand-in-glove in getting things done in the world of politics. Instinctively, she and her team knew that Poilievre had to take the energy of the Trucker Freedom Convoy and make it his own. Whatever flak the mainstream media fired back, it was but a small price to pay for the win. And winning was the game that had to be played.

Described as "a ruthless, no-holds-barred politico willing to turn on allies the moment she's crossed,"[476] allegedly she brought down O'Toole and put Poilievre in his place by her behind-the-scenes machinations. Politico quotes sources as saying she is a "force of nature," who has mastered the "dark arts" through a long time of political experience from working with Stephen Harper and Doug Ford.

Byrne's political savvy comes down to her "rare, deep understanding of what everyday voters, especially conservative-minded folks, care about."[477] While politicians often forget the "little guy" when they get in power, Byrne does not. She understands what's necessary to get the hearts and minds of the person on the ground.

---

474 Catherine Lévesque, "As 'moderate' Conservatives meet, suspicions of anti-Poilievre plotting grow," *National Post*, July 20, 2022, accessed May 12, 2023, https://nationalpost.com/news/as-moderate-conservatives-meet-suspicions-of-anti-poilievre-plotting-grow
475 Jenni Byrne and Associates, accessed May 12, 2023, https://jennibyrne.com/.
476 Andy Blatchford and Nick Taylor-Vaisey, "Jenny Byrne is just getting started," *Politico*, September 10, 2022, accessed May 12, 2023, https://www.politico.com/news/2022/09/10/jenni-byrne-is-just-getting-started-00056012.
477 Ibid.

Poilievre's leadership campaign has all the markings of Byrne's political acumen in "winning the ground game." "[I]t's the art of identifying voters, sharpening the message, cutting down opponents, funneling resources to the right places, mobilizing volunteers and getting out the vote." His negative attacks on the opposition proved effective. While the media says he skirts too close to the "conspiracy theories" of his base on such issues as the World Economic Forum, he nevertheless said no cabinet minister of his will ever go to a WEF meeting.[478]

While Byrne may be "Pierre's most-effective weapon," I believe that her instincts saw the opportunity in the Trucker Freedom Convoy as the most effective political wave of small-town, no-nonsense Canadians to hit the shores of Parliament Hill in a long time. She worked her strategic skills to Poilievre's benefit in riding that wave, first as victory for leadership of the Conservative Party, and second, given her political knowhow she, her team, and Poilievre's own political instincts could conceivably ride the wave to 24 Sussex Drive and the prime minister's office.

In truth, the small-town men and women the truckers represent have been rejected by the Cathedral. Therefore, the field is wide open for politicians to fill the vacuum and carry the truckers' freedom flag. In doing so, they'll bring out those trucker supporters who have never voted or who haven't voted in a long time.

The Trucker Freedom Convoy had a way of separating the political wheat from the political chaff. This protest movement puts the politicians to the test to see if they truly walk the talk. The prime minister is soon to learn that this "fringe minority with unacceptable views" has a political electoral brigade of its own that is slowly marching toward Parliament Hill, with the beat of the ballot soon to be dropped in deciding the next prime minister.

The Trucker Freedom Convoy is a defining moment in Canadian politics and its lessons are marching on.

---

478 GaffleBab, "Pierre Poilievre DENOUNCES World Economic Forum," YouTube, August 29, 2022, 1:07, https://www.youtube.com/watch?v=EroPanMlhCo.

# 14. Exposed the Lies of the Prime Minister

"I AM STILL mad at myself for that—for being convinced, at one point in time, that the prime minister was an honest and good person, when, in truth, he would so casually lie to the public and then think he could get away with it."[479]

Jody Wilson-Raybould's account of her time as a member of Parliament and in Justin Trudeau's cabinet, *Indian in the Cabinet*, was published in the fall of 2021. The timing couldn't have been better. The prime minister had called an unnecessary election for September 20, 2021. Rather than getting the majority he longed for, Trudeau ended up in virtually the same place with a minority of seats in the House. Canada was $600 million worse off with the election expense.

Wilson-Raybould's descriptions of interactions with the prime minister and his staff reminded the Canadian electorate of the Trudeau government's multiple scandals and conflicts of interest. Her story no doubt played a part in denying him a majority government.

*The Globe and Mail* reported that Trudeau placed undue influence on Wilson-Raybould to lift the prosecution of SNC-Lavalin. Trudeau

---

[479] Jody Wilson-Raybould, *Indian in the Cabinet*, (Toronto: HarperCollins Publishers, 2021) 229–30.

responded that the story was "false."[480] We now know unequivocally that Mr. Trudeau himself was false and spreading "disinformation."[481]

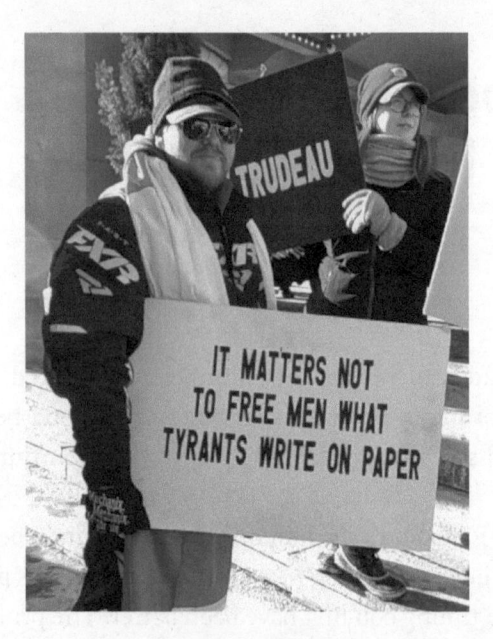

*It Matters Not*

The propensity for falsehood is a hallmark of Mr. Trudeau's government.[482] That predisposition was evident during the Trucker Convoy. It

---

480 Elizabeth Thompson, "Trudeau under fire over claim he pressured justice minister to intervene in SNC-Lavalin fraud case," CBC News, February 7, 2019, accessed May 12, 2023, https://www.cbc.ca/news/politics/trudeau-snc-lavalin-fraud-corruption-1.5009578.

481 John Ibbitson, "Justin Trudeau and things that are not so," *The Globe and Mail*, August 16, 2019, accessed May 12, 2023, https://www.theglobeandmail.com/politics/article-justin-trudeau-and-things-that-are-not-so/

482 Brian Lilley, "Trudeau again claims Jody Wilson-Raybould's story false: 'I did not want her to lie. I would never do that. I would never ask her that. That is simply not true.'" *Toronto Sun*, September 11, 2021, accessed May 12, 2023, https://torontosun.com/opinion/columnists/lilley-trudeau-again-claims-jody-wilson-rayboulds-story-false; Diane Francis, "Justin Trudeau's track record of failure: The Trudeau Liberals have a track record of dismal leadership, yet this country has so much talent and potential," *Financial Post*, September 17, 2021, accessed May 12, 2023, https://financialpost.com/diane-francis/diane-francis-justin-trudeaus-track-record-of-failure.

was as if there were alternate realities: one that was on the ground in a few streets of downtown Ottawa adjacent to Parliament Hill,[483] and the other in the minds of Mr. Trudeau and his associates, which was parroted by the mainstream media.

As I mentioned earlier, I spent three full days in Ottawa over two weekends during the convoy protest. What I saw when milling among the crowd was nothing—absolutely nothing—like what the mainstream media and Mr. Trudeau said was going on. That experience more than anything else told me that something unhealthy was happening in the media narratives about the convoy.

I remember the first two days of the protest as being very noisy. The blaring of the horns was a bit much, to be honest. Strangely enough, as time went on, I did get accustomed to it. Like living near a train track. Eventually, you ask, "what train?" Somehow, the mind seems to filter out background noise. By far, the majority of the trucks were parked along Wellington Street from about the Supreme Court to the Chateau Laurier.

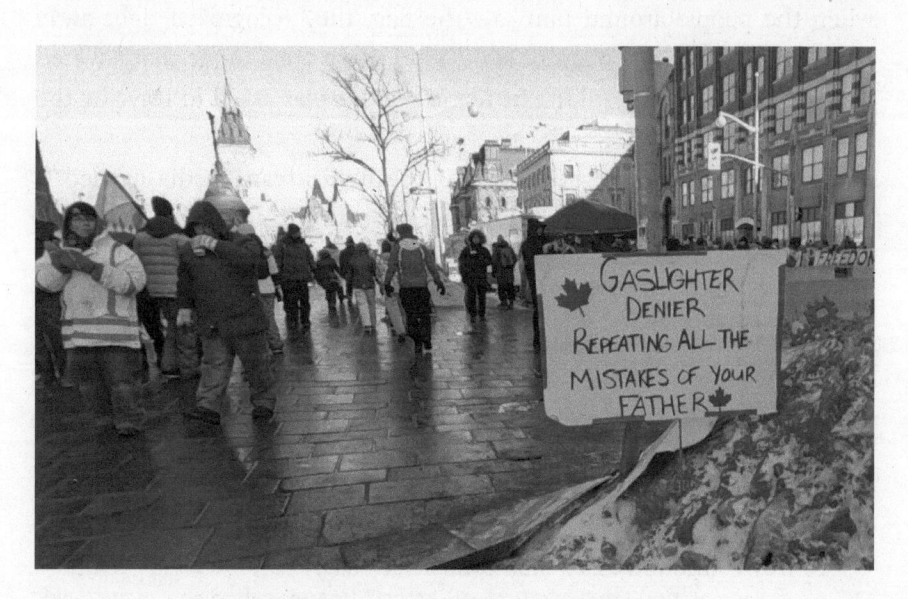

*The Gaslighting Propensity Of Guess Who?*

---

483 One friend of mine told me, "I cannot stress enough how minimally disruptive the Freedom Convoy was to life in Ottawa. It was literally several city blocks of the geographically largest city in the country."

Before the Truckers arrived in Ottawa, Trudeau said they didn't represent Canadians.[484] The mainstream media presented the truckers as an extreme group that was going to create mayhem in Ottawa. They did cause inconvenience for sure. Indeed, there was some hardship. For example, Henry Assad closed three of his downtown cafés. "It's been horrendous," said Assad. "Big machinery spewing diesel fumes and honking days on end ... they're impeding on everybody else's right to live peacefully."[485]

Sometime during the first days there were two incidents that the mainstream media reported on and used to paint the entire convoy with the same brush. One involved a person with a Nazi flag. The picture I saw in the media was taken from the opposite side of the Rideau Canal, facing the Chateau Laurier. The individual was among a crowd of people climbing the stairs. I saw not a single Nazi flag myself when I was there, nor did I hear of any others being waved throughout the rest of the protest.

The second involved a young man carrying a US Confederate flag with a transport truck in the middle of it. The video I saw online showed that when the people around him saw the flag, they recognized right away that this person was a plant of some kind. He wore a toque that covered his entire face, so he couldn't be identified. He was asked to leave by the crowd, and he did.[486]

Those two incidents were all that the mainstream media needed.[487] Trudeau, speaking from an "undisclosed location" as he left Ottawa for

---

[484] *Global News*, "Trudeau says 'fringe minority' in trucker convoy with 'unacceptable views' don't represent Canadians," YouTube, January 27, 2022, 1:32, https://www.youtube.com/watch?v=vDfMybczw1k.

[485] Julie Gordon, "Ottawa's sleepy core transformed into protest street party," Reuters, February 17, 2022, accessed May 12, 2023, https://www.reuters.com/article/us-health-coronavirus-canada-trucking-ot-idCAKBN2KN0AI.

[486] Angelo Isidorou, "Canadian trucker convoy protestors confront masked man with Confederate flag, tell him to leave," PM., January 30, 2022, accessed May 12, 2023, https://thepostmillennial.com/canadian-trucker-convoy-confront-masked-man-confederate-flag.

[487] Nazi flags at the Trucker's Protest, https://finance.yahoo.com/news/nazi-flags-truckers-protest-152500396.html; Daniel Otis, "Obscene slogans spotted at trucker convoy sold on Amazon, Facebook," CTV News, February 3, 2022, accessed May 12, 2023, https://www.ctvnews.ca/canada/obscene-slogans-spotted-at-trucker-convoy-sold-on-amazon-facebook-1.5766921; Andrew Cohen, "The Ottawa occupation is the October Crisis revisited.

safety reasons, stated, "freedom of expression, assembly and association are cornerstones of democracy, but Nazi symbolism, racist imagery and desecration of war memorials are not. It is an insult to memory and truth. Hate can never be the answer. Over the past few days Canadians were shocked and frankly disgusted by the behavior displayed by some people protesting in our nation's capital."[488]

There was only one flag of each type present, And both were unwanted by the protesters as a whole. At the POEC hearings, Brendan Miller, the lawyer representing the convoy organizers, claimed that it was a former journalist who held the flag.[489]

*Blacklock's Reporter* obtained a secret memo from Canadian Security Intelligence Service (CSIS) that discounted government claims that the convoy was infiltrated by Nazis: "A lone swastika flag spotted outside Parliament was offensive but not representative of protesters who considered themselves 'patriotic Canadians standing up for their democratic rights' ... Only a small, fringe element supports the use of violence or might be willing to engage in it."[490]

In parliamentary debate after the invocation of the Emergencies Act government MPs did their best to tarnish the Freedom Convoy with the Nazi image. Consider, for example, Ya'ara Saks (York Centre), who proclaimed, "How much vitriol like "honk honk," which is a term for "Heil Hitler," do we need to see by these protesters on social media?" Even "honk

---

Justin Trudeau must be bold," *The Globe and Mail,* February 8, 2022, accessed May 12, 2023, https://www.theglobeandmail.com/opinion/article-the-ottawa-occupation-is-the-october-crisis-revisited-justin-trudeau/.

488 WION, "Canadian PM Justin Trudeau slams protestors," YouTube, February 2, 2022, 2:21, https://www.youtube.com/watch?v=agvl5uPKqv4.

489 Christopher Nardi, "Executive accused of carrying Nazi flag to discredit Freedom Convoy denies being in Ottawa," November 23, 2022, *National Post*, accessed May 10, 2023, https://nationalpost.com/news/politics/executive-accused-of-carrying-nazi-flag-at-freedom-convoy-not-in-ottawa; See also, Glen McGregor, "'Freedom Convoy' lawyer sued over Nazi flag claim," CTV News, December 21, 2022, accessed May 10, 2023, https://www.ctvnews.ca/canada/freedom-convoy-lawyer-sued-over-nazi-flag-claim-1.6204577.

490 "Nazi Flag Overblown: Memo," *Blacklock's Reporter*, October 11, 2022, accessed May 10, 2023, https://www.blacklocks.ca/nazi-flag-overblown-memo/.

honk" on social media was Nazified! After all, as Saks blazoned, "…. This is about something much deeper, darker and uglier that is threatening the stability of the House, the work that we do as legislators ... and the democracy that we have to uphold."[491]

A day earlier, the prime minister answered a question from Conservative MP Melissa Lantsman (Thornhill), a Jewish descendant of Holocaust survivors, with a Nazi slur. Incredible. His first response to her question was that her party can stand "with people who wave swastikas. They can stand with people who wave the Confederate flag."[492]

The House of Commons erupted in a roar that made the honking truck horns sound like crickets. The now former Speaker, Anthony Rota, rebuked the "the Right Honourable Prime Minister, to use words that are not inflammatory in the House."[493] Mr. Trudeau refused to apologize for such outlandish provocation.

Ironically, in September 2023, Rota invited the House to recognize an aged Ukrainian veteran, Yaroslav Hunka, sitting in the parliamentary gallery during the visit of Ukrainian President Volodymyr Zelenskyy.[494] Hunka was not only from Rota's federal constituency but served in the Waffen-SS Galicia Division under the command of the Nazis in WWII. In other words, a Nazi, was in fact honoured by the Canadian Parliament. Video of all the MPs including the Right Honourable Prime Minister giving Mr. Hunka not one but two standing ovations circled the globe. Immediately, social media burned with indignation at the spectacle.

Of course, it goes without saying that the MPs did not know of Mr. Hunka's past. They followed Rota's lead. The problem was Mr. Hunka was not properly vetted. At first blush one could surmise that Mr. Rota thought, if he was indeed responsible, that it was great to have a member of his constituency who fought the Russians in World War II as a great

---

491 House of Commons Debates Official Report (Hansard), Volume 151 No. 033 Thursday, February 17, 2022, at p. 2420.
492 House of Commons Debates, Official Report (Hansard), Volume 151 No. 032, Wednesday, February 16, 2022, at p. 2309.
493 Ibid.
494 "Moment Canada's House of Commons gave standing ovation to veteran later revealed as Nazi," The Telegraph, accessed October 4, 2023 https://www.youtube.com/watch?v=LbuWNyyo7ql

prop for Mr. Zelenskyy's address. However, any student of history would know Russia was on our side toward the end of that War – the Nazis were fighting Russia! Huge questions remain. Was it Rota who invited Hunka? Or, was it the Prime Minister's Office? After all, given the PMO's hyper vigilance over everything around Parliament Hill, it is hard to believe it was simply Speaker Rota's gaffe. Surely a visit of a war time leader would mandate a thorough vetting of all who would be within an earshot of the protected dignitary. Will we ever know what happened?

What we do know is rather than take any ownership the prime minister skirted the firestorm for days. He even avoided the House of Commons for a couple of days so three days later he said the incident was "deeply embarrassing" but then he pivoted to warning about "Russian misinformation."[495] No apology. I do not think it a coincidence that it was not until CBC's "At Issue" panel called on the prime minister to apologize[496] that he in fact did so the very next day. Not an apology of his government's mishandling of the affair but "on behalf of Canada's Parliament."[497]

On top of this, government House Leader Karina Gould (Burlington) sought unanimous consent to strike Anthony Rota's comments about Yaroslav Hunka from the record! Her motion was to remove the event from the "appendix" of the Commons Debates and from "any House multimedia recording."[498] Thankfully, the opposition knocked it down as soon as it was presented. It was a move that only O'Brien in Orwell's *1984* could appreciate. Reality is indeed stranger than fiction.

My point is this: the prime minister and his colleagues had no problem roasting the entire Freedom Convoy 2022 with the "Nazi" brand over the

---

[495] Nadine Yousif, "Trudeau calls praise for Nazi-linked veteran 'deeply embarrassing'," BBC, September 26, 2023, accessed October 4, 2023, https://www.bbc.com/news/world-us-canada-66919862

[496] CBC News, "At Issue | Is the Speaker's resignation enough?" September 26, 2023, accessed October 4, 2023, https://www.youtube.com/watch?v=d0w6fstgQrA&list=PLvntPLkd9IMdQ15d846WkdNgHHuUISVDe&index=3

[497] John Paul Tasker, "Trudeau apologizes after man who fought in Nazi unit was praised by parliamentarians at Zelenskyy event," CBC, September 27, 2023, accessed on October 4, 2023, https://www.cbc.ca/news/politics/yaroslav-hunka-fallout-1.6979628

[498] House of Commons Debates Official Report (Hansard), Volume 151 No. 223, Monday, September 25, 2023, p. 16897.

flimsiest of excuses but when he was amid an absolutely blunderous display of incompetence in giving two ovations to a member of the Waffen-SS Galicia Division he sought to avoid, deflect, blame, and ultimately erase it from the official record. Is there any wonder why we cannot but be nervous about his increased control over the internet and his definitions of "disinformation"? Is there any doubt why we cannot accept his defaming response to the hardworking, freedom loving supporters of the Freedom Convoy?

There can be no doubt that if you followed the mainstream media reports, and you believed the words of the prime minister, you would have a very dim view of the convoy. You would ask, how could our country tolerate these protesters with the hateful flags? How is it that tens of thousands of Canadians lined the streets, stood on overpasses, and waved Canadian flags in support of the truckers?

A friend of mine who works in construction carried out renovations in a client's house, and the conversation turned to the trucker protest. When the client found out that my friend had actually attended the protest, she couldn't handle the fact that there was a trucker sympathizer in the house! The client left the house to do a walk-about to calm down, so convincing was the media and the prime minister. The client informed my friend that seeing a Canadian flag on the back of a pickup truck "makes me nervous!"

Understanding the world through the Trudeau lens, which is also the mainstream media lens, there's no question that a sizable group of Canadians became very fearful of the truckers. "I did feel that this [fear Canadians had] threatened my life and livelihood," a trucker told me. It was "not a phantom threat, but a real threat."

The truckers were characterized as anti-everything-that-is-good. They represented an opinion opposite the "progressive" views of the Cathedral and therefore had to be discredited. As Bruce Pardy explained, "Let's just look at the double standards: If you're burning churches or you're blocking railways, but you're doing it for a progressive cause then that's okay. But if you're a trucker convoy protesting vaccine mandates, well, that is beyond acceptable civilized behaviour, and you must be crushed."[499]

---

[499] Barry W. Bussey Interview with Bruce Pardy, "You Must Be Crushed," First Freedoms Foundation, accessed May 12, 2023, https://firstfreedoms.ca/you-must-be-crushed/.

It was in Trudeau's interest to paint as dark a picture as possible. Given what we know about the government's manufacturing of opinions to be published in national papers to support their narrative as seen in the Jody Wilson-Raybould affair,[500] it's conceivable that the PMO was in contact with the various op-ed writers to call upon the government to be "bold" in dealing with the truckers. It's not without precedent and, given the prime minister's proclivity to doubling down on his positions, it's certainly probable.[501] The bouncy castles were too much! He had to go all in for the Emergencies Act powers. Those truckers had to be stopped.

As already noted, to invoke the Emergencies Act in line with its intent, there has to be a general emergency such that it cannot be handled under current law, requiring extreme measures to meet the emergency. These criteria were not met. Not only was the media's take a misrepresentation, but it was simply false that the police asked for the Act to be invoked.[502]

The Truckers' Convoy exposed Mr. Trudeau's dramatic skills of ignoring the truth by claiming:

- the truckers were violent extremists—they were not.
- the convoy was unsafe—it was not.

---

500 Simon Houpt, "'Write op-eds saying that what she is doing is proper.' What the Wilson-Raybould testimony reveals about the politics of newspaper opinion pieces," *The Globe and Mail*, February 28, 2019, accessed May 12, 2023, https://www.theglobeandmail.com/arts/article-what-the-wilson-raybould-testimony-reveals-about-the-matrix-of/

501 This despite newspaper editors who say that they, not politicians, decide on op-eds. That is rather doubtful given the millions of dollars the Trudeau government gives to the newspapers. There is an applicable adage that comes to mind: "He who pays the piper plays the tune." See Kathy English, "Newspaper editors, not politicians, determine which op-eds are published, *Toronto Star*, February 28, 2019, accessed May 12, 2023, https://www.thestar.com/opinion/public_editor/2019/02/28/newspaper-editors-not-politicians-determine-which-op-eds-are-published.html. Sorry Kathy, that does not pass the smell test. Your, "the *Star* strives to include a diverse range of voices and viewpoints on its opinion pages" is simply not true. As I was told personally, my voice was not needed—I was too conservative for your opinion pages. Unless you have suddenly changed. I do not think so.

502 Sarah Ritchie, "Emergency Preparedness Minister: police did not ask for Emergencies Act," CTV News, June 15, 2022, accessed May 12, 2023, https://www.ctvnews.ca/politics/emergency-preparedness-minister-police-did-not-ask-for-emergencies-act-1.5946705.

- the convoy was bigoted and racist with Nazi flags—it was not. Even if the flag holders turn out *not* to both be plants, to suggest that two incidents were indicative of the whole is ludicrous.
- the funding for the truckers came from Russia—it did not.
- the funding for the truckers came from America—some of it did, but the vast majority came from Canadians.[503]
- responding to the convoy required emergency powers—it did not.
- the police asked for the emergency powers—they did not.

The truckers' protest was a reminder that we ought to live as Aleksandr Solzhenitsyn admonished his compatriots in the Soviet regime to live.[504] We can no longer afford to live by lies. The truckers were emboldened to speak up and not be fooled by the consistent lying currently emanating from Ottawa and then proclaimed in the government-funded media.

Like Solzhenitsyn, and like the example of the Truckers, let us refuse:
- to say that which we do not think;
- to write, sign, or print a single phrase that distorts the truth;
- to utter a phrase in private or public that is a lie;
- to use any creative art or scientific endeavour that depicts or broadcasts a false idea;
- to cite out of context a quotation to please someone or further his interests if he doesn't share completely the idea quoted;
- to raise a hand to vote for that with which we do not sincerely agree;
- to be forced to attend a meeting to which we are called upon to distort a matter;

---

503 Sarah Turnbull, "GoFundMe head testifies over Freedom Convoy fundraising, says most donors were Canadian," CTV News, March 3, 2022, accessed May 12, 2023, https://www.ctvnews.ca/politics/gofundme-head-testifies-over-freedom-convoy-fundraising-says-most-donors-were-canadian-1.5804094; "Fed Convoy Allegations False," *Blacklock's Reporter*, March 4, 2022, accessed May 12, 2023, https://www.blacklocks.ca/fed-convoy-allegations-false/.

504 Alexander Solzhenitsyn, "Live Not By Lies," https://web.archive.org/web/20201118134739/https://www.orthodoxytoday.org/articles/SolhenitsynLies.php

- to subscribe to any media outlet that distorts or conceals primary facts;
- to do anything or allow to be done to us anything that we know or suspect to be a lie.

As Solzhenitsyn put it, we have the choice to be free or to accept slavery and conform while saying "I am in the herd, and a coward. It's all the same to me as long as I'm fed and warm."

It's not easy to stand against the lies. We will not, as Solzhenitsyn pointed out, be the first to take this path. We will join that brave few who in times past were willing to put it all on the line. "This path will be easier and shorter for all of us if we take it by mutual efforts and in close rank," he said, "if there are thousands of us, they will not be able to do anything with us. If there are tens of thousands of us, then we would not even recognize our country."[505]

The truckers' protest taught us to be true to what is right rather than bow to what is false. This is key to our own and children's future happiness.

---

505 Ibid.

# 15. Revealed That Non-Violent Protest Works

THE NIGHT BEFORE she was arrested, Tamara Lich gave a stirring address to her supporters. By that time, it had become evident that the prime minister, if he were to use the Emergencies Act powers, had to do it quickly because the truckers, the police, and the City of Ottawa were working through the most contentious issue of the protest—the trucks in the residential areas.

In truth very little of the City of Ottawa was occupied during the protest. As Dr. Don Hutchinson observed, "[t]here were ... political motivations for framing messaging about the situation that unfolded primarily at Parliament Hill and its immediate surrounds." The reality was that "roughly 3 km2 area of the 2,790 km2 city was designated as 'the red zone.'" Only 15,000 of Ottawa's 1,100,000 residents live in those 3 km2. But it gets better. When the Emergencies Act was invoked the demonstration area within that red zone came out to "one and a half kilometre (one mile) stretch of Wellington Street, and the off-site staging area at the RCTG park some five kilometres (3 miles) away."[506] Clearly things were moving in the right direction it was exceedingly evident this was not an emergency.

Investigative reporter Andrew Lawton observed that Trudeau realized that his window of opportunity to claim any legitimacy for the emergency powers was closing. So, he acted before the agreement between police and city resolved all the issues with the truckers.

---

506 See Dr. Don Hutchinson's report to the Rouleau Commission at: http://www.donhutchinson.ca/wp-content/uploads/2022/10/Submission-to-Rouleau-Commission-Don-Hutchinson.pdf

The non-violent trucker protest was having its effect. The more the prime minister talked about the "fringe minority" with "unacceptable views," the more the Canadian public could see the opposite through livestream on social media—children playing in the street, and the warm relations everyone shared. The more animated the prime minister became with his false rhetoric, the more nakedly unhinged his position was becoming.

The invocation of the Emergencies Act powers was ultimately so far over the top that it created a caricature of the entire Trudeau response to the protest. It was comedic in the age-old "juxtaposition of the incongruent." It was funny—in a dark humour sort of way. The more the "emperor" yelled, the less sane he appeared.

Of course, those who did not support the Freedom Convoy maintained that it was violent. While they would admit that it was not physically violent it was "violent" none the less in their minds. Such was the position of Josh Greenberg, a professor at Carlton University who has expertise, among other things, "Activism and Social Movements."[507] The Trucker Convoy was not a peaceful protest in his mind.

Greenberg wrote, "By what common understanding of the term does what we are seeing on the ground, on TV, in our social media feeds qualify as 'peaceful protest?'" "Is it merely the absence of physical violence and injury? That's not unimportant but is insufficient as a definitional threshold."[508]

What would be a "definitional threshold" of "peaceful protest" when people, who were penned up in their homes for so long during the pandemic, lost jobs, had family and friends disown them, lost houses and cars, and then when finally, they had an opportunity to express their frustration they did so in a manner without smashing windows, burning cars, or punching faces? That is more than sufficient to warrant the nomenclature of "non-violent" and "peaceful protest."

---

507 https://carleton.ca/sjc/profile/greenberg-josh/
508 Adina Bresge, "Calling the Ottawa protests 'peaceful' plays down non-violent dangers, critics say," The Canadian Press, January 31, 2022, accessed September 5, 2023, https://www.theglobeandmail.com/canada/article-calling-the-ottawa-protests-peaceful-downplays-non-violent-dangers/

If we are left with low thresholds of "violence" being triggered only for some unsavory comments or signs, then we are in real trouble.

As the Trucker Convoy gained attention from the average Canadian, one by one the provinces began lifting their draconian COVID lockdowns and vaccine mandates. Even the Quebec premier decided against imposing the "vaccine tax" he had been waving around for some time, I believe out of concern that his province would see the same sort of protest that would make it difficult to crack down on and still be seen as "the good guys."

Saskatchewan Premier Scott Moe noted that "[v]accination is not reducing transmission. An unvaccinated trucker does not pose any greater risk of transmission than a vaccinated trucker."[509] Meanwhile, Alberta Premier Jason Kenney said that "[t]he threat of COVID-19 to public health no longer outweighs the hugely damaging impact of health restrictions on our society."[510]

Those were significant wins for the protest.

Unfortunately, the prime minister's petulance against the truckers only meant that he would double down despite premiers calling for his relaxing of the federal health restrictions.[511] He was not going to give in, even when his mandates were anything but scientific. It became an issue of pride at that point.

Invoking the Emergencies Act meant that a violent end to the protest was inevitable. What violence the truckers wouldn't do during their three-week protest, the police would carry out over their three-day removal of the truckers from Ottawa.

---

[509] Theresa Kliem, "Sask. Premier says province will end proof of vaccine policy in 'not-too-distant future'," CBC News, January 29, 2022, accessed May 12, 2023, https://www.cbc.ca/news/canada/saskatchewan/scott-moe-proof-of-vaccination-twitter-1.6332514.

[510] Lisa Johnson, "COVID-19: Alberta's vaccine passport program lifted as of midnight Tuesday," *Edmonton Journal*, February 9, 2022, accessed May 12, 2023, https://edmontonjournal.com/news/local-news/covid-19-kenney-to-announce-albertas-plan-to-lift-restrictions-at-5-p-m.

[511] Charlie Hart, "Jason Kenney Is Calling on the Feds to End Vaccine Mandates & COVID-19 Tests for Travel," Narcity, March 7, 2022, accessed May 12, 2023,https://www.narcity.com/jason-kenney-calling-for-end-vaccine-mandates-covid-19-tests-for-travel.

With the police moving in and arresting fellow convoy organizer Christopher Barber, Tamara knew she was next. The night before she was arrested, Tamara Lich made a video address to her supporters.[512] "I just wanted to come on again and say first of all, thank you; second of all, to say please keep that love in your heart. Don't give in." She noted that "there's been a lot of joy and a lot of happiness." Overcome with emotion her tears flowed. She said, what is "transpiring against my fellow Canadians breaks my heart, it is breaking my heart, you guys. I just want you to stay strong and I want you to continue to be unified and spread the love."

She called upon those supporting the truckers to be kind and show love to the reporters on the streets. "We don't have to agree with what they're doing but it upsets me when I see people upset with them." Even though it was frustrating to see reporters put a negative spin on the convoy, Lich maintained that "we still have to have love in our hearts. Please show respect to them."

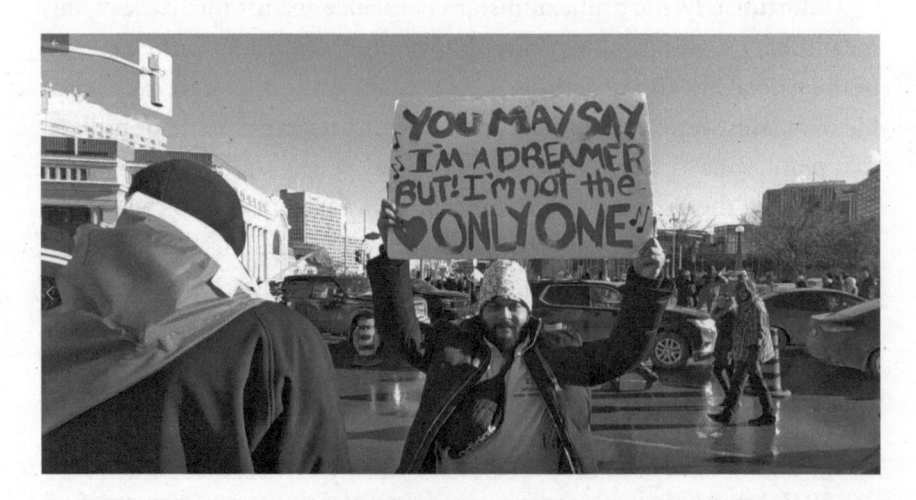

*Dreamers For Freedom*

Then she reminded everyone of the importance of respecting "our police officers" as they "are probably just trying to feed their families. I said

---

[512] *Western Standard*, "Freedom Convoy 2022 organizer Tamara Lich says she will likely be behind bars by the end of Thursday," YouTube, February 17, 2022, 12:52, https://www.youtube.com/watch?v=Yrfoy6eG49U.

it from the start, and I'll say it again, please pray for them and forgive them for they know not what they do."[513]

In a sign of true magnanimity, Tamara called upon her supporters to pray for Prime Minister Justin Trudeau—the same man whose ego had unnecessarily created this entire crisis. Recognizing that "there's a lot of rightful anger at our government" she reminded everyone that Justin Trudeau is a father of "three beautiful children" and while, "we don't have to like what he does[,] I'm gonna ask you to pray for him too ... I pray that you all find forgiveness in your hearts. I pray that you all find love even when we don't understand it."

She went on to admit her expectation that the following day she would be arrested. She was, and without incident, as she did not resist, while the Ottawa snow gently fell.[514]

"I think it's inevitable at this point. I'll probably be going somewhere tomorrow where I'll be getting three square meals a day," she announced. "That's okay. I'm okay with that. I want you to know that I'm not afraid. I'll probably get some sleep finally. Just please stay peaceful and please take care of each other and know that this too shall pass."

"There will be a tomorrow," she reminded her listeners, "and we will get through this ... The only way that this is going to succeed is if we always come from a place of love. I've always said, as human beings, we make choices from one of two places: we make choices from love, or we make choices from fear. That's it. That's the bottom line."

She warned those who opposed the convoy "are trying to provoke us. I mean, you hear their language. You hear the language and the verbiage that they're using and that is not coming from us. I know you guys all know that, but we can only win this with love, and we can only win this together and it's time to stand together." She called upon her supporters to "come to Ottawa and stand with us," but if they could not then "pray

---

513 Canadian Rights Reviews, "Tamara Lich, personal video message," YouTube, February 16, 2022, 13:18, https://youtu.be/xK92HRvDUWc?t=220.
514 Publica News, "Tamara Lich is arrested—'Freedom Convoy' Live Update from Ottawa," YouTube, February 17, 2022, 1:44, https://www.youtube.com/watch?v=OUpu-mKnLBE.

for us." There were many "brave men and women" who planned to stay "to fight for your freedom as long as they possibly can."

Tamara explained how she grew to become family with so many people through the experience. She said, "I know we're gonna have summer vacations together. We're gonna have Christmas together and I can't wait."

The video reveals, yet again, her tears. "But it's not tears of sadness," she said, then emphatically, "It's definitely not tears of fright." Rather, "I'm just so damn proud of all of you—every single one of you, not just in Canada but all around the world. Who knew? Who knew that this was going to take off in this way? So, please try not to be angry. Keep love in your heart. Stay strong. Stay unified and stay proud because we are so proud of you. The love we have felt in the last nineteen days, well before then actually ... it feels like it's been a year across this country with the likes of nothing I have ever seen before and that was you guys, that was all you.

"Don't you worry, I'll be back. I want you to keep fighting the good fight, and I want you to look out for each other. I want you to have each other's backs. I think you're all amazing and I hope one day that all the people that are here on the ground, that have worked so hard, they're all heroes. All of them ... Tomorrow is a new day and I'm ready. I am not afraid and we're gonna hold the line. Thank you. I love you guys. See you soon."

The next day she was arrested. As the police arrested her someone yelled "Hold the line!" She repeated it. Then another was yelling at the officers but she "asked them to stop and to be respectful."[515]

Taken to the Elgin police station two female officers searched her in the parking lot "in the dark and freezing cold." Once inside they took her photo and fingerprints, and weighed her. They put her in a cold cell, with no blanket. Wet from the melting snow she spent the night on the concrete floor that was "sucking what little warmth I had out of my body."[516]

The next day in handcuffs and leg shackles she was carted to the detention centre where they made her strip down, open her mouth and all her "nooks and crannies." "They even asked me to wear a mask while I was doing it," she tells. "Picture me bent over with my ass in some cop[']s face, but I'm wearing a mask for her protection. What a reminder of

---

515  Tamara Lich, 167.
516  Tamara Lich, 168.

the nonsensical public health "science" bullshit that we were so tired of putting up with."[517]

Asked if she was vaccinated, she said no and if she wanted a vaccine she said, "No thanks" and if she would take a COVID test. "[N]o thanks." "I have never taken a COVID test. If I don't feel sick I don't see why I should have to. And I'm not just going to take it because the state wants me to."[518]

They gave her bed sheets and extra prison clothes and led her to what she called the "dungeon." "It was solitary confinement," she recalls. "It was a dark cell, with high walls, with a teeny little window way up at the top. The place was covered in disgusting graffiti—swear words, drawings of naked women, all kinds of gross comments."[519]

She slept.

The truckers' emphasis on non-violence is a testament to the clear-minded thinking of Tamara Lich and her fellow organizers. Violence only begets more violence. Throughout the millennia, the principle of non-violent protest has shown itself to be an effective tool in bringing about social change.

The non-violent philosophy of Jesus Christ was evident in Tamara's video address. Her call to respect the police and to "pray for them and forgive them, for they know not what they do," references the statement of Jesus on the cross.[520] Likewise, the reference to pray for the prime minister reflects the common teaching of Jesus to pray for one's enemies.[521]

During the Montgomery, Alabama bus protests in 1954, Martin Luther King, Jr. was asked to be the fledgling movement's spokesperson. "In

---

517 Tamara Lich, 171.
518 Tamara Lich, 171.
519 Tamara Lich, 171.
520 Luke 23:33–34: "And when they had come to the place called Calvary, there they crucified Him, and the criminals, one on the right hand and the other on the left. Then Jesus said, 'Father, forgive them, for they do not know what they do'" (NKJV).
521 Matthew 5:43–45: "You have heard that it was said, 'You shall love your neighbor and hate your enemy.' But I say to you, love your enemies, bless those who curse you, do good to those who hate you, and pray for those who spitefully use you and persecute you, that you may be sons of your Father in heaven; for He makes His sun rise on the evil and on the good, and sends rain on the just and on the unjust" (NKJV).

accepting this responsibility," said King, "my mind, consciously or unconsciously, was driven back to the Sermon on the Mount and the Gandhian method of nonviolent resistance. This principle became the guiding light of our movement. Christ furnished the spirit and motivation while Gandhi furnished the method."[522]

Like the non-violent activists of the past, the truckers tapped into a long tradition of nonviolent confrontation with the authorities. That doesn't mean that there weren't those who advocated for violence. In every crowd you'll have rowdy people. In every crowd you're going to have violent slogans (I've already spoken about my personal distaste for the "F*ck" signs). Just because there's a Peter in the group willing to be violent for his leader doesn't mean the leader and the movement as a whole are violent. It means that Peter had some spiritual maturing to do. Peter was one of the disciples of Jesus who swung his sword at one of the crowd who came to arrest Jesus. Jesus told him to "[p]ut your sword in its place, for all who take the sword will perish by the sword."[523] To characterize the Ottawa truck protesters as "Nazis" is beyond the pale. It is a smear used in an attempt by vested interests against the truckers to ignore the facts and propagandize a hatred for the trucker protest.

As non-violence proved effective in other protest contexts throughout the millennia, so too it proved effective in Canada. It showcased to the country and the world that non-violence brought change without a hardening of the heart. While the prime minister continued using incendiary language, Tamara Lich called upon the truckers and protesters to pray for him. The contrast could not be more stark.

The prime minister's over-the-top invocation of emergency powers was a "jumping the shark" incident that was seen for what it was—an outrageous abuse of power to show the truckers who was boss and to show the Canadian public[524] that he was "saving" them from a "January 6" incident at

---

522 Martin Luther King, Jr., "Pilgrimage to Nonviolence," Stanford, April 13, 1960, accessed May 12, 2023, https://kinginstitute.stanford.edu/king-papers/documents/pilgrimage-nonviolence.
523 Matthew 26:52 NKJV.
524 "Canada Under the Emergencies Act: What Does it Mean? Interview with Iain T. Benson, Phil Horgan, and Jay Cameron," First Freedoms Foundation,

their doorstep.[525] The non-violence stance of the truckers elicited sympathy. There was no blood on the streets due to the truckers or their supporters. Blood did flow, however, from their mistreatment at the hands of police.

The truckers gained the sympathy of the average Canadian and an ever-increasing number of elected Canadian politicians. There can be no doubt that had there been a violent turn of events instigated by the truckers, there wouldn't be much sympathy going their way. Nor would there be as much admiration from around the world.

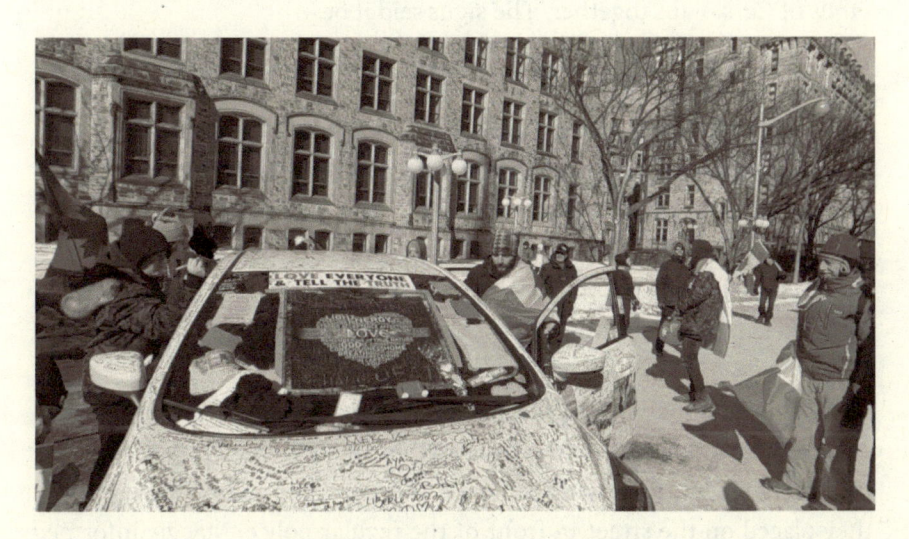

*Messages of Love Tattooed This Car*

Tamara Lich and her fellow organizers made the right call—hold the line but in a spirit of love and forgiveness. It showed without question the true non-violent nature of the protest, and it was a winning method that, despite the unacceptable approach of the government, has done much to heal the fractured country that was pushed into a vaccine mandate and lockdowns regime that had more to do with politics than science.

---

accessed May 12, 2023, https://firstfreedoms.ca/canada-under-the-emergencies-act-what-does-it-mean/.

525 Alex Boutilier & Rachel Gilmore, "Far-right groups hope trucker protest will be Canada's 'January 6th'", *Global News,* January 25, 2022, accessed June 5, 2023, https://globalnews.ca/news/8537433/far-right-groups-trucker-protest-jan-6/.

A police helicopter flew overhead, keeping an eye on the crowds as I walked along Wellington Street. Uniformed police were present, and I'm sure there were many plainclothes police as well. There were several officers in parked cars. The cars were running—not only to keep warm but to be prepared just in case they needed to take off at a moment's notice.

The mood on the street was akin to the Ottawa Winterlude festival in those pre-COVID days in February. The celebratory mood was in stark contrast with the seriousness of the cause that had brought so many thousands of Canadians together. The signs said it best:

"Freedom Is Essential"
"This Ends When We All Say No!"
"Member of the small fringe minority of unacceptable views"
"Freedom Not Fear"
"Our Future Is Now: Fight For It"
"It's All For Nothing If You Don't Have Freedom"
"It Matters Not to Free Men What Tyrants Write on Paper"

Maggie Braun stood on the frontline with the other trucker protesters as the riot police made the final arrests. In a moving symbolic act, the protesters were armed with copies of the Canadian Bill of Rights[526] that they placed on the street in front of the regular police. Maggie informed the officers in front of her that if they moved forward, they would be trampling the Bill of Rights with their boot and she would not move. A man next to her laid down his prayer mat, another gave her a Bible. "The whole scene was actually quite calm," she recalled. "They switched out the regular police with the riot police." She remained in a prayer stance on the street and her back was stomped on by the riot police with a rifle pointed at her head. She was handed off to an Ottawa police officer.

---

526 The Canadian Bill of Rights (SC 1960, c. 44) was passed during the John Diefenbaker Government in 1960. It remains law but is not a constitutional document as is the Canadian Charter of Rights and Freedoms, being the Constitution Act, 1982, Schedule B to the Canada Act 1982, 1982, c. 11 (U.K.), which came into force on April 17, 1982 under the P.E. Trudeau Government. The Canadian Bill of Rights applies only to the federal law and federal government actions.

She and the officer looked behind at the scene. The copies of the Bill of Rights were swirling up with a blast of the wind. "He cried," Maggie remembers. "He dropped a tear and he told me, 'The protesters won this today. You proved you were peaceful today to the end and the truth will come out.'"[527]

The entire protest was safe, non-violent, and meaningful. Canada got the message. The world got the message: these people had enough of the belittling and the disrespect shown them by their own government who denied them medical choice and mobility.

They rightly opposed. They rightly did so non-violently. And so it must be in the future encounters with arbitrary power. The truth will come out.

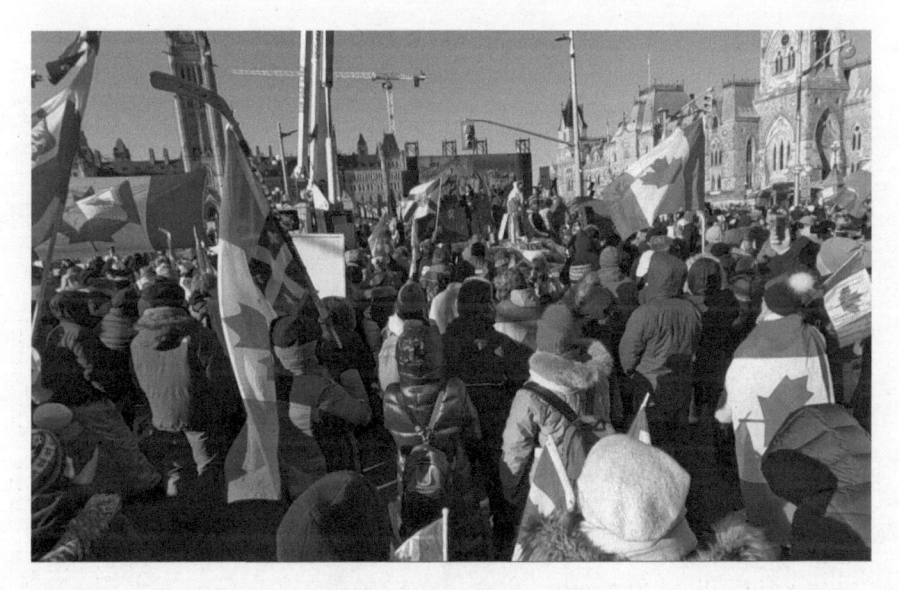

*Peaceful Protest Remains Effective*

---

527 Maggie Braun interviewed by Barry W. Bussey on July 20, 2023, for Freedom Feature, https://firstfreedoms.ca/part-one-one-womans-story-on-how-to-make-a-difference-interview-with-maggie-braun/

# 16. Awakened the People to Faith and Freedom

THE TRUCKER CONVOY struck a deep emotional and spiritual chord among a lot of Canadians.[528] That shouldn't surprise us. Human beings are naturally drawn to religion, even as children.[529] As adults, it's not uncommon to return to our natural religious curiosity, especially when we face rough times. The three years of the COVID-19 pandemic were rough for many who refused to be "vaccinated," as they lost jobs, houses, family, and friends. Not only did they lose economically but also socially, as the country turned against them, from the prime minister to their very own family members. Never in the history of Canada have we seen such widespread vitriol against a marginalized group based on their private medical decision on vaccination.

The anguish of losing so much for standing on the principle of conscience was met with a torrent of callous ridicule. "That was your decision! Your loss is your fault" was a familiar refrain the unvaccinated heard repeatedly. It was a dispiriting, dark, and painful realization that very few of their acquaintances held the same convictions. That's the reality for conscientious people willing to buck the popular trend. Familial relationships and friendships developed over decades were blown out, just like candles in the wind.

---

[528] See my discussion, "Totalizing Crisis—Freedom Feature with Peter Stockland," First Freedoms Foundation, accessed May 12, 2023, https://firstfreedoms.ca/totalizing-crisis-freedom-feature-with-peter-stockland/.

[529] Justin L. Barrett, *Born Believers: The Science of Children's Religious Belief*, (New York: Free Press, 2012).

The abandonment was real.

When the Trucker Freedom Convoy 2022 rolled across the country and into the nation's capital, the dispirited unvaccinated and those who supported their right to choose were hopeful that things would change. It was an answer to many prayers.

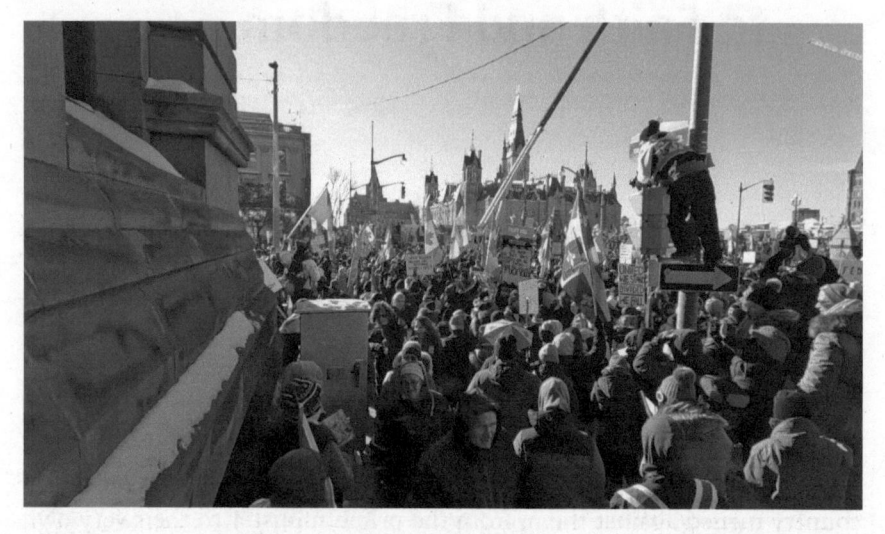

*Crowds Desired Encouragement And Camaraderie*

The vaccinated had no idea what a symbol of hope those trucks were to the "unvaccinated" who had lost so much. How could they? The vaccinated didn't lose so much materially. In fact, most, if not all, the vaccinated kept their jobs or were bailed out by the government's CERB program. Some, such as the federal bureaucrats, even got pay raises. Life for them was comparatively good.[530] Really good, if money is any indication.[531]

Many troubled souls sought solace in their religious faith. With Christianity being the majority faith by nearly two-thirds in Canada (as of

---

[530] Franco Terrazzano, "A tale of two downturns: A report on government pay raises during the pandemic," Canadian Taxpayers Federation, January 2022, https://www.taxpayer.com/media/Report-pandemic-pay-raise.pdf.

[531] Andrew Kozak, "Over 45,000 more federal workers receiving six-figure salary than before the pandemic," True North, August 10, 2022, accessed May 12, 2023, https://tnc.news/2022/08/10/federal-workers/.

2011),[532] it's not surprising that the Christian faith saw the most expression during the convoy protest.

If we look at the history of the struggle for human rights and freedoms in our free and democratic societies, we'll begin to appreciate the religious context in which those rights emerged. For example, freedom of conscience has been called by the Supreme Court of Canada a "prototypical right," since that freedom blazed the trail for other rights.[533] It was in the religious tumult of the Reformation and aftermath of the English Civil War that religious conscience found itself as the bedrock for freedom of speech, expression, assembly, and so on.

If we limited our news to the mainstream media, we'd think that religion is only a force for great evil and chicanery, duping people from their hard-earned money. The call for religious freedom is now referred to by its detractors as a demand for the "right to discriminate."[534] Our sophisticated society has made light of religion, misrepresenting religious adherents as being judgmental and gullible. Yet by now I think we have enough information to conclude that there is a profound judgmentalism combined with a horrendous lack of critical thinking in the legalistic progressive ideology that has motivated much in our current political reality.[535]

The Trucker Freedom Convoy raised the profile of religion in a way that was fascinating to watch. As I made my way through Ottawa, I came

---

532 "Two-thirds of the population declare Christian as their religion," Statistics Canada, accessed May 12, 2023, https://www150.statcan.gc.ca/n1/pub/91-003-x/2014001/section03/33-eng.htm.

533 Barry Winston Bussey, "Blazing the Path: Freedom of Conscience as the Prototypical Right (2020)." *Supreme Court Law Review* 2nd Series, volume 98, 2020, SSRN, accessed May 12, 2023, https://ssrn.com/abstract=3698265.

534 For a discussion on religious freedom in the current context see, "Reasonable Limits for Religious Freedom in Canada—Interview with Professor Dwight Newman," First Freedoms Foundation, accessed May 12, 2023, https://firstfreedoms.ca/reasonable-limits-freedom-feature-with-dwight-newman/.

535 Daniel N. Gullotta, "If Conservatives are the New Punks, are Progressives the New Puritans?" Law & Liberty, September 7, 2022, accessed May 12, 2023,
https://lawliberty.org/book-review/if-conservatives-are-the-new-punks-are-progressives-the-new-puritans/.

across several groups praying and others singing hymns or preaching on the streets.

Such sermonizing reminded me of the preaching I read about at the time of the American Revolution, when many preachers across the thirteen colonies spoke about the right of the people to revolt against the English Crown.[536] Religious fervour has a unique relationship with political events. This is especially true when the political events cross over into the religious domain. Of course, there's often no clear line between what is or is not "political" or "religious." What is for some a totally "political" issue is for others a totally "religious" issue. In recent years there has been an explosion of issues that were once considered "religious" but are now considered "political." Here I think of the institution of marriage. Has there been a more political/religious issue? Yes, perhaps abortion. The list can go on—medical assistance in dying (MAiD), conversion therapy, and sexuality, to name but a few more.

My point is this: we shouldn't be surprised or concerned that religion found expression at the Trucker Freedom Convoy. Why? Because religion and political freedom movements have worked in tandem throughout history, and like running water, our human condition will continue to lead us on the well-worn paths of the past no matter what current political philosophy rules the day. It's inevitable in the struggle for freedom.

I wasn't at all surprised or alarmed by the overt religious presence among the crowd. The religious activity I saw at the convoy was positive. Indeed, I suggest it was reassuring. It was a relatively small part in the overall mix. It wasn't a giant worship service, but it was present and not uncommon. I will speak more on this religious aspect of the convoy below as I describe my discussion with former MP, pastor and dentist, Dr. Harold Albrecht.

Within that framework, Pastor Henry Hildebrandt's sermon on January 30 to the protestors on Wellington Street, in front of the Centre Block of Parliament, fit with what was happening on the ground. He pointed to the Peace Tower and proclaimed, "Look in that window in the south of the Peace Tower. It says that 'Freedom is the sure possession of those alone

---

536 See Ellis Sandoz, ed., *Political Sermons of the American Founding Era 1730-1805* (Indianapolis: Liberty Fund, 1991).

who have the courage to defend it.'" He continued, "Pastor, should you be preaching Jesus? Yes! God giveth freedom!"[537]

When dealing with issues of conscience, like the vaccine mandate, it's not surprising to hear these kinds of religious idioms and metaphors come into currency.[538] Artists in support of the truckers published material with a distinctly religious theme.[539] "Truckers fight, Jesus saves" was another sign I saw. I'm not sure about the theological implications, but it's evidence that there was a mixing of the political reality with the spiritual desire for validation of the cause.

While in Ottawa, I encountered a street evangelist telling the story of salvation in Jesus and handing out free copies of the Bible. Another preacher was prophetic, using biblical illustrations to urge Canada to put away "corrupt leaders." He referenced the New Testament account of how Jesus raised Lazarus from the dead.

---

[537] Pastor Henry Hildebrandt, "Live—Prayer for Unity at Parliament Hill, Ottawa," YouTube, January 30, 2022, 46:00–, https://www.youtube.com/watch?v=liF2u2ikBCA.

[538] For an interesting discussion see, "Wake Up! A Storm is Brewing—Interview with André Schutten," First Freedoms Institute, accessed May 12, 2023, https://firstfreedoms.ca/wake-up-a-storm-is-brewing/.

[539] Artist Hannah Dieleman's picture of the Trucker Convoy going through the departing waters brought to mind the opening of the Red Sea story in the Book of Genesis. See https://www.facebook.com/photo.php?fbid=10159676630197674&set=pb.715897673.-2207520000.&type=3 accessed June 20, 2023

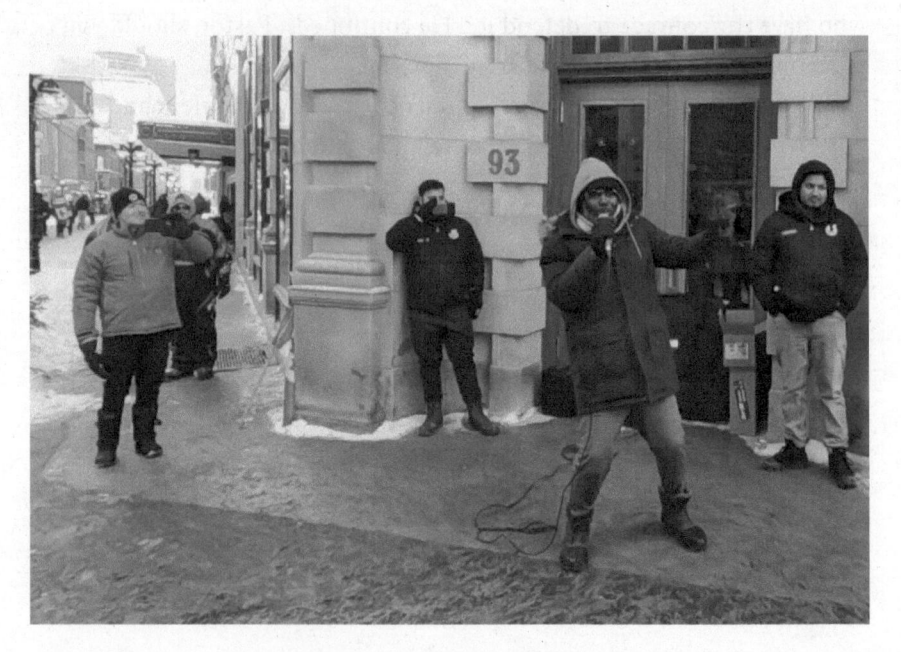

*Canada! Rise Up! Said The Preacher*

The transcript from my video recording of the preacher reveals the deep religious and prophetic connection with the Trucker Freedom Convoy:

> But Martha said to Jesus, "Lord if you came on time my brother would have lived but even now, I know you are the Resurrection and the Life. Anyone who believes shall live though they die."
>
> You know there's a connection between Lazarus and Canada.
>
> For so long, under bad leadership, Canada looked like it was dead. For so long, under bad government, Canada looked like it was sick, [like it] was in a tomb. But people like myself, we pray for Canada. We said, "God, heal our land! God, we want to see change! Lord, remove the corrupted leadership. People are hurting." It looked like it was taking so long but GOD HAS SHOWED UP ... God was listening to our prayers!

The Bible says that the writing of God interceded for his people. And God looked at Canada like this [*the preacher looks down to the ground*]! God looked down on Canada. I believe Jesus declared, "Canada shall be saved"!

The Bible tells us when Jesus came to the tomb of Lazarus Jesus did not say, "Oh my God, what are we going to do? Lazarus is dead." Jesus never said, "Angel Gabriel, we are finished!" He never said, "Father, why has thou forsaken Lazarus?" Jesus never said, "Oh my, I can't raise him up." Jesus walked to the tomb. He called in a loud voice, "Lazarus! Lazarus! [*at this point the crowd of forty or so gathered around are in sync with the preacher*] Rise up!"

And the Bible says there was a rattling in the grave. And Lazarus, he came out of the tomb, walking!

I believe right now, Jesus, like Lazarus, he says, "Canada, rise up!" [*Preacher then gets the crowd many times to chime in. Preacher says "Canada" and the crowd answers "Rise up" over and over.*]

*The preacher: Canada!*

*The crowd: Rise up!*

*Canada!*

*Rise up!*

*Canada!*

*Rise up!*

And this is how we can stand on guard for thee! When the people who are obsessed with Jesus, when the people who love Jesus, when we rise up for righteousness. We stand for righteousness. We stand up for what is just! Then we are standing on guard for thee.

God wants us to be about His business. To preach the gospel, to cast out demons, to raise the dead, to heal the sick, to advance the kingdom. He said to teach everything He was commanded by the Father, Son and Holy Spirit. The gospel is a symbol. It is the birth, the death, the resurrection of Jesus Christ.

God is on a mission to seek and save the lost. Canada, God is saying to rise up! and Canada has to rise up because of the resurrection power ....

We are in the middle of an awakening. This is God's wake up call! Because, you know why? Because when people keep doing evil, eventually, people are awakened to the truth.

I met a couple of young people who were working in tandem with the street preacher by handing out tracts. One of them, Ryan, told me he was there to proclaim freedom, "but freedom through Jesus Christ." He loved what was going on all around him. "I love to see so many Canadians out and about fighting for freedom, all of us doing it in the same kind of spirit." He said, "But for me here, I believe that freedom is in Christ ultimately, so that's why I'm here."

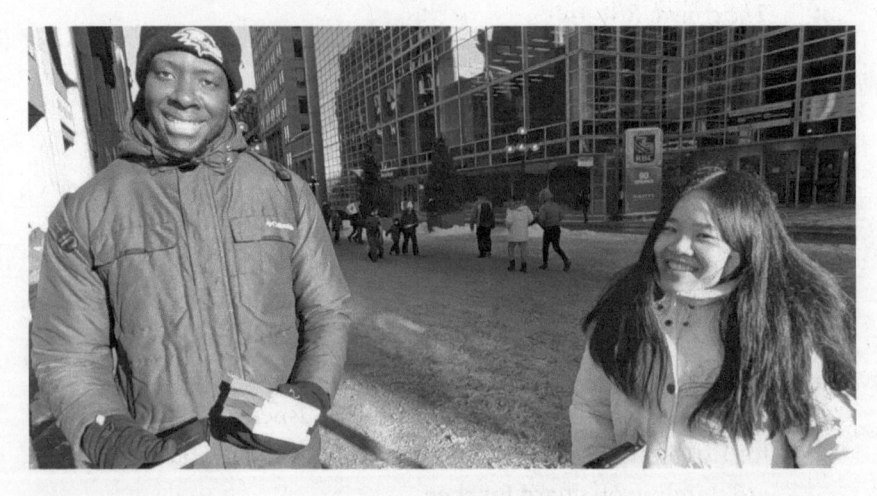

*Freedom Is In Christ Ultimately*

As to the street preacher, "He's trying to get a crowd [and] to talk to anyone who will listen. We want people to be free, not only on the outside but in their hearts as well."

Of course, not all protestors were "into the religious thing," but many were. Christian groups came from around the country to get involved in the protest—not just to fight for political freedom, as Ryan noted, but for freedom of the heart.

Among the Christian "missionaries" was Harold Albrecht, former member of Parliament for Kitchener-Conestoga. He was part of a religious group that went on prayer vigils throughout the protest, praying that peace would prevail.[540] Prior to entering politics, Mr. Albrecht not only practised dentistry but served as a pastor. "It was my pastoral work that led me into political work," he noted. He encouraged his members to be part of prayer vigils supporting prolife or marriage rallies. In time he felt he should get involved politically. "I believe that as Christians we are called to be stewards of God's creation and government is a creation of God—it's not man's idea. If we're going to be stewards of His environmental creation of the beauty of our natural resources, we need to also be stewards of our government and to be sitting at the table where important decisions are being made for our country. If we're not at the table, we have no one to blame but ourselves.

"It strikes me that it's extremely important for everyone to have an opportunity to serve in the public arena. Christians are no different than any other group that needs to have that voice as well."

Throughout his time in Parliament, Mr. Albrecht wasn't shy about his Christian faith. "You cannot deny your faith," he told me as he went on to quote Sir Thomas More, with words to the effect that "public statesmen who forsake their private conscience for the sake of their public duties lead their country on a short route to chaos." Albrecht concluded, "I'm not prepared to give up my faith to preserve my political career."

During our interview, he expressed concern with where the prime minister "is going now ... he is literally driving a wedge between people of

---

540 "Time for Faith—Interview with Harold Albrecht," First Freedoms Foundation, accessed May 12, 2023, https://firstfreedoms.ca/time-for-faith-freedom-feature-with-harold-albrecht/.

faith" on a host of issues, of which the vaccine mandate is but one. This government not only denies but defies "the principles that we've come to enjoy and appreciate in our country and have led us to where we are. It's very troubling," says Albrecht, "especially for people of faith."

Albrecht desires that "pastoral leaders across the country [be] more engaged in the political spectrum and I don't mean they should take on a partisan view, but they should be willing to address issues and political issues. Every issue is political in some form or another and politics is not necessarily partisan ... This current division of vaccinated and unvaccinated" is but an example.

"I think we need to stand strong for the freedom [of] people to make a decision that's informed by their conscience in scripture," says Albrecht, "... and to stand up for the person who is potentially losing a job like the truckers are, like many nurses have, like many university professors have, like many university students who have lost their ability to continue their education have, even if [they're] double-vaxxed. As believers I think we should be standing up for those who are being negatively impacted by these very divisive measures."

Albrecht continued in his conversation with me,

> The whole spirit of our age right now, when it comes to the vaccine, has really put a lot of people's back up because it's a spirit that is not at all what we have been used to in our society. I mean a society that has championed freedom of choice, suddenly to be not only making life difficult because ... you're losing jobs, losing positions in the university, but then to be labeled and dehumanized as racist, misogynist, anti-science, fringe with unacceptable views, this kind of language is genocidal in the sense that it is attacking a group of people.

His criticism struck a chord with me, as it's exactly how I, and many people I know, feel about the circumstance. He carried on. "Basically, saying they're unworthy. These are people that we can agree to disagree with." Then he quoted the prime minister, "'Should we even tolerate these people?'" and points out, "that is extremely divisive and that's one of the reasons I participated in a prayer vigil and a ... number of prayer walks on Parliament Hill ... in support of the cause of protecting someone's right to work."

Albrecht is motivated by a deep spiritual commitment that goes back to a teaching in Old Testament law, in Deuteronomy 24:6, which says you cannot take a tool of trade as surety for a debt, for the simple reason that the tradesperson won't be able to work to pay the debt. "To have the prime minister of our country take a person's livelihood away because of a decision they've made that is in good conscience, informed by belief, informed by faith, is one of the most dehumanizing things we could possibly do."

He wasn't at all pleased with the mayor of Ottawa's call to confiscate the trucks that were towed away. "Not only are you taking someone's ability to work away from them," said Albrecht, "but now you're taking their whole assets. The assets that they have accumulated over a lifetime of hard work and commitment. You're taking that away because of a protest that was held on the problem [to begin with]."

"I think it's criminal," says Albrecht, "I cannot get over how quickly Canada has descended into, and I don't use this term lightly, but a 'fascist' mindset. A mindset that says you do not even have the right to exist and provide for your family because you will not comply with the government directive."

Albrecht referred to what many of us in the pursuit for freedom have heard. Many people shared how their family members didn't speak to them for over a year because of their vaccine status. Young lawyers shared with him the struggle they have in some of the top-named law firms in downtown Toronto. They described "the absolute vitriol that is thrown out around the water cooler, discussions against those who do not accept the government's position resulting in people who are very nervous about even voicing their opinion. It's like, who do you trust? It's almost like the government is requiring each individual, not to be an individual standing up for your rights and your freedoms ... freedom of speech and so on but simply you are now an arm of the state. You are to snitch on your neighbor, snitch on your family. It truly is remarkable that we have descended so low and so quickly."

But as Albrecht noted, it doesn't stop there but has continued into the Christian churches. "God is grieved by this division," Albrecht said, "and I hope and pray that we can get beyond that and stand up for those who are voiceless as we're called to do all through Scripture."

Standing up for the vulnerable and the voiceless was one of Albrecht's motivations throughout his career, whether as a parliamentarian, a dentist, or a pastor. "That's why I take so seriously this current situation, the overreach of government initially, but especially with the Emergencies Act and some of the things that happened in downtown Ottawa."

For five days Albrecht walked the streets of Ottawa. "I can tell you that I have never seen more smiles, more happy people, more joyful and hope-filled people than I did in those five days."

His experience mirrored mine. He didn't see any negative incidents and wished that the mainstream media were more balanced. "I went on numerous walks around the Parliament buildings with groups of people who are passionate about their faith in Christ, who wanted to see God's intervention. And I believe we did see God's intervention in the fact that it was a largely peaceful protest. I'm thankful that I had that opportunity to be part of that."

Albrecht raises an interesting point. He's convinced that part of the reason the convoy protest was as peaceful as it was stemmed from the religious influence of the people praying at the protest for Divine intervention. Believers like me may find this plausible. However, even for the non-believing atheist, there's a reasonable explanation of why that would be the case. Just consider being in the presence of a deeply spiritual grandmother. Suddenly, you have difficulty swearing or doing something that would offend her. Could it not be that many were prevented from doing any mischief because of the sizeable presence of people of faith praying and singing hymns? I witnessed people kneeling on the streets, praying earnestly for the peacefulness of the protest and the safety of everyone there.

Albrecht, like me, was troubled by the "F-bomb" flags against Trudeau. "I denounced them," Albrecht told me, "but having said that, ninety-nine per cent of what I saw was positive. It was [a] celebration of Canada and a celebration of the freedoms that we've come to enjoy and appreciate, and

I want to do all that I can to support my brothers and sisters in defending those freedoms."

He participated in "the Jericho Walk," which went around the Parliament precinct every day. Each morning the organizer would give a brief introduction as to what the Jericho Walk was about. Albrecht recounted, "She would say, 'This walk is a respectful walk. We don't want any disrespectful flags as part of this walk.' I observed on one day, a person who was carrying a flag that was inappropriate ... You can imagine what it was...and he quietly and respectfully rolled up his flag and put it away. I think that's where we need to stand. We need to stand for the cause but ... denounce the negative aspects that are there."

On his spiritual walks, he saw groups of people engaged in prayer and worship. These "people of faith," most double-vaccinated, were standing up for those who had lost their jobs.

Mr. Albrecht spoke to several truckers personally and found many were out of a job. "Think of the implications of that for a young family," said Albrecht. "I talked to one guy that was probably under forty, thirty-five I'm guessing, who said, 'I have no work. That's why I'm here. I have no work.' And to hear politicians glibly say at the end of their speeches in Parliament, 'You've been here long enough it's time to go back to work.' Well, how ridiculous is that statement when the very reason they were there in the first place is because they had no work to go back to, right? They [the politicians] lost sight of that."

The many people of faith who came to Ottawa made a difference in Albrecht's mind. Many of them led others to a faith in Christ. "And that is what is really the ultimate source of our freedom. They were led to Christ. That's got to be our living hope."

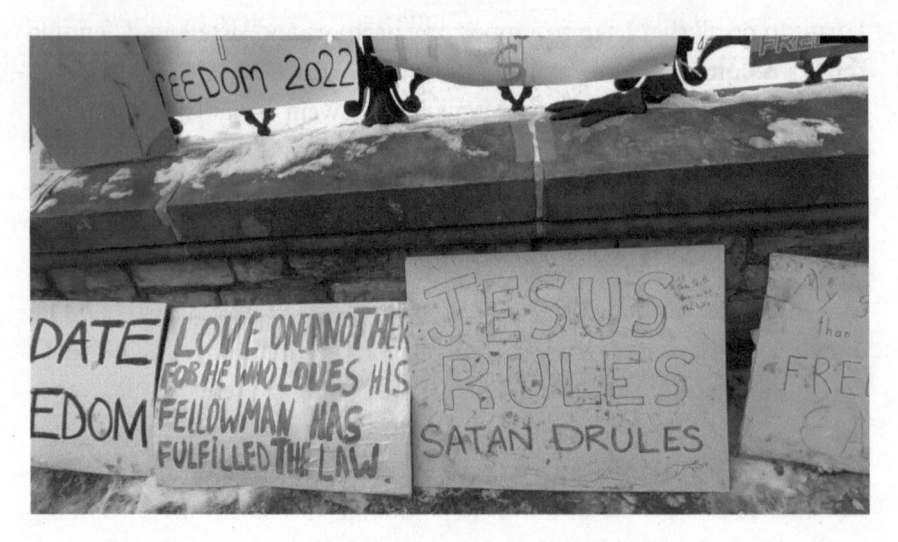

*Religious Messages Abounded*

While politics is important, Albrecht told me that having people of faith around the table didn't mean that they "always [got] the solution we had hoped to achieve. But [we knew] that the result was ... less drastic in terms of its potential negative impact than it would have been had we not been at the table." At the end of the day, it was faithfulness to one's duty. "God had not called us to be *victorious* in every battle, but He had called us to be *faithful* in every battle.

"I've never believed and still do not believe, that politics is the hope of the world," said Albrecht. "Jesus Christ is the hope of the world. The message of the local church is... the freedom that He offers us and the direction that He gives us in our life for full and meaningful relationships.

"So whether Trudeau is prime minister or Biden is president, or Trump is president or Harper is prime minister, none of those factors matter to me as much. Because He [Jesus] lives I can face tomorrow. Because He lives all fear is gone. Because I know who holds the future. Life is worth the living just because He lives."[541]

---

541 Albrecht was quoting from the hymn, "Because He Lives" written by Bill and Gloria Gaither (1971), accessed May 12, 2023, https://hymnary.org/text/god_sent_his_son_they_called_him_jesus.

The centennial flame was put out during the protest. But Albrecht noted that a person told him "'They put out the centennial flame, but a flame has been lit in the lives of the Canadian people that will not go out.' I don't mean that in a sense of ongoing protests, but it was a flame of hope ... We see many times where God's people and the cause of righteousness was being denigrated and looked like it had lost and along comes a little group, in Gideon's case 300, and defeated armies that were much more powerful.

"When you look at some of the decisions of the last number of years in terms of going against God's principles this is a beautiful picture that God is in control. He will keep us safe, maybe not physically. [I think of the words of that] great song 'A Mighty Fortress is Our God,' 'the body they may kill but God's truth abideth still.' So that's my ultimate source of hope and I want to be known as one who not only talks about it but lives it out in my personal life and that doesn't keep me from being involved.

"Too many people have said in these past two years but especially in the last two months ... oh God's in control, God's in control, God's in control. I agree a hundred per cent, but the implication of many of them ... is 'we shouldn't get involved.' I think that is absolutely wrong." Using the illustration of tending to a garden, Albrecht said it isn't enough that God is in control of the garden; the gardener must attend to it. "I can trust Him to provide the sun and the rain and thank Him for the good soil but if there's no garden at the end of the year, it's not because God wasn't faithful, it's because I didn't do my job."

At the end of the interview, Mr. Albrecht read a paragraph from a document he'd received shortly before our conversation:

> Is it really so surprising that communists and fascists from the Soviet Union to present-day China fear people of faith? They know that faith poses a moral challenge to their unchecked authority. Faith gives our lives a moral structure. To the state it says, "this far and no farther." Without faith the government has no vision. Without family, government has no foundation.

"I think that answers part of the question," concluded Albrecht, "why so many people of faith were engaged in this freedom movement."

My time following and being with the Trucker Freedom Convoy 2022 convinces me that Harold Albrecht is spot on. "I am convinced," says Albrecht, "that we are in the middle of an awakening. This is God's wake-up call! Because, you know why? Because when people keep doing evil, eventually, people are awakened to the truth."

"Canada!"

"Rise up!"

Canadians suffering during the pandemic reached out to their political leaders for help; instead of receiving sympathy, they were ridiculed or rejected. Is it any wonder that so many turned back to their spiritual roots to find meaning, comfort, and hope? Their faith made them whole. The fight was bigger than each individual and collective. It had a metaphysical component that allowed everyone to take solace that immediate victory was not the goal—but being a faithful presence during the storm that Canada was going through was the objective. That was met.

The truckers woke up the deep spiritual reservoir that played a major role in building our country in the first place—and played a significant role in keeping the protest peaceful and will continue to play a role in the future.

# Conclusion

THE EBBS AND flows of politics are much like the ocean's tidal movements. I grew up near the ocean in Newfoundland. The first time I ever thought of the tide was when I went with my father and grandfather in the early summer to get capelin, which is a small, smelt-like fish that literally rolls onto the beach with the waves at high tide where they spawn. It was a time of great delight as a child to get the buckets and buckets of these fish. And how easy it was compared to the other fishing I would do—like spending all day trouting in the rivers and ponds for a few measly trout! (Mind you, I like the taste of trout better!)

The rejoicing over the capelin coming to shore is much like the feeling of jubilation that occurs for the political partisans of the winning party on election night. It's exhilarating. When the tide comes your way, it lifts all boats. It also comes with financial and material rewards and power.

Power is an opiate for any political leader.

The person holding the office of Canadian prime minister gains an immense amount of power. Technological advances in social media and security tracking have meant a rapid growth in influence and power. It's not surprising that a relatively young, politically cunning, and astute prime minister, who is also an ideologically driven scion of one of Canada's most famous prime ministers, would become addicted to such power and seek to change Canada into his image.

Most Canadians in 2015 were willing to give Justin Trudeau the benefit of the doubt. They expected that he would be surrounded by knowledgeable, seasoned, and competent helmsmen and helmswomen, who would help him steer the Canadian ship of state to peaceful and productive shores. However, he and his close associates got rid of the "old guard" immediately. Canada lost the wisdom that those older statesmen and stateswomen had to offer. Justin Trudeau and his inner circle knew more than all the seasoned Liberal insiders. "It's 2015" after all! The arrogance that accompanied this government is truly baffling. Individuals with no experience or expertise were put in charge of huge government departments and expected to do well simply because they met the new "woke" identity qualifications. Arrogance is no substitute for competence, as our now one trillion-dollar plus debt and untold pain and suffering of the COVID-19 mismanagement testify.

The Trucker Freedom Convoy exposed Trudeau's lack of appreciation for our forebears' democratic legacy. It exposed a raw viciousness, a fanged bite of political power not seen in the history of this country. Lying about the nature of the trucker protest to the point of implementing the most draconian laws meant for existential threat to the body politic but used in peacetime to control a political protest is not who we are. Freezing bank accounts for having the "wrong political opinion" is not peace, order, and good government—it is sheer madness.[542]

Canadians saw it. Indeed, the world saw it in real time, not in the commentary of mainstream media but in the accompanying video and from the private independent media and social media.

There has developed a line of thinking amongst the Cathedral that they are the arbiters of what is truth. Power does that. They have the truth. They impose it. They get to define the meaning of words. They get to control speech. In other words, they get to rule on what is and is not appropriate to think. If you have the temerity to challenge their truth, you will pay the price. You are the "fringe minority with unacceptable views". You do not deserve to be part of the society of the "right thinking people." Therefore, censorship, dismissal from gainful employment, freezing of bank accounts, dismissal from university, in short, everything is on the table to mete punishment for "wrong think." As Professor Pardy noted, "you must be crushed." The thought of a free and open exchange of ideas and debate, and the questioning of authority to discover the truth

---

[542] "Comply or Else—Interview with Jeffrey Tucker," First Freedoms Foundation, accessed May 12, 2023, https://firstfreedoms.ca/comply_or_die_jeffrey_tucker_brownstone_institute/.

of things is dismissed as "extremism" and somehow "undemocratic!" It is "racist", "misogynist". How then does the Cathedral deal with such people? So far has the political goalposts been moved from the Charter's notion of a "free and democratic society."

The Truckers Freedom Convoy, a protest of the working class was not simply a movement against the elite imposition of an unjustified vaccine mandate, it was a direct challenge to the Cathedral's claim to have the power to define truth. That challenge has forever changed Canada. Even with the Trudeau government's doubling down on its draconian measures against the unvaccinated, those that dared to challenge the Cathedral, the government no longer has the leverage over the people it once had during the COVID pandemic. Fear is gone.

The benefit of the doubt has been shattered. Already Mr. Trudeau and his government are viewed by Canadians as no longer trustworthy. The tide on this government is going out. The tide of the Cathedral's monopoly on power is going out. It's as inevitable as the ocean.

Liberal partisans can no longer pretend that the fall of the Trudeau mystique has not occurred. The hero worship, indeed, the cult-like figure that Trudeau has become among his supporters is partly to blame. The religious fervour of "my leader can do no wrong" made it possible for Mr. Trudeau, a fallible human being like the rest of us, to fall victim to ego and fame. It is a modern-day Greek tragedy unfolding before our eyes. If Liberal partisans, as well as Mr. Trudeau, can't admit to themselves that they were wrong in how the Truckers were treated by the government, then we have a serious problem in this country.

Hero worship, the cult of personality, imposing the Cathedral's definitions, would be our downfall but for the autoignition of the human spirit to be free.

It's not only true for Liberal partisans but all partisans, whether Conservative, or NDP and any other partisan group, because we are human. Humans will forever make mistakes. That's why we were given the democratic institutions we have. The definition of what it means to be human – the ravaging thirst to be free to think and debate has been our guide throughout the millennia. The Parliament, the judiciary, the executive, the media, the academics, and average citizens all have a part to play in keeping us on the straight and narrow of what works best for a free and flourishing society. As inheritors of a political system that has given much to Canadians, we must relearn our history. We must relearn what it means to be free from the tyranny of the Cathedral. Our future depends upon it.

The Truckers experienced, in only a wee point in time, what it is like to be in a place where freedom is of little importance to the leader of the land. The petulant response of power showed us all we need to know. Democracy is only as strong as the weakest politician. Free and democratic societies require an electorate that is educated in its ideals with sufficient courage to hold government to account. Failing that it is but a castle made of sand and water.

I believe that during the COVID-19 pandemic, our institutions, by and large, failed to hold the government accountable to our democratic ideals. The Cathedral has so infiltrated our system. It was the Canadian truckers who took to the road and went to Ottawa to make noise that held everyone accountable. They, in my view, saved Canada from the tyranny of the Cathedral during that critical hour of our country's history.

Our institutions have long claimed the honour of being democratic guardians. In this case, they were not. They were missing in action during the COVID-19 pandemic—as noted in the pages of this volume. More can be written about the individual institutions and the peculiarities of their failures to protect our Canadian democracy, but that would take a book on each account.

Suffice it to say that the truckers stopped the Cathedral's momentum in its tracks and shamed the elites in their institutions. And it is up to us to stop that momentum from being forced into action again, and to ensure it does not swing back too far the other way. Those in the Cathedral have, for the most part, doubled down and tried to paint the truckers as malcontents without a cause as they, the elites, had everything under control. Except that they did not "have everything under control." They enjoyed their taxpayer-paid time off during the lockdowns. They didn't lose their homes. They got their raises as they worked from home. They claimed to be on the "right side" of the vaccine debate. They scoffed at the lowly trucker who dared to say, "No! I am not taking the jab! I defy your authority over my body."

The Cathedral claimed the vaccine would bring us all back to normal—there would be no transmission etc., etc. Then when that was not the case, they changed the narrative: "We did not say there would be no transmission with the vaccine but that it would limit the symptoms." While the elites basked in the ever-changing narrative of what was the "science of the day," the average blue-collar worker driving a truck had enough.

The progressives among us define what is "reasonable." As Professor Bruce Pardy notes, "the range of what is considered reasonable has been narrowed to progressive ideals alone."[543] Whatever falls outside of their ideals is defined as "unreasonable" and not "worthy of respect."

It will remain the spoken narrative of the Cathedral that the truckers were wrong, they overstayed their welcome, they were racists, they were misogynists, etc., etc., but the average Canadian is no longer cowering in fear of the official narrative. They no longer worry about being alone. They know they are not alone. They know that their first instinct to question the coerced narrative of the government and the media was correct. They have nothing to apologize for—only that they should have spoken up sooner for individual freedom.

If there's a lesson for all of us, it is this: Question authority. Don't let the official narrative be the first and only narrative you listen to or believe. Recognize that everyone is fallible and will tend to tell a story that fits their own interests. Scientists—the "experts," the media, the politicians, the academics—are human like the rest of us and are prone to make "gut decisions" and then reason why their decision was right. As Professor Jonathan Haidt observes, we're all prone to decide first and reason later, rather than the other way around. The sooner we learn that the sooner we'll be humble enough to listen to our neighbour with a different view than ours in our search for truth.

---

543 Bruce Pardy, "Supreme Court undermined by chief justice condemning freedom convoy," *National Post*, June 2, 2022, accessed May 12, 2023, https://nationalpost.com/opinion/bruce-pardy-supreme-court-undermined-by-chief-justice-condemning-freedom-convoy.

"In a country like ours," Philip Slayton, retired lawyer, university professor, and accomplished author, told me,[544] "the price of freedom is every citizen—you, me, and everybody else—paying close attention. Asking intelligent questions. Overall, Canadians, unlike, for example, Americans and many Europeans, tend to be far too deferential to authority. They look at the authority and they say, 'Well, you know they're judges or they're cabinet ministers, or they're this or they're that, or they're something else. I have to pay attention. I have to accept what they say and do what they tell me to do.'" To which Slayton emphatically said, "Wrong! You don't have to do those things. At least not without questioning, not without inquiry, not without criticism, not without demanding to be convinced that this is the right course of action."

"So, at the end of the day," said Slayton, "it's every citizen's obligation to do these things if we are to preserve the freedom of democracy in this country."

"Democracy," said the Hon. Brian Peckford, "once you get it, it's hard to keep it. It will involve the people being involved all the time. People get lazy as the society grows, flourishes, prospers. People get lazy and leave it up to everybody else. I think we failed our democracy. The people have failed our democracy as much as our leaders have because we haven't held them accountable."[545]

The trucker protest matters to this country present and future. They held our leaders accountable for that one, brief, shining moment. They questioned authority. I'm more convinced of this every day when I see those in power continue to bumble their way through their lies and mischaracterizations. The government has, to date, failed to be a good liar. One must have a good memory to lie, otherwise one lie gets tripped up by a subsequent lie, as the story can never be consistent. Just imagine Justin

---

544 See "Our Role in Guarding Freedom—Philip Slayton Interview," First Freedoms Foundation, accessed May 12, 2023, https://firstfreedoms.ca/our-role-in-guarding-freedom-philip-slayton-interview/.
545 "We Have All Failed Our Democracy—Brian Peckford," First Freedoms Foundation, accessed May 12, 2023, https://firstfreedoms.ca/we-have-all-failed-our-democracy-brian-peckford/.

Trudeau's outright mischaracterization, while giving testimony at the POEC hearing, that he did not call the unvaccinated names!

We must never cover up the falsehoods (like Karina Gould's recent attempt with the Hunka affair) but own them. I would even go a step further. The mistakes of the prime minister are our mistakes. We elected him. And who knows—if we were in the same position as him, we might have done the exact same thing. It's this realization of human nature that is missing from our national discourse. We must be critical of ourselves and our human institutions. Failure to be critical will lead to our demise and despotism. As Pardy noted, in order "[t]o defeat COVID collectivism, we must reject the nanny state."[546] That state that thinks it knows it all.

The truckers, and in particular Tamara Lich, have held up a mirror of who we are. We are the mounted police trampling an eighty-year-old Indigenous lady. We are the police handcuffing the non-violent grandmother Tamara Lich. We are the lying government, the non-sympathetic justice system. We are the uncaring and faceless bureaucracy. We are the conflicted government-supporting media. We are the virtue signalling and rarely truthful prime minister. We are the judgemental vaccinated against the unvaccinated and vice versa. We are all those things and more. Yes, human beings have a fallen nature. It is why when we do something good, we celebrate it – it is out of the norm. That basic premise underlies our political and social institutions that, until recently, served us well.

The truckers in the end showed who Canadians are—the line between good and evil runs through each Canadian heart. We are the vaccinated who came out to support the unvaccinated. We are the Canadians standing on the roads and overpasses waving Canadian flags in support of the convoy, giving the truckers food at the gas stops. We are the Canadians who came in the tens of thousands for a carnival of freedom on Parliament Hill amid brutally cold weather and fellowshipped together and rejoiced in our humanity. We were the Canadians who got on our knees to pray for our prime minister and his government even though we lost our jobs and family because of him.

The Great Canadian Trucker Protest, in truth, kept Canada from losing its way entirely.

---

546 Bruce Pardy, "Anatomy of the Administrative State," https://brownstone.org/articles/anatomy-of-the-administrative-state/

We have turned the corner. Our democracy is on the way back from the brink and will remain so if we commit to holding the line and keeping up the fight for truth, democracy, rule of law and our first freedoms of speech, religion/conscience, and the inviolability of the person. We have our children and grandchildren to live for. To them we owe a much better country than the one the Trucker Freedom Convoy 2022 protested.

It's time for us to appreciate what we have in our collective Canadian citizenship: a free people, free to speak without fear, free to worship God in our own way, free to stand for what we think is right, free to oppose what we believe is wrong, free to choose those who govern our country. This heritage of freedom we pledge to uphold for ourselves and all mankind.[547]

We saw first-hand in the political engine of this country what happens when the populace's freedom is under pressure. The Canadian government's compression of freedom reached auto-ignition of the citizenry. Truckers crossed the country to Ottawa to say, "Enough is enough!" Tens of thousands joined the protest and its ramifications remain for the long haul.

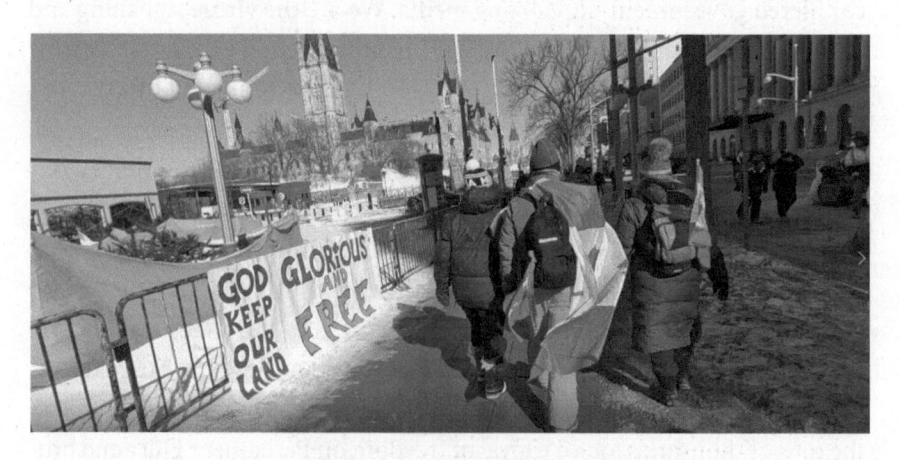

*May God Keep Our Land Glorious And Free!*

---

547 This is a take on John Diefenbaker's statement, "I am Canadian, a free Canadian, free to speak without fear, free to worship God in my own way, free to stand for what I think right, free to oppose what I believe wrong, free to choose those who govern my country. This heritage of freedom I pledge to uphold for myself and all mankind" (John Diefenbaker, House of Commons Debates, 1 July 1960).

# Epilogue: Trying to Make Sense of Canada after Rouleau

HOW DOES ONE characterize the promise of a free and democratic society after reading Mr. Paul Rouleau's report on the Trudeau government's use of the Emergencies Act last year? The report lays out the groundwork for future governments to declare a national public order emergency without having to meet a stringent set of guidelines.

Rouleau's decision is akin to the parent recognizing the inappropriateness of a wayward child's misuse of the family car in knocking down a pedestrian. After a few words of reproof, the parent hands over the car keys for the child to go cruising with friends, hoping against hope things will be better next time.

First, despite Mr. Rouleau's report, I remain firmly convinced that Prime Minister Trudeau did not meet the conditions to invoke the Emergencies Act. Further, Rouleau's decision has no legal weight.

Mr. Rouleau wasn't asked to determine whether the government acted lawfully in invoking the Emergencies Act. He was simply to inquire "into the circumstances that led to the declaration being issued and the measures taken for dealing with the emergency."

The POEC had all the trappings of a court—witnesses were called, and they had to affirm or swear that they would tell the truth and so on. But it was not a court. Mr. Rouleau's decision is not a binding legal precedent. Only the Federal Court of Canada can judicially review decisions made by the federal cabinet. There are two cases in that court now dealing with that question. And it will be that court and, if appealed, the Supreme Court of Canada, that will decide whether the government acted within the law. Rouleau pre-empted the Federal Court by ruling that the government met the legal threshold of the Act.

The Emergencies Act defines a public order emergency as one that "arises from threats to the security of Canada and that is so serious as to be a national emergency." Threats to the security of Canada are defined in the *Canadian Security Intelligence Service Act* as "espionage or sabotage," "foreign influenced activities," a movement to overthrow the government or the "threat or use of acts of serious violence against persons or property for the purpose of achieving a political, religious or ideological objective."

Was the trucker protest in Ottawa such a security threat? Were they seeking to overthrow the government? Honestly? The government tried its best to raise the profile of the very few in the crowd wanting the governor general to dismiss Trudeau. The government pointed to such talk as if the entire trucker protest was an organized coup attempt. It would be like saying because I'm from Newfoundland and I'm vegetarian, so that means everyone in Newfoundland is vegetarian. It's simply laughable. It nevertheless served the government's narrative that the truckers were the "fringe minority with unacceptable views."

During the POEC hearings, Chrystia Freeland, our minister of Finance and deputy prime minister, told of seeing a lady walking by a truck in Ottawa, who was startled when the trucker blew his horn. The lady gave the trucker an obscene gesture, and then the trucker blew the horn again. Freeland said, "It was just this small, young woman, and this big truck, and a person in it. And she was mad, and I just thought, you know, there are dozens and dozens of these things happening every day, and you know, God forbid that one of them should actually flare into violence and physical harm."[548]

I would agree that such an experience is unpleasant for anyone, and the trucker as described was being obnoxious. But does that kind of thing rise to a national threat such that near dictatorial powers are to be used against that trucker? I say no.

---

548 POEC, Volume 30, p. 76.

The government consistently referenced the threat of violence, but there were no actual threats of violence. Not one. Instead, there was government innuendo that something untoward might happen. Nothing did, of course, but there were bouncy castles and street hockey games and people handing out hot chocolate and donuts, and there were speeches on the flatbed of a truck with a huge crane hoisting the Canadian flag. The scariest stuff would have to be the truck horns and the obscene Trudeau flags. There was nothing that justified the government reaching the threshold of the Act to take dictatorial powers and freeze bank accounts of those who held different opinions than it.

Mr. Rouleau's willingness to let the government off sets a horrible precedent for the future.

Second, the prime minister of Canada holds an extremely powerful office, with little check on that power. That means that what the prime minister wants, he or she usually gets. Everyone around him or her will do what it takes to ensure that his wishes and desires are carried out. Why? Because their job and career advancement are dependent on the prime minister's approval.

Political parties are wrapped up and identified with their leaders, especially in the Liberal Party today. This symbiotic relationship becomes even more solidified when the leader keeps winning elections. It's a cult-like phenomenon. The leader can do no wrong because he keeps winning.

As we saw with Jody-Wilson Raybould, so we see with the Trucker Freedom Convoy in 2022. Those within Mr. Trudeau's circle worked together to solve his desire to invoke the Act. The POEC hearings made it clear that the political culture surrounding Mr. Trudeau's inner circle did everything in its power and influence to see that his desire to end the protest expeditiously was carried out. In other words, the prime minister's office, the Privy Council, members of the cabinet, CSIS, the RCMP, and the government's legal advisers were engaged in an atmosphere of satisfying the prime minister's goals and objectives regarding the convoy.

Not surprisingly, the prime minister has at his disposal a substantial bench strength of clever lawyers able to think outside of the traditional legal box of statutory interpretation. The rule of thumb in interpreting statutes is first, you take the statute at face value. You accept the plain meaning of the words. In most cases, the plain meaning resolves the case. However, if the Act is ambiguous, extrinsic matters may be referred to as surrounding circumstance to understand the Act. For example, you look at the state of the law prior to the statute. You ask: What mischief is the Act meant to correct? Why did the Act come into being? Did any government commissions address the Act? Were there any judicial decisions on the Act? And so on.

From the POEC testimony of the prime minister and others, it became clear that the legal minds counselling the prime minister fully understood that if you take the Emergencies Act at face value, the government had no authority to invoke the emergency powers. That's when somewhere in the inner circle a legal theory was hatched to provide the prime minister the legal cover.

It must be said that I don't have any inside information. No one has leaked anything to me. I'm just a lawyer of thirty years, who has advised clients for a living and sat across the table from many government lawyers. I understand the dynamics of trying to provide the best counsel possible to clients who are looking for a way to legally accomplish a task.

Those lawyers put their arguments in a memo that was given to the prime minister's office. However, it truly baffles me that the government of Canada didn't supply the POEC with a copy of that memo, as it was their legal justification for invocation of the Emergencies Act. Think about that—we are supposedly a free and democratic society with a government that is to be open and transparent to the people. This same government now claims that they don't have to reveal the legal advice that supported giving them powers to arrest citizens without a warrant, freeze bank accounts, bring out the riot squad, and forcefully remove peaceful protesters.

Mr. Rouleau didn't see that legal memo, which is truly remarkable. It's even more remarkable that he said it didn't matter: "I do not need to see the legal advice itself," he said, "in order to accept the evidence that they believed their conclusions to be justified in law."

Think about this for a minute. The most draconian power of the government is justified simply because the government says, "Yeah, we had a legal opinion that we were acting within the law, but we won't let you see it."

We do have a glimpse of the legal argument the government came up with based on the testimony of the government officials, including the prime minister. However, that testimony isn't sufficient. When we're dealing with absolute power, I submit that we can't simply accept the "say so" of those wielding the power. It makes no sense.

Third, the legal argument the government came up with goes like this: the Emergencies Act was a product of the 1980s and needs to be modernized. The Emergencies Act references the definition of a security threat under the *CSIS Act*. The contexts of the two Acts are different. CSIS decides whether there's a security threat under that Act. But declaring a public order emergency under the Emergencies Act is the responsibility of the cabinet and the prime minister. The decision is therefore a political one. As long as the cabinet and the PM have reasonable grounds that there is a "threat of serious violence," the threshold is met in the context of a Public Order Emergency.

I encourage you to read Mr. Rouleau's decision and decide for yourself. For me, it simply doesn't add up to a convincing position at all.

While Mr. Rouleau's report isn't legally binding, it is, nevertheless, another example of the modern judicial proclivity to support government actions, even though the strict reading of the law is ignored. What is terribly wrong in this approach is the complete lack of respect for the law over a "political necessity" that was seen to be of more importance than staying within the legal guardrails.

There is a cruel irony to consider. At the same time that the peaceful Trucker Freedom Convoy in Ottawa was being rounded up by a violent police force, over in British Columbia a group of environmental protestors attacked a pipeline construction site. Hundreds of thousands of dollars worth of damage was done. For the government, it was the non-violent Ottawa protest that warranted the Emergencies Act.

Fourth, our Charter of Rights, our Constitution, as well as our statutory or legislative law, are meaningless if politicians hold them in contempt and interpret them based on whatever whim catches their fancy. Those politicians without integrity can severely damage helpless, average citizens by such assaults to their legal rights. This is why we desperately need men and women of personal integrity in our public offices. We need to remember that those we put in office reflect our principles. If the politician is without integrity, we only have ourselves to blame. We put them there.

Finally, if we are to read the Emergencies Act as written, we know that the government did not meet the test. The Freedom Convoy was not a national security threat. Every time there was a court order, whether in Windsor, Coutts, or even in Ottawa, the truckers complied. The blockades ended in Windsor and Coutts, and they stopped the horns in Ottawa.

The Emergencies Act says the powers can be invoked if the government "believes on reasonable grounds, that a POE exists." But that requires no legal authority to act in other ways. However, Mr. Rouleau accepted the government's statement that it had the ability to interpret the definition itself, according to its own set of criteria. The government had all the authority it needed to remove the Trucker Freedom Convoy in Ottawa. It didn't need the emergency powers. But Rouleau basically said, in essence, "No problem—if you think there was a threat, then there was."

As Prime Minister Trudeau said, "What if someone had gotten hurt? What if a police officer had been put in the hospital? ... What if, when I had an opportunity to do something, I had waited." He said he was "absolutely, absolutely serene and confident" that he made the right choice in invoking the Emergencies Act.

Sadly, Mr. Rouleau agreed with Mr. Trudeau. We have now reached a new low standard to declare a national emergency. Rest assured that if we Canadians do not speak up now, we can expect that the action of Mr. Trudeau will be the new touchstone. Of course, it will be up to an actual court of law to determine whether the government acted within the law. But now the courts have the opinion of a very respected, retired Justice Rouleau, who said he is of the view that Trudeau met the test to declare a POE.

Rouleau didn't stop there. He recommended that the definition of a public order emergency be "modernized in order to capture the situations that could legitimately pose a serious risk to the public order, now and in the foreseeable future." It truly is incomprehensible that we are at this place in Canada when a government can not only reinterpret the law, granting itself dictatorial powers, but can also be supported by such an eminent, retired judge to bring in legislation to redefine the Emergencies Act!

Do you think it will take Mr. Trudeau and his government very long to bring in new legislation to do that very thing? Not at all. Further, there can be no doubt that such a move will be fully supported by Mr. Jagmeet Singh and the New Democratic Party. Passing such legislation will further justify and legitimize the abuse of power we have witnessed. It has the potential to be the new normal.

Canadians, is that what we want? Do we really want a government who, on a whim, can take away our freedoms with the stroke of a pen?

## Why Rouleau Didn't Have All the Information Needed to Rule on Emergencies Act Invocation.[549]

The report from the Public Order Emergency Commission shows that Commissioner Paul Rouleau was missing key information he needed to make his ruling, in which he said he found "with reluctance" that the use of the Emergencies Act to clear convoy protests was justified.

On the one hand, the report is critical of everyone involved—the police, social media, and the government. On the other hand, it lets the federal government claim a victory. It is, however, a pyrrhic victory, as we will soon see.

There is also the issue of perception. There have been reports of Justice Rouleau's past work with the Liberal Party. That's not to take away from Mr. Rouleau personally, but in such delicate matters, justice must be seen to be done. Let it suffice to say that Prime Minister Trudeau would have better served the Canadian people had he appointed a judge with a Conservative past.

Indeed, anyone who watched the hearings saw firsthand the multiple incidents where government officials redacted documents, and ministers, such as David Lametti, refused to answer questions because of claimed privilege. It's disappointing that Mr. Rouleau refused to hold the government to account for such lack of transparency. His recommendations reveal that, as a commissioner, he had his hands tied behind his back. He didn't have all the information he needed.

---

[549] What follows was previously published with The *Epoch Times* Barry W. Bussey, "Why Rouleau Didn't Have All the Information Needed to Rule on Emergencies Act Invocation," *The Epoch Times,* February 19, 2023, https://www.theepochtimes.com/barry-bussey-why-rouleau-didnt-have-all-the-information-needed-to-rule-on-emergencies-act-invocation_5068814.html

With that impediment, however, he did not cry "Foul!" and hold the government accountable. Instead, his ruling effectively whitewashes the abuse of power and lowers the bar for future governments to impose draconian measures against those with whom they disagree.

The Trucker Freedom Convoy was a pivotal moment in Canadian political history, when the average Canadian who was adversely affected by Mr. Trudeau's demonizing and overreach recognized that they had the wherewithal to peacefully protest. Not even the commission's contradictory and confusing report will take that realization away. In other words, the "fringe minority" class awareness has not dissipated but is now awakened to ensure that government abuse does not continue.

Rouleau's recommendations, and particularly numbers 37–49, are evidence that all was not well in his assignment. For example, Recommendation 37 says the *Emergencies Act* (EA) should be amended to allow any future inquiry to be pursuant to Part 1 of the *Inquiries Act*, which allows the inquiry to be open-ended in getting to the bottom of the matter. That was not done for his inquiry. Note the litany of other recommendations that reveal Rouleau's uncomfortable position of being asked to review the government's actions but then not be given the tools to do so.

Consider the following recommendations:

> 38—EA should be amended to allow the inquiry to "examine and assess the basis for the declaration and the measures adopted." This was not clear for Rouleau in the current situation.

> 39—The commissioner "should be consulted as to the substance of the terms of reference for the inquiry." In other words, no longer should the Prime Minister's Office dictate the terms of the inquiry but all future commissioners should be free to go wherever the evidence leads.

> 40—EA needs to be amended "to require the Government deliver to the commission a comprehensive statement setting out the factual and legal basis for the declaration and measures adopted, including the view of the Minister

of Justice of Canada as to whether the decision to proclaim an emergency was consistent with ... the Emergencies Act, and ... with the Charter." Here is the shocker: Mr. Trudeau's government did not disclose this very important information to the commissioner. Rouleau obviously was not pleased and hence the recommendation, yet he still let the government off the hook.

41—EA should be amended to require government elected officials and bureaucracy to maintain "a thorough written record of the process leading to a decision to declare a public order emergency." That was crucial information not given to Rouleau.

42—Government should collect all its "documents and information as soon as the declaration of emergency is made" and give them to the inquiry at the outset of its work. Again, not done.

43—All of the inputs to cabinet and ministers should be given to the inquiry. Not done.

44—There should be no redactions on government documents (aside from national security confidentiality). Rouleau was given a host of redacted documents.

45—Create a "working group" to deal with the government's claims of keeping documents confidential. Government kept Rouleau in the dark on a host of documents.

46—EA should be amended to allow the commissioner to appoint a judge to resolve any claim of privilege by government. Obviously, Rouleau was frustrated with the government's constant claim of privilege.

47—A Federal Court judge should be appointed to determine the government's claims of privilege on an expedited basis. Rouleau was forced to accept the government's claims of privilege at face value. As a result, scads of material were denied his review.

48—EA needs to be amended to give the inquiry power to order anyone to hand over all information. Rouleau did not have that.

49—EA needs to be amended so that a parliamentarian cannot claim parliamentary privilege to refuse to testify. Doug Ford got off the hook on this one.

These recommendations, in my view, suggest that Rouleau did not have the information he needed to properly carry out the inquiry.

No wonder he said that it was "with reluctance" that he decided the government met the threshold to invoke the Emergencies Act. It appears to me that Rouleau recognized the inadequacies of the commission's investigatory powers, yet he gave the government a pass in the most serious abuse of power ever seen in a federal government.

It behooves us as Canadians to remain vigilant in these uncharted waters of increased government power.

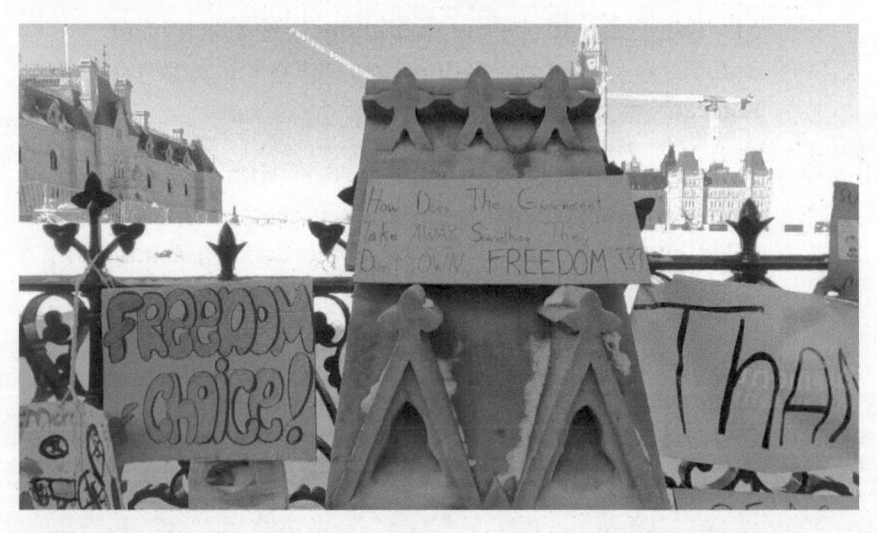

*How Does The Government Take Away Something They Don't Own: Freedom*

# ACKNOWLEDGEMENTS

MICHAEL R. J. Clark said, "Barry, a person with your experience and knowledge should write a book about the truckers." From that discussion my mind started the process of Winston Churchill's oft quoted trance a writer finds himself in, "Writing a book is an adventure. To begin with it is a toy and an amusement. Then it becomes a mistress, then it becomes a master, then it becomes a tyrant. The last phase is that just as you are about to be reconciled to your servitude, you kill the monster and fling him to the public." Indeed, such has been my experience. So, thanks Michael for being the spark that got me going.

Given the nature of this work I was keenly aware that I did not want to be overbearing in my judgement. I am by nature strongly opinionated. Therefore, I had to temper my passionate positions with wise counsel. My greatest counsellor is my wife LaVonna, who is freer than most to share with me what is on her mind. Then my daughter—who read the manuscript with care and gave meaningful suggestions—comes in at a close second. My long-term writing assistant Amy Ross was of great help in getting my trajectory right and reading and editing the early drafts of the manuscript. Then there were others with whom I discussed and debated at length and who took the time to read the manuscript—Law Professor Bruce Pardy, former Newfoundland Premier Brian Peckford, Stephen LeDrew, Jonathan Martin, Daniel Freiheit, Tom Theordore, Robert Carrier, David Crofton, Dr. Don Hutchinson, Renata Jasaitis, and Professor Iain Provan. Each made me think and as a result I made changes. Truly, writing a book is not a lone adventure.

My good friend Law Professor Iain Benson came in at the last-minute with great suggestions for the title. He rightly said that my advertised working title was not suited. Between his "long haul" analogy and my son-in-law's suggestion of "210° Celsius" the title came to be.

David Crofton was a tremendous assistance as he meticulously combed the manuscript in his editing. So too did the unknown editors at Friesen Press. Christoph Koniczek and Kayla Lang of Friesen Press and their team did great work to bring the book to completion.

I thank Anna Flores and Renata Jasaitis for their assistance with the companied **210° Celsius Study Guide** that will allow me to continue the conversation about what this experience means for Canada in the long term.

Finally, I thank all those First Freedoms Foundation (Canada) (www.firstfreedoms.ca) supporters who gave us a much-needed boost to get this work off the ground. It took longer than I expected but it is here now. I hope that this work will be of benefit to help us all learn from our mutually uncomfortable experience. Thank-you to the FFF Board of Directors, Jonathan Martin, Iain Provan, Caroline Walters, and Robert Yeager, for your help, assistance and support as we venture together in bringing important conversations before Canadians and the world on our First Freedoms—speech, religion and conscience, inviolability of the person in the context of the rule of law and democracy. We have much work to do.

# A book with a difference!
# Are you ready to accept
# the call to action?

**SCAN ME**

This book is not meant to be read and put back on the shelf to collect dust. Barry invites you to join him in an ongoing conversation about our First Freedoms. He has recorded a video for each chapter so that you may continue the dialogue with your friends. A companion **210° Celsius Study Guide** is available at a nominal cost so that you and your friends can dig deeper into how we can flourish as a truly free and democratic society.

Simply scan this QR code with your smartphone or tablet and start a study group today and be ready to answer the call to change Canada for the better!

Printed in Canada